Acute and Critical Care
Clinical Nurse Specialists

Synergy for Best Practices

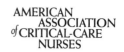

AMERICAN
ASSOCIATION
of CRITICAL-CARE
NURSES

Acute and Critical Care
Clinical Nurse Specialists

Synergy for Best Practices

Mary G. McKinley, MSN, RN, CCRN
Partner, Critical Connections
Maxwell Center
Wheeling, West Virginia

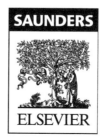

SAUNDERS

ELSEVIER

SAUNDERS
ELSEVIER

11830 Westline Industrial Drive
St. Louis, Missouri 63146

Library of Congress Control Number: 2007924080

Executive Publisher: Barbara Nelson Cullen
Senior Developmental Editor: Jennifer Ehlers
Publishing Services Manager: Gayle May
Project Manager: Tracey Schriefer
Cover Designer: Paula Ruckenbrod
Text Designer: Paula Ruckenbrod

Printed in the United States of America

Last digit is the print number: 9 8 7 6 5 4 3 2 1

Contributors

Foreword
Dorrie K. Fontaine, RN, DNSc, FAAN
Associate Dean for Academic Programs
School of Nursing
University of California–San Francisco
San Francisco, California

Chapter 1
Mary G. McKinley, RN, MSN, CCRN
Partner, Critical Connections
Maxwell Center
Wheeling, West Virginia

Chapter 2
Deborah G. Klein, RN, MSN, CCRN, CS
Clinical Nurse Specialist
The Cleveland Clinic
Cleveland, Ohio

Chapter 3
*Roberta Kaplow, RN, PhD, CCNS,
CCRN, AOCNS*
Clinical Nurse Specialist
DeKalb Medical Center
Decatur, Georgia

Chapter 4
Kathleen Vollman, MSN, RN, CCNS, FCCM
Clinical Nurse Specialist/Educator/
Consultant
ADVANCING NURSING LLC
Northville, Michigan

Brenda Lyons, DNS, FAAN
School of Nursing
Indiania University
Indianapolis, Indiana

Chapter 5
Marla J. De Jong, RN, PhD, CCNS, CCRN
Co-Editor, *AACN Advanced Critical Care*
San Antonio, Texas

Chapter 6
Christine Schulman, RN, MSN, CCRN
Clinical Nurse Specialist Trauma and
Critical Care Nursing
Clinical Faculty
School of Nursing
Oregon Health and Science University
Portland, Oregon

Chapter 7
Karen K. Carlson, RN, MN, CCNS
Critical Care Clinical Nurse Specialist
Carlson Consulting Group
Bellevue, Washington

Chapter 8
Jan Foster, RN, PhD, CCRN
President, Nursing Inquiry and Intervention, Inc
The Woodlands, Texas
Texas Woman's University
Houston, Texas

Chapter 9
Mary Fran Tracy, RN, PhD, CCRN, CCNS, FAAN
Critical Care Clinical Nurse Specialist
School of Nursing
University of Minnesota
Minneapolis, Minnesota

Ruth Lindquist, RN, PhD, APRN, BC, FAAN
Professor and Senior Associate Dean
School of Nursing
University of Minnesota
Minneapolis, Minnesota

Chapter 10
Linda J. Bell, RN, MSN
Clinical Nurse Specialist
American Association of Critical-Care Nurses
Aliso Viejo, California

Ramón Lavandero, RN, MA, MSN, FAAN
Director of Development and
Strategic Alliances
American Association of Critical-Care Nurses
Aliso Viejo, California
Adjunct Associate Professor of Nursing
Indiana University
Indianapolis, Indiana

Chapter 11
Elizabeth M. Nolan, RN, MS, APRN
Clinical Nurse Specialist, Cardiovascular Center
University of Michigan Hospitals &
Health Centers
Ann Arbor, Michigan

Chapter 12
John F. Dixon, Jr., RN, MSN
Baylor University Medical Center
Dallas, Texas

Chapter 13
Mary Lou Sole, RN, PhD, CCRN, CCNS, FAAN
Professor
University of Central Florida
College of Health and Public Affairs
School of Nursing
Orlando, Florida

Chapter 14
Marcia Bixby, MS, CCRN
Beth Israel Deaconess Medical Center
Boston, Massachusetts

Karen Giuliano, RN, PhD, FAAN
Clinical Research Specialist
Philips Medical Systems
Bothell, Washington

Chapter 15
Karla A. Knight, RN, MSN
Writer, Nursing Spectrum
Boston, Massachusetts

Connie Barden, RN, MN, CCRN, CCNS
Clinical Nurse Specialist
Mercy Medical Center
Miami, Florida

Gladys M. Campbell, RN, MSN
Executive Director
NWONE
Seattle, Washington
Independent Consultant
Portland, Oregon

Preface

In today's health care environment, clinicians must focus on providing quality care through best practices in a cost-effective manner. Advanced practitioners are faced with the challenge to excel in clinical practice as well as in system analysis and insight—to be not only clinical experts but also organizational experts, whose skills are needed beyond the boundaries of the critical care unit to any general care areas where complex and acutely ill patients receive care. Such patients require strong clinical skills as well as advanced skills in analysis and problem solving.

This book will be valuable to practicing clinical nurse specialists (CNSs) and to CNS students, given the resurgence in admissions as health care organizations have increased demand for advanced practitioners with the knowledge and skills that CNSs provide.

In three parts, this book seeks to give acute and critical care CNSs the knowledge and practical tools to employ those best practices, which result from a framework comprising the scope of practice and standards of professional practice developed by the American Association of Critical-Care Nurses (AACN), the AACN Synergy Model for Patient Care, and the spheres of influence as defined by the National Association of Clinical Nurse Specialists.

The book also will help CNSs to integrate the standards with measurement criteria, including the necessary content for achieving certification as a clinical nurse specialist in acute and critical care.

Part I introduces the concepts, provides some historical perspective, identifies the competencies for the CNS, and discusses the Synergy Model framework and spheres of influence in which CNSs practice. Part II identifies the dimensions of practice for the CNS in acute and critical care using the Synergy Model as a basis for expert practice. Each dimension of practice is highlighted with methodology to assist CNSs in implementing their role. Case studies illustrate the spheres of influence and how the standards of professional performance fit within the dimensions of practice. This section includes discussion questions to guide critical analysis of the issues surrounding the dimensions of practice. Part III focuses on professional development opportunities for the CNS, practice and professional issues, and future trends facing CNSs in acute and critical care.

Mary G. McKinley, RN, MSN, CCRN
Editor

Acknowledgments

Many people helped in the publishing of this book. First and foremost, thanks to the contributors—those talented and expert-level nurses who were gracious, patient, and understanding throughout the process of editing and publishing. Second, many AACN members unselfishly gave their time to participate in the Advanced Practice Work Groups, and their contribution to advanced nursing practice is reflected here. The multitalented AACN national office staff members assisted in ways too numerous to mention—from the generation of initial ideas to the nitty-gritty of reviewing chapters. Linda Bell, Carol Hartigan, Ramón Lavandero, and Ellen French, your help has been invaluable. To the folks at Elsevier who have been patient and understanding—Barbara Cullen, Julie Vitale, and Jennifer Ehlers—my many thanks. To Harriette Kelly, librarian extraordinaire, many thanks for all your assistance.

To those nurses who have given me so much in my career and have assisted in my professional development: the staff in the intensive care unit and coronary care unit at Ohio Valley Medical Center, my former CNS colleagues Cathy Robinson and Alicia Taylor, and Sara Smith, thank you for your support.

And, finally, thanks to my family. To my mother and dad for all they gave me and to my brothers and their families who every Thanksgiving challenge my thinking and vocabulary skills with our annual Scrabble match, please accept my many thanks. To my wonderful and loving children—David, Amy, Elizabeth, and Bennett—as well as my grandchildren—Jackson, Davey, Maxwell, Thomas, and Annie—I am so blessed to have you all in my life. To my husband David, who believes that I can do anything and promptly gives me the push to do it, your patience, love, and support have been a blessing to me in this endeavor and in so many others.

Table of Contents

Acute and Critical Care
Clinical Nurse Specialists

Synergy for Best Practices

Evolution of the Clinical Nurse Specialist in Acute and Critical Care

Mary G. McKinley

OVERVIEW

To understand the challenges facing clinical nurse specialists (CNSs) in acute and critical care today, one must understand the historical development of both critical care and the CNS role. The growth of critical care and the CNS role is a complex story of opportunities, challenges, and struggles within the larger context of the profession of nursing and the health care needs presented in acute and critical care units. From the very beginning, the role of the CNS within the specialty has been influenced by social, economic, technological, and theoretical changes within nursing and health care. The purpose of this chapter is to highlight the historical development of critical care and the growth of the role of the CNS in acute and critical care. Additionally the development of the scope of practice and standards of professional performance for the CNS in acute and critical care will be reviewed.

CRITICAL CARE NURSING

The concept of critical care is modern, but its roots are deep, having its origin as far back as the work and writings of Florence Nightingale. In *Notes on Nursing*, she states, "We kept the sickest patients close to the nursing desk while moving those requiring less nursing care to the end of the ward" (Nightingale, 1860). In this way she advocated that patients who needed the most care be closest to the nurse's desk where they could be watched constantly. Critical care nursing is concerned with human responses to life-threatening problems (Medina, 2000). These life-threatening problems require continuous in-depth assessment and intense therapeutic measures and interventions. To understand the current idea of critical care it is important to understand the concepts that serve as a foundation for this nursing specialty and the factors that have influenced change within the health care environment.

The first concept is that the patient who needs critical care is one who is at risk. These patients are physiologically unstable or in danger of dying. The second concept is that the person who requires intensive care is one in whom there is an expectation of recovery or hope for recovery. It is these two concepts that form the basis of critical care (Fairman, 1998).

In analyzing the impact of the first concept on the development of critical care, it is important to review that this patient population is one that is vulnerable or at risk. The patient and his or her needs have always been the focus for nursing in critical care. Therefore these susceptible patients require intensive nursing support. The polio epidemic of the 1950s gave rise to nursing units where polio victims could receive specialized care. By the nature of their illness, these high-risk patients required intensive nursing care, sometimes including mechanical ventilation support via the iron lung. In the 1960s the need arose for specialized nursing care for patients following surgery and spurred the development of recovery rooms where nurses were specially trained to assist patients recovering from anesthetic agents. At the same time, Dr. Lawrence Meltzer worked to establish a coronary care unit in which nurses were educated in depth about the diagnosis and treatment of cardiac arrhythmias so they could better care for this at-risk group of patients (Fairman, 1998). This increased knowledge led to nurses administering medication and defibrillating patients according to protocols. Inherent in the role of nursing is providing continuous care and intensive support. Often the support needed is physiological in nature, but there are also psychosocial implications that can impinge on the health and well-being of the individual requiring intervention by the nurse. Therefore nursing in critical care requires an active role by the nurse to provide the interventions necessary to support the patient through this crisis state.

The second concept focuses on patients who have an expectation or hope for recovery, however slim. This concept has been altered by medical research. Federal budget appropriation for medical research increased dramatically between 1945 and 1960, resulting in a surge of research in many specialized areas and providing for dramatic innovation in health care (Chitty, 2005). Patients who once were thought to be "hopeless" could now routinely be treated and recover. New approaches to patient care from pharmacological to surgical procedures changed the definition of "hopeless" forever.

Two methods provide the foundation for the practice of acute and critical care nursing. These are watchful vigilance and a method of sorting. Watchful vigilance or observation (i.e., gathering of the sickest patients together for intensive observation or watchful vigilance) is based on Florence Nightingale's advocation that patients who need the most care be in close proximity to the nurse. Critical care units of today use both physical design and technology to provide watchful vigilance with open units and video and cardiac monitoring for continuous observation of patients.

The second foundational method is to sort or triage patients according to the stability or their condition. The more recent use of highly specialized units attests to the value of this foundational concept. In the 1950s caring for polio patients in iron lungs could more effectively and efficiently be done if those patients were located on a centralized location with nurses who were specially trained in caring for these patients. Likewise, Dr. Meltzer found that the unique care of and concerns for cardiac patients would be more effectively addressed if patients were located within a unit designed to monitor these patients and nursing staff educated to meet their advanced care needs (Fairman, 1998). Today specialized units exist for many different patient populations (e.g., neurological, neurosurgical, burn, trauma, surgical, or medical patients). Table 1-1 is a breakdown of specialized critical care units from a study completed by AACN in 2006. This table shows how specialized units break down in a sample of 300 hospitals surveyed (Kirchhoff & Dahl, 2006).

TABLE 1-1

Types of Specialized Critical Care Units

Type of Critical Care Unit	Percentage of Total Sample (N = 300 Units)
Intensive care units	53
Medical-surgical	8
Combined intensive/ coronary care	8
Cardiovascular/surgical	7
Coronary care	5
Neonatal	5
Pediatric	4
Medical	4
Surgical	4
Neuro-neurosurgical	3
Trauma	2
Burn	2
Postanesthesia care units/recovery rooms	10
Progressive care units	30
Telemetry	12
Step-down	7
Intermediate care	6
Progressive care	5
Other types of critical care units	4
No answer	3

Data from Kirchhoff K., Dahl N. *American Journal of Critical Care*, Jan 2006.

The multiple factors that have influenced the growth and development of critical care include technology and social and economic forces.

Technology

A recent influence on the rapidly increasing growth of critical care units is the explosion of technology and availability of treatments for patients who are unstable but for whom there is hope of recovery. It wasn't too long ago that many of the patients cared for in critical care units would not have been expected to survive. The treatments, procedures, and pharmacological agents simply weren't available. For example, at one time patients with acute heart disease were admitted to the hospital and placed on bed rest. Little was available to help patients with this life-threatening disease. Care for these patients has advanced to include a vast array of pharmacological and surgical procedures and treatments that can actually change the course of disease for these patients. These advances have dramatically impacted the health care environment and fostered the continued growth and development of acute and critical care nursing.

Social

Early hospitals were seen as places where the seriously ill patient went to die. The availability of technology and treatment has shifted the focus of the public viewing hospitals as institutions where recovery was expected. Sicker patients entered hospitals and expected to receive higher levels of care, with the expectation of a high level of recovery. This expectation came about because of the ability to treat illnesses that previously were untreatable. The focus of hospital care shifted to cure and recovery from illness. The average age of patients in the hospital increased. Chronic debilitating illnesses that previously would have been given little hope of treatment were now treatable and could survive. As more and more of these sicker, severely ill patients came into the hospital, demands placed on nursing staff increased. Nurses faced more and more complex patients, treatments, and procedures. Often the nursing staff was ill prepared to take care of these complex and vulnerable patients. Even today, despite the advances of technology, situations occur in which critical care cannot provide the reasonable expectation of recovery for patients. In those instances, nurses in critical care can support patients and families in end-of-life decision making and palliative care.

Economic

Post World War II hospitals underwent financial and architectural changes that influenced change within the overall health care system. Greater numbers of patients held some form of voluntary insurance and could afford hospital care. Hospitals no longer relied on charitable donations but looked to insurers and individual clients for revenue. This change in financial perspectives altered the way that communities and hospitals interacted. Hospitals now had to struggle to attract patients. Hospitals advertised renowned physicians, advanced technologies, and high-quality accommodations. The public demanded more services and expected care to be completed in an atmosphere that was more personal than impersonal large wards. The demand for a homelike atmosphere replaced the twenty- and thirty-bed wards.

Thus from 1950 to 1970 huge changes were taking place in health care and hospitals. Medical knowledge and technology were growing tremendously, government and private funding and support were increased, patient needs were becoming increasingly complex, and society's values and demands for quality health care were intensifying, all of which combined to stimulate a reorganization of nursing care (Fairman, 1998). Critical care units were an outgrowth of this reorganization.

Every day nurses were confronted with increasingly complex patients whose needs exceeded the availability, knowledge, and authority that they had. The frustration that nurses experienced led nurses to find a better way to care for these vulnerable patients. Building on models that existed served as a basis for early efforts at critical care nursing, from the precedent of the recovery room model introduced following World War II to the development of polio units in the 1950s to care for paralyzed patients in iron lung respirators. Wartime necessity also provided models to improve approaches in providing care to the severely wounded soldiers who had special needs. Rapid transport and close proximity of field hospitals (medical and surgical hospital [MASH] units) enabled medical teams to triage patients so that those who were unstable could receive more intensive care in the field hospitals close to the front lines. This experience assisted in the evolution of emergency services on the home front. Trained emergency personnel could assist in getting seriously ill and injured patients into the health care system sooner. These critically ill patients required ongoing care and support within the hospital system.

Thus from the 1950s intensive care units emerged as permanent specialized areas in which to care for critically ill patients. This growth was expanded in the 1960s when the defibrillator and electrocardiographic monitoring was refined and the concept of the coronary care unit (CCU) was developed. Nurses in these early units learned to recognize arrhythmias and were permitted to administer drugs or defibrillate patients according to written protocols (Chitty, 2005). These early CCU nurses set the stage for a more autonomous practice for critical care nursing. As Lawrence Metzer, Rose Pinneo, and Roderick Kitchell published in their guide to intensive coronary care (the *Yellow Manual*), "Intensive coronary care is above all a system of specialized nursing care and, its success is predicated almost wholly on the ability of the nurse to assume a new and different role"(Fairman, 1998). By 1969 critical care had exploded, with more than half of the nations' not-for-profit hospitals claiming to have an intensive care unit.

In 1969 the American Association of Critical-Care Nurses (AACN) had its start as the American Association of Cardiovascular Nurses. This association began with the focus of developing educational standards, establishing a central bureau of information, and disseminating knowledge about critical care. The founders were expert nurses in the area of cardiovascular nursing, and thus the initial focus was on cardiovascular disease. However, it was quickly recognized that this focus was somewhat limiting, and by 1972 the group changed its name to the American Association of Critical-Care Nurses. This broadened title reflects the philosophy of the association of being inclusive and centering on meeting the needs of the nurses and ultimately the patients in intensive care. Focusing on the shared interest in a concept of nursing care as opposed to a specific organ or system was new to nursing and health care organizations but provided the broader basis for membership. In 1972 the membership grew to 9200, which demonstrated that the broad concept–based association was meeting the needs of nurses working with this vulnerable patient population. This growth has continued; the current membership is 65,000. AACN is the world's largest nursing specialty organization.

So from its beginning, critical care has had the needs of the patient and the abilities of the nurse as its focus. The patient who requires critical care is one who is physiologically unstable or at risk or in danger of dying, whereas intensive care is directed with the expectation or hope of recovery and positive outcomes (Fairman, 1998). Within this context, the dynamic interaction between and among acutely and critically ill patients and their families, acute and critical care nurses, and the health care environment defines the scope of practice for acute and critical care nursing (Medina, 2000). This synergistic relationship demands a knowledgeable and highly educated nurse. As the growth of critical care has occurred, the demand for nurses with specialized skills and knowledge has also increased.

CNS IN ACUTE AND CRITICAL CARE

The idea of specialization is also not new to nursing. The first issue of the *American Journal of Nursing*, published in 1900, had an article entitled, "Specialties in Nursing" (DeWitt, 1900). But the focus on specialization brought about the need for advanced education in the concepts needed by nurses working in these units. However, the idea of a specialist in clinical nursing prepared at the master's level represented a significant variation from the traditional view of nursing. Initially nurses in specialty areas learned their skills on the job, not in school (Fairman, 1998). Nurses collaborated with physicians and

with other nurses working in similar settings to learn about innovations and gain support and encouragement for specialized practice. But the need for education and consultation went beyond this limited collaboration. This was especially true in the new specialty of critical care. Nurses working in these new critical care areas needed immediate, highly knowledgeable resources to assist in increasing their knowledge and providing care for these complex patients. The role of the CNS in acute and critical care developed from this need for advanced knowledge and high level care.

Changes in governmental perspectives assisted in supporting the growth of a new role in nursing. In 1963, a major legislative mandate occurred for funding of graduate nursing education via the Division of Nursing in the United States Public Health Service. The Professional Nurse Traineeship Program was expanded at this time to include CNS education. The intent of this funding was to ensure that better educated and more experienced nurses would deliver direct patient care rather than to prepare nurses for only administration and teaching, as had been the pattern for the previous generation (Fairman, 1998). This legislative directive provided a major impetus to develop graduate program content in advanced clinical nursing.

The specialty of psychiatric nursing is credited with being the first to develop graduate level clinical education and CNSs. In 1954, Peplau designed the first master's degree program for CNSs in psychiatry. This educational program was developed in response to the vast increase in clinical specialty knowledge, rapid development of patient care technology, and public need. The role was used in acute and tertiary psychiatric care settings. Although the first master's-prepared CNSs appeared in psychiatric–mental health, the role quickly spread to maternal-child health, oncology, and cardiopulmonary nursing (Hamric, 1996). A graduate level course in oncology nursing was developed in 1947. In the mid-1970s critical care CNS programs were offered at the master's level.

Unfortunately the title has been somewhat misused by organizations and nurses who call themselves CNSs without benefit of this educational background. Nurses in administrative or education positions, as well as nurses with extensive experience but no master's degree, sometimes call themselves CNSs. This has led to confusion about the role and the education needed for it.

In 1980 the ANA identified two primary criteria for the specialist in nursing practice: "(1) an earned graduate degree that represents study of scientific knowledge and supervised advanced clinical practice and (2) eligibility requirements for certification through the professional society or completion of the certification process" (ANA, 1980). Graduate education prepares the nurse for expert practice, and certification identifies the nurse at a level of expert competence. The requirement of graduate level education is the minimum that associations believe is appropriate for those working as CNSs.

IMPLEMENTING THE ROLE OF THE CNS IN ACUTE AND CRITICAL CARE

The reaction to the role of the CNS was mixed. Early CNSs in critical care often had to figure out exactly what their jobs were. This was a new "on the job" training model. Many nurse administrators, nurse educators, and nursing staff were skeptical of the role. One concern was that these advanced practice nurses were too medically focused, abandoning the caring role of nursing. But these early pioneers experimented with new roles and made adaptations in their practice and education based on the experiences they had or the environment in which they practiced.

The CNS role is now recognized as an advanced nursing practice role within a specialized setting. Other advanced practice roles include acute care nurse practitioners, nurse midwife, and nurse anesthetists; and, while there are commonalities in advanced practice, there are also differences based on the unique contributions each brings to patient and family care.

The ANA's support and commitment to the development of the CNS role was illustrated by the creation of the Council of CNSs in 1982. The function of this group was to collect and analyze documents and information about the role. The ANA group defined a role statement in 1986 emphasizing the requirement for the CNS to have a patient-based practice and discussing factors influencing the implementation of the role. The ANA defined the role as a "nurse who has become expert in a defined area of knowledge and practice in a selected clinical area of nursing" (Council of Clinical Nurse Specialists, 1986). The role was designed as an avenue for professional advancement for nurses who wished to remain in clinical practice at the bedside rather than enter administrative or academic practice. This role statement became a foundational document for the development of specialty-specific statements.

In the arena of critical care, the AACN published a detailed description of the critical care clinical specialist defining the expectation of the master's prepared expert practitioner in 1987 (AACN, 1987). In their "Competence Statements for Critical Care CNSs in 1989," AACN described the advanced knowledge and skills needed by the CNS working in critical care. These documents focused on the traditional functions of the CNS as practitioner, educator, consultant, researcher, and manager (AACN, 1989). From this perspective the CNS exemplifies professional nursing practice and functions collaboratively and autonomously to achieve high-quality patient outcomes. This served not as a job description but as a description of the advanced knowledge and skills needed by the CNS in critical care.

The focus on roles was seen as a way to establish the CNS position within organizations. It was also designed to provide flexibility in implementation. A CNS in critical care might be hired by an organization because of an acute need for expanded education or because of a need for further research development. Unfortunately the flexibility often led to organizations seeing the position as too broad and sometimes allowing the individual to develop his or her own position.

However, the versatility and ambiguity of the role definition approach to CNS practice has been both a bane and a blessing for those in the CNS position (Hamric, 1996). Although it seems that the flexibility is desirable, it has led to many variations in implementation, which has created confusion in the overall understanding of the position. If the position focus is education, is research excluded from the role? What are the measures of the impact of the position if so many variations in implementation exist? It is difficult to justify a position when there is ambiguity and lack of performance criteria. A stable framework with clear and realistic expectations is needed to enhance the position of CNS in organizations.

In 1998, the Board of Directors of AACN approved the development of the *Scope of Practice and Standards of Professional Performance for the Acute and Critical Care Clinical Nurse Specialist* (Bell, 2002). The purpose of this document was to clarify the role of the CNSs working in this area for the patients and families, public, organizations, employers, educators, and regulatory and legislative bodies. The advanced practice work group was given the charge to develop and write the scope and standards document. This describes the role of the CNS and provides a framework for a minimum level of competent and professional practice for the CNS in acute and critical care. Foundational to the work were the concepts of the nursing process, the AACN Synergy Model for Patient Care, and the Statement on Clinical Nurse Specialist Practice and Education from the National Association of Clinical Nurse Specialists. The advanced practice work group maintained the Association's focus on the patients and families in acute and critical care as the driving force for the development of the standards statements. It was the goal of the group to facilitate the transfer of the standards into the daily practice of CNSs working in the current practice environment. The Standards are included in Appendix A.

The Scope of Practice document includes the role of the CNS in acute and critical care as a facilitator of care to improve outcomes for this patient population. The CNS achieves this purpose by working within the three spheres of influence of patient/family, nursing personnel, and organizational systems. The key elements of CNS practice include demonstrating clinical expertise, integrating care across the continuum, using research-based evidence to improve outcomes and care in a cost-effective manner, facilitating learning based on the needs of the learner, collaborating with other disciplines to provide interdisciplinary best practices, assisting patients and families in navigating the complex health care system, creating environments that assist in the development of caring practices and serving as a strong patient advocate. This role occurs in any setting in which patient care requirements include complex monitoring high-intensity nursing interventions or continuous nursing vigilance within the full range of high-acuity care. The patients within this scope include those who are at high risk for actual or potential life-threatening health problems. The CNS works with and through nursing personnel and other members of the health care team within the system to achieve optimal outcomes. Graduate education in the specialty of acute and critical care is required to assist the CNS to integrate the collaborative model of care into a coordinated patient management plan. Competencies in the educational program should be developed within the spheres of patient/family, nursing staff, and organizational system. A three-level educational system is identified as delineated in *The Essentials of Master's Education for Advanced Practice Nursing* (American Association of Colleges of Nursing, 1994). This includes graduate nursing core content, advanced practice nursing core content, and CNS specialty content. The advanced practice nursing core curriculum includes courses in advanced health/physical assessment, advanced physiology and pathophysiology, and advanced pharmacology so that the graduate is prepared to formulate differential diagnoses by systematically comparing and contrasting assessment findings; and to prescribe, order, and/or implement pharmacological and nonpharmacological interventions, treatment, and procedures within the framework of state licensure and hospital privileges. The clinical experiences must include a minimum of 500 hours in direct clinical practice within the educational program. The regulation of the CNS practice is accomplished through statues, rules, and regulation of state nurse practice acts, certification, peer review, and self-regulation. The ANA Code of Ethics supports the ethical component of the CNS role for nurses, as well as the AACN Ethics of Care based in the principles of beneficence, justice, and respect for persons.

The Standards of Practice for the Acute and Critical Care CNS follows the format of the nursing process: assessment, diagnosis, outcome identification, planning, implementation, and evaluation. Each of these standards highlights measurement criteria that assist in the operationalization of the standards into practice. The Standards of Professional Performance include quality of care, individual practice evaluation, education, collegiality, ethics, collaboration, research, and resource utilization. Provided within the document are specific examples to describe the practical application and integration of the standards into clinical practice.

The Synergy Model highlights the specific nurse competencies that the CNS embodies. It is through the integration of the Standards and the actualization of the Synergy Model that the CNS accomplishes the desired high-quality outcomes of practice. Each of the competencies is highlighted in this book with examples and methods of how the CNS could implement these competencies within their practice.

In a parallel process the AACN Certification Corporation developed an advanced practice certification program for acute and critical care CNSs. Through this process a job analysis and role delineation study was completed by the AACN and Professional Examination Services (PES). In 1998 a team of content experts met with PES psychometricians and the AACN

Certification Corporation staff and used the Synergy Model as a framework to construct an examination for the CNS working in critical care. This expert group served as the examination committee and item writers for the first examination.

The first critical care CNS certification examination was administered in January 1999. Before this examination a nurse who wanted to be certified as a CNS would have taken the medical-surgical CNS examination offered by American Nurses Credentialing Center (ANCC). The critical care CNS examination, with its test plan based on a job analysis study of current practice in the critical care setting, was more applicable to the health care environment.

The development of the role of the CNS in practice requires examination of the implementation of the Standards of Practice and Performance, as well as the integration of the principles of the Synergy Model. By examining the historical perspectives of critical care and the role of the CNS, foundations for practice in the role can be developed and nurtured. CNSs have seen many challenges and opportunities; there are many more to come.

References

American Association of Colleges of Nursing. (1994). *The essentials of master's education for advanced practice nursing*. Washington, DC: Author.

American Association of Critical-Care Nurses. (1987). *The critical care clinical nurse specialist: Role definition position statement*, Newport Beach, CA: Author.

American Association of Critical-Care Nurses. (1989). *AACN's competence statements for differentiated nursing practice in critical care*. Newport Beach, CA: Author.

American Nurses Association. (1980). *Nursing: a social policy statement*. Silver Spring, MD: Author.

Bell, L. (Ed.). (2002). *Scope of practice and standards of professional performance for the acute and critical care clinical nurse specialist*, Aliso Viejo, CA: American Association of Critical Care Nurses, 2002.

Chitty, D. (2005). *Professional nursing concepts and challenges*, Philadelphia: Elsevier Saunders.

Council of Clinical Nurse Specialists. (1986). *The role of the clinical nurse specialist*. Silver Spring, MD, American Nurses Association.

DeWitt, K. (1900). Specialties in nursing. *American Journal of Nursing 1*, 14-17.

Fairman, J., & Lynaugh, J. (1998). *Critical care nursing: A history*, Philadelphia: University of Pennsylvania Press.

Hamric, A.B., Spross, J.A., & Hanson, C.M. (Eds.). (1996). History and overview of the CNS role. *Advanced Practice Nursing: An integrative approach*, Philadelphia: Saunders.

Kirchhoff, K., & Dahl, N. (2006). American Association of Critical-Care Nurses' national survey of facilities and units providing critical care, *American Journal of Critical Care, 15*, 13-28.

Medina, J. (Ed.). (2002). *Standards for acute and critical care nursing practice*. Aliso Viejo, CA: American Association of Critical-Care Nurses.

NACNS Research and Practice Committee. (1998). *Statement of clinical nurse specialist practice and education*. Glenville, IL: National Association of Clinical Nurse Specialists.

Nightingale, F. (1860). *Notes on nursing*. (First American Edition). New York: D. Appleton and Company.

From Novice to Expert

CNS Competencies

Deborah G. Klein

Implementing the clinical nurse specialist (CNS) role in the critical care setting is a challenge even for the most experienced CNS. The complexity of the role, as well as the pressure to be cost-effective and produce positive outcomes can be frustrating and overwhelming. Understanding CNS competencies and the different phases of the CNS role development can be helpful to the CNS student, as well as the novice and experienced CNS. This chapter discusses CNS competencies, phases of the CNS role development, and strategies to enhance role effectiveness.

CLINICAL NURSE SPECIALIST COMPETENCIES

The AACN Synergy Model for Patient Care describes a patient-nurse relationship that optimizes patient outcomes (Curley, 1998). When patient needs are matched with nurse competencies, optimal outcomes occur. CNS practice can be described by the Synergy Model's eight nurse dimensions (clinical judgment, advocacy/moral agency, caring practices, collaboration, system thinking, responses to diversity, clinical inquiry, and facilitator of learning) through three spheres of influence (patient/family, nursing personnel, and organizational systems). Certification programs based on the Synergy Model provide a way to measure practice. Application of the Synergy Model to the role of the CNS is discussed in detail in other chapters of this book.

Hamric (2005) proposed a framework for describing primary criteria and competencies (knowledge and skills) for advanced practice nursing that are applicable to the role of the CNS (Fig. 2-1). The three primary criteria for advanced practice include an earned graduate degree with a concentration in an advanced nursing category, professional certification of practice at an advanced level within a given specialty, and a practice that is focused on patients and their families. Advanced practice nursing is further defined by a set of core competencies that have been described in the literature (American Association of Colleges of Nursing, 1996; AACN, 2002; American Nurses Association [ANA], 1995, 2003; Davies & Hughes, 1995; National Association of Clinical Nurse Specialists [NACNS], 2004; Spross & Baggerly, 1989). These core competencies are:

1. Direct clinical practice
2. Expert coaching and guidance of patients, families, and other care providers
3. Consultation
4. Research, including implementation of evidence-based practice, evaluation, and conduct
5. Clinical and professional leadership, including the role of a change agent
6. Collaboration
7. Ethical decision-making skills

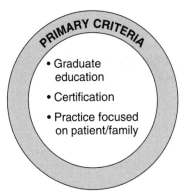

FIG 2-1 Primary criteria of advanced practice nursing. (In A.B. Hamric, J.A. Spross, & C.M. Hanson (Eds). 2005. *Advanced Practice Nursing.* (3rd ed.). Philadelphia: Elsevier Saunders).

The essence of CNS practice is clinical expertise based on advanced knowledge of nursing science. The dimensions of the CNS role are expert clinician, consultant, educator, and researcher. A CNS must master direct clinical practice, expert coaching and guidance, consultation, and research of core competencies to integrate the CNS role dimensions. The remaining competencies of clinical and professional leadership, collaboration, and ethical decision-making are present throughout the core competencies.

The CNS cares for and improves outcomes of patients through the three spheres of influence—the patient/family, nursing personnel, and organizational systems (AACN, 2002; NACNS, 2004). CNS practice within these three spheres of influence in combination with mastering the seven competencies is essential for a CNS to be successful.

The first core competency is direct clinical practice and is central to all the other competencies. Direct care or direct clinical practice refers to CNS activities involving patient-nurse interactions. The CNS may be involved with a patient whose diagnosis or care is complex, unique, or problematic. A CNS's clinical expertise is directly related to the patient population. For example, a CNS may be a clinical expert in pediatric critical care and involved in caring for a child with a complex congenital heart disease or planning a patient's complex hospital discharge.

Involvement in direct patient care provides opportunities for the CNS to demonstrate clinical competence; maintain clinical expertise; identify staff learning needs; role model appropriate clinical behaviors; evaluate resource utilization; and identify problems that interfere with care and develop a plan to resolve these problems, including staff education, revisions to policies or procedures, or conflict mediation among staff members. For each clinical situation, the CNS uses a comprehensive approach, advanced knowledge, expert skill, and discriminative judgment.

Another example of CNS direct clinical practice is when a CNS selects a patient population in which there are recurring problems or poor outcomes. The CNS collaborates with other health team members to develop and implement standards of care, procedures, or quality improvement plans. The CNS is often the champion and coordinator of such efforts of implementation and evaluation. The evaluation of technology and how it impacts patients and resources is another example of direct clinical practice. CNS clinical practice interventions should result in improved clinical outcomes, patient/family satisfaction, improved staff knowledge and skills, health team collaboration, appropriate resource allocation, and organizational efficiency (Sparacino, 2005).

The next competency is expert coaching and guidance. Expert coaching is dependent on the interaction between technical, clinical, and interpersonal competence and self-reflection (Spross, 2005). It is both formal and informal. A CNS is a role model for staff nurses by focusing on continuously improving clinical practice and integrating new knowledge. As a result, the CNS influences the development of the competent, proficient, and expert nurse and enhances accountability and autonomy. As the staff nurse integrates new knowledge and skills into his or her practice, the CNS is able to move to new or more complex responsibilities.

The CNS is both a resource and a process consultant. As a resource consultant, he or she provides relevant information that enables the staff nurse and others to make decisions based on alternatives. As a process consultant, the CNS facilitates change so that decisions can be made in specific and future situations. CNS consultation can be measured by outcome achievement and documentation of specific process activities. Consultation can be both internal (within the institution) and external (outside the institution, including specialty organizations, other health care providers, and other health care systems).

The research competency includes the interpretation and use of research, evaluation of practice, and participation in collaborative research. Inherent in the CNS role is the analysis and evaluation of research and application of research findings into clinical practice. Evidenced-based practice is seen in clinical protocols and procedures, administrative policies, educational materials, and clinical pathways. Evaluation of practice incorporates documentation of activities, peer review, staff evaluation, and outcomes management. Such information can be used to demonstrate CNS contributions to quality patient care, cost-effectiveness, and improved patient satisfaction. Participation in collaborative research can facilitate quality improvement, strengthen evidenced-based nursing practice, and enhance CNS research skills. The CNS is the clinical expert, understands the clinical issues, and has access to patients. The nurse researcher is the research expert, knows research methodology, and has access to resources that support the research.

Clinical and professional leadership, collaboration, and ethical decision-making are common threads that weave throughout the core competencies (Sparacino, 2005). Leadership is integral to the CNS role. Through clinical leadership and influence, strategies for change are implemented, and nursing practice and patient care improve. The CNS identifies the need for practice changes and is able to lead the process for change through the development and implementation of clinical

protocols and procedures, practice guidelines, and quality and performance improvement initiatives. The CNS is able to manage clinical projects, chair multidisciplinary committees, and influence institutional policy decisions. In addition, the CNS serves as an advocate for patients, families, and nursing staff, providing support, listening, and explaining decisions when needed. The CNS also helps the priorities and perspectives of other disciplines to enhance communication and as a result benefit patients.

Collaboration is a second common thread since there are many people who interact with the CNS. The CNS collaborates with nurses, physicians, other health care providers, patients, and families. The CNS has a good understanding of the knowledge and skills of other health care team members and is actively involved in multidisciplinary rounds and teams. Effective CNS collaboration is the result of clinical competence, effective communication, mutual trust, collegiality, and a favorable organizational structure (Hanson & Spross, 2005; Sparacino, 2005).

Ethical decision making involves a moral obligation that includes respect for individual uniqueness, personal relationships, and the dynamic nature of life as interrelated and interdependent (AACN, 2002). Behaviors that demonstrate the ethical influence of CNSs include fostering autonomy; advocacy for patients, families, and other nurses; assisting patients and family in addressing end-of-life issues with dignity; and mentoring nurses and other professionals to deliver safe care (NACNS, 2004). The CNS can educate nurses in ethical decision making through patient care conferences, ethics consulting, ethics rounds, and multidisciplinary ethics committees (Scanlon, 1994; Clark & Taxis, 2003).

These competencies develop over time. A new CNS does not graduate from a program fully prepared to implement all of them. However, it is critical that graduate programs provide exposure to each competency in didactic content and practical experience so that new graduates can be tested for initial credentialing and have a base on which to build their practice (Hamric, 2005).

EDUCATION

Graduate education should provide knowledge, skills, and clinical experiences to prepare the CNS to practice at an advanced level, regardless of the clinical setting or patient population. A blueprint for graduate nursing programs, the *Essentials of Master's Education for Advanced Practice Nursing* (American Association of Colleges of Nursing, 1996) recommended a core curriculum of theory, research, ethics, health policy, and professional role development. Recommended clinical specialty courses for advanced practice nurses included advanced physical assessment, advanced pharmacology, physiology, and pathophysiology. In 2004, the NACNS further described 13 additional core content areas for developing CNS competencies that include components of the Synergy Model (AACN, 2002):

1. Theoretical foundations for CNS practice
2. Phenomena of concern within the CNS specialty
3. Design and development of innovative nursing interventions and programs
4. Clinical inquiry/critical thinking using advanced knowledge
5. Technology, products, and devices
6. Teaching, mentoring, and coaching
7. Influencing change
8. Systems thinking
9. Leadership development for multidisciplinary collaboration
10. Consultation theory
11. Measurement
12. Outcome evaluation methods
13. Evidence-based practice and research utilization

The clinical practice component of CNS education is crucial. There should be sufficient opportunities to apply knowledge and skills and to begin the transition from competent to expert in the selected area of clinical practice. The clinical practice content should be divided

into two components: practice that refines skills and a "residency" that integrates the advanced practice concepts of consultation, education, and clinical leadership (Sparacino, 2005). The NACNS (2004) and AACN (2002) further support 500 hours of clinical practice and incorporation of the conceptual framework of the three spheres of influence (patient/client sphere, nurses and nursing practice sphere, and organization/system sphere). The National Council of State Boards of Nursing (2002a, 2002b) state that clinical experience should be directly related to the graduate student's specialty and supervision provided by a person licensed for the same APN role.

One of the challenges in curriculum design in advanced practice nursing educational programs preparing both CNSs and nurse practitioners (NPs) has focused on the similarities and differences in the core curriculum. A core curriculum that includes common areas of CNS and NP knowledge, domains, and competencies is practical. However, others argue that content for each is different since the NP has a medical-focused practice (primary care, physical assessment, and history taking) and the CNS has a nurse-focused practice (Lyon, 2004). Supporters of combined education cite the preparation of clinicians who are flexible and better prepared for broader practice opportunities (Stark, 2000).

Prescriptive Authority

Historically CNSs have not needed or demanded pharmacological prescriptive authority to influence positive patient outcomes. However, recent changes in health care delivery systems have prompted some CNSs to reevaluate prescriptive authority in their practices. For CNSs whose roles involve managing specialty care of patients with complex health needs, the option of prescribing pharmacological agents may promote autonomy, efficiency, reduced fragmentation of care, cost-effectiveness, and more comprehensive care (Tucker, 2003).

Credentialing and licensure for prescriptive authority occur at the state level. Pharmacology requirements vary from state to state, although most states require a graduate pharmacotherapeutics course and clinical supervision prescribing during the advanced practice nursing educational program, as well as yearly continuing education credits thereafter to maintain prescriptive privileges. Prescriptive authority may be regulated by the board of nursing, by the board of nursing and the board of pharmacy, or by three boards: the board of nursing, pharmacy, and medicine. It is the responsibility of the CNS to know and comply with the requirements for prescriptive authority in his or her state.

On graduation, the CNS is expected to have a clear understanding of the CNS role. In addition, it is beneficial for graduate students to learn marketing skills, interviewing skills, regulatory issues (e.g., scope of practice, certification), organizational issues (e.g., placement of the CNS within the organization, supervision of the CNS, authority and accountability of the CNS) and how to develop and use CNS outcome indicators (Hamric, 2003).

CNS ROLE DEVELOPMENT: THEORETICAL PERSPECTIVES

Role theory is a collection of concepts and hypotheses that suggest how people behave in a particular societal role. A role is composed of functions performed while a person occupies a certain position in society (Biddle & Thomas, 1979). Professional role development is a dynamic, ongoing process that, once begun, spans a lifetime. Anyone entering a new role experiences the process of role development before being able to function with maximum effectiveness.

Models of Role Development

The process of role development has been conceptualized by several authors. Dreyfus and Dreyfus (1986, 1996) have described the acquisition of knowledge and skill as a progressive movement through stages of performance from novice, advanced beginner, competent, proficient,

to expert. According to the Dreyfus model, the movement from novice to expert is incremental but not always linear or occurring in steps. Plateaus, setbacks, and stagnation can occur, as well as rapid steps forward. The competent level is a critical step in the development of expertise. Some individuals do not advance to the expert level because they do not become engaged in their practice. In addition, it takes time and practice for new skills to become embodied in practice.

At the proficient level, intuition replaces analytical reasoned responses. Expertise develops over time through personal encounters, with the resulting fine tuning of intuition or deliberative rationality (Dreyfus & Dreyfus, 1986). Deliberative rationality is described by Dreyfus and Dreyfus as a reflection on goals and possible ways to achieve these goals. It is used in distinguishing a novel situation or a situation in which the initial understanding may be incorrect from a situation in which experience can be trusted.

Brykczynski (2005) demonstrates a typical advanced practice nurse (including the CNS) role development pattern using the skills acquisition model (Fig. 2-2). One important implication of this novice-to-expert model for advanced practice nursing is that even experts can perform at lower skill levels when they enter a new situation. Hamric and Taylor (1989) believe that experienced CNSs starting a new position experience the same role development phases as new graduate, but over a shorter period of time.

For example, a critical care nurse who also is a preceptor for new graduates decides to return to school to become a CNS. As a graduate student, this nurse has a new role as novice student learning new skills. However, if he or she is still working as a registered nurse in the critical care unit, he or she may be functioning at the competent, proficient, or expert level. Once graduating, the new CNS may experience a time of limbo, when he or she is interviewing for CNS positions and meeting certification requirements. Even after starting a CNS position, progression through role implementation is not linear since there is movement

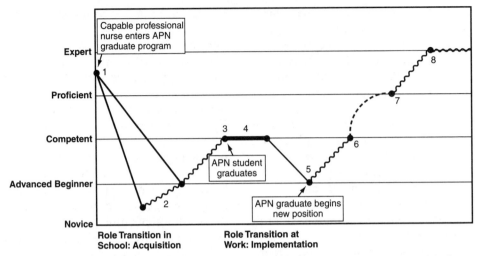

FIG 2-2 Typical advanced practice nurse (APN) role development pattern. (In A.B. Hamric, J.A. Spross, & C.M. Hanson [Eds]. (2005). *Advanced Practice Nursing,* ed. 3. Philadelphia: Elsevier Saunders).

back and forth as the CNS acquires new skills (see Fig. 2-2).

Benner (1984) used this model in her observational and interview study of clinical nursing practice situations from new nurses and their preceptors within the hospital setting. Although Benner's work did not focus specifically on the CNS, the process of skill acquisition and role development that she describes can be applied to the developing CNS.

Benner describes the *novice* as a beginner with no experience in the situation in which he or she is expected to perform. Behavior is governed by rules determined to be necessary to guide performance. However, it is difficult for the novice to be successful because the rules cannot give the most relevant tasks to perform in an actual situation. For example, a critical care CNS with graduate work and experience in adult critical care would be at the novice stage if he or she were to work in a neonatal intensive care unit.

In the second stage, *advanced beginner,* the nurse demonstrates marginally acceptable performance. The nurse has been involved with enough situations to recognize, either alone or with a mentor or preceptor, recurrent, meaningful patterns. However, the nurse still focuses on the rules and tasks that have been taught.

Assistance from a preceptor is needed to help set priorities. For example, a new critical care CNS is often enthusiastic and eager to implement changes. Without experience in the components of the CNS role, the new CNS may attempt to implement all role components simultaneously (e.g., start a unit-based research project, develop and implement a new continuous renal replacement therapy educational module, and implement weekly multidisciplinary patient care conferences) without the support of the nurse manager or the critical care unit staff. A preceptor or mentor would be helpful in assisting this new CNS in setting priorities and focusing on strategies that would facilitate timely implementation and enhance role development.

The third stage of skill acquisition is the *competent* nurse. Competence develops when the nurse begins to see actions in terms of conscious goals or plans. The plan establishes perspective and is based on conscious, abstract, and analytical thought about the problem. Deliberate planning helps achieve efficiency and organization. The competent nurse lacks the speed and flexibility of the proficient nurse (the next higher stage of development) but can manage more complex patient situations than the advanced beginner. In addition, competent nurses have enough experience and knowledge to recognize incompetence. They may become anxious and take on more responsibility than they can handle. A critical care CNS at this stage would be able to identify a clinical need, develop a plan to address that need, and successfully implement and evaluate the plan with the support of the nurse manager and nursing staff (e.g., a family support group or a hemodynamic monitoring review class).

The *proficient* nurse perceives situations holistically based on experience. This nurse knows what events to expect in a given situation and how plans must be modified in response to these events. The proficient nurse recognizes when the expected normal picture does not occur. For example, he or she is able to recognize deterioration in a patient before explicit changes in vital signs occur and is able to respond appropriately. Decision making is more precise. The proficient CNS is a recognized, trusted, clinical expert who is consulted by the nurse manager and staff as well as other departments within the institution. For example, a critical care CNS with expertise in cardiac transplantation may move from the competent stage with a strong clinical, consultation, and education focus to the proficient stage with a focus on new program development and research related to cardiac transplantation patients.

The fifth and final stage is *expert* nurse. The expert nurse has an extensive background of experience and an intuitive grasp of each situation because of an understanding of the total situation. Clinical performance is highly proficient. Analytical problem-solving methods are used when faced with a new situation or when the initial grasp of the problem proves to be incorrect. Expert nurses are not just engaged in use of knowledge; they are developing clinical knowledge (Benner, Tanner, & Chesla, 1992). Expert nurses provide consultation for other nurses. They recognize early clinical changes in a patient and can effectively make a case for further medical evaluation. In the critical care unit, the nurses have the opportunity to compare

their observations and develop consensus about conclusions with other nurses to further enhance performance. Critical care CNSs move into the expert stage when they can describe clinical situations in which their interventions made a difference. For example, a critical care CNS recognizes that ventilated tube-fed patients are lying in a supine position with a backrest elevation less than 30 degrees, thus increasing the risk of pulmonary aspiration of gastric contents and pulmonary bacterial colonization. Data are collected to determine how frequently this is occurring. On the basis of the results, a protocol is developed that focuses on the care of ventilated patients receiving tube feedings (i.e., backrest elevation 30 to 45 degrees, frequency of mouth care, frequency of checking tube-feeding residuals, frequency of turning, changing ventilator tubing only when needed). Nursing staff is educated on the protocol, and, as a result of this planned intervention, the critical care CNS is able to demonstrate a decreased incidence of pulmonary aspiration of gastric contents and pulmonary bacterial colonization.

Other models of CNS role development have been developed that have additional validity for critical care CNS role development (Table 2-1).

Baker's Model
In phase 1, *orientation*, the new CNS has just completed a graduate program or is new to the institution. Time is focused on becoming familiar with a new work situation, including the institution's functioning, personnel, and policies. The CNS is often enthusiastic and optimistic with feelings of anxiety and confusion. These feelings may interfere with conceptual knowledge. The CNS is eager to prove himself or herself as clinically competent and hopes to affect change through role modeling. One of the major tasks of this phase is to clarify the role to oneself first and then to others. This phase may be shortened in an institution where a CNS has been used effectively or if the CNS is experienced in the CNS role.

In phase 2, *frustration*, the CNS is often shocked by the overwhelming multitude of responsibilities and the anxiety that resistance

TABLE 2-1

Phases of CNS Role Development

Phase	Baker (1979)	Hamric & Taylor (1989)	CNS Characteristics
1	Orientation	Orientation	New CNS; optimistic; enthusiastic; anxious, confused, eager to prove self as clinically competent and to make change; clarifying role to self and setting
2	Frustration	Frustration	Overwhelmed with responsibilities and priorities of role; conflict between graduate school values and real-world values; unrealistic high performance expectations; feelings of confusion, anger, depression, isolation, and frustration; resistance encountered
3	Implementation	Implementation	Rethinking and reclarifying role to self and setting; modifying activities in response to feedback; implementing specific projects with tangible results; perspective returns; secure in role; consultation role expanded
4	Reassessment	—	Mutual respect between CNS and staff; role functions evaluated, reorganized or further developed; enthusiasm and optimism renewed; risk taking, creative, challenged
		Integration	Self-confident; wide recognition and influence in specialty area; challenged; congruence between personal and organizational goals and expectations
5		Frozen phase	Self-confident; conflict between personal goals and organizational goals and expectations; angry, frustrated
6		Reorganization	Organization experiencing major changes; pressure to change role that is incongruent with own conception of CNS role and goals
7		Complacent phase	Settled, comfortable in role; questionable impact on organization; practice constructed to meet selected, narrowly focused needs

to change evokes. The new CNS often has unrealistically high performance expectations. He or she begins to realize that one person cannot perform all role functions described in the literature, much less simultaneously. Conflict between graduate school values and real-world values become apparent. These conflicts may be due to adjustment to change, territoriality, interpersonal differences, or the way a particular CNS implements the role (Page & Arena, 1991). Role confusion may affect CNS performance and impede integration into the system. Feelings of inadequacy, confusion, anger, depression, isolation, and frustration may temporarily freeze the CNS in this phase. The CNS wonders about personal worth and believes that perhaps an imposter will soon be discovered.

Baker (1979) describes phase 3, *implementation*, as a period of organization and reorganization and of rethinking and clarifying one's position on the staff and health care team. As the CNS interacts with others, he or she begins to modify the approach in response to feedback received from the nursing staff and other health care professionals. Trust may be substituted for the pervasive feeling of constantly being tested. The CNS is effectively able to implement and balance new subroles. The consultant role is increasingly used and may surpass the more tangible role of educator. Consultation for clinical expertise is more frequently requested if the CNS remains patient oriented and highly visible on the patient units. Focusing on specific projects and visible tasks with tangible results can be rewarding. The desire to be all things to all people decreases as the CNS becomes more comfortable directing others to more appropriate resources. Enthusiasm and optimism return as positive feedback is received and expectations realigned. This security is a sign of developmental progression, enabling the CNS to believe that the role is finally gaining cohesiveness (Page & Arena, 1991). Lack of structure or self-goals, time management, and evaluation of progress may be stressful for those who are used to teamwork or following the directions of a leader. This phase is critical because it can lead to either positive or negative resolution.

In phase 4, *reassessment*, the energy and time spent building relationships and learning the system decrease, allowing for exploration of new areas of interest. Role functions are evaluated, reorganized, or further developed. Mutual respect between the CNS and staff has developed, and administration supports the role. New directions and goals are formulated.

Hamric's and Taylor's Model

Hamric and Taylor (1989) found in their study that CNSs with more than 3 years' experience used descriptors that fell out of Baker's phases. They identify four additional phases of role development: integration, frozen phase, reorganization, and complacency. CNSs in the *integration*

phase rated themselves at an advanced level of practice. There was congruence between personal and organizational goals and expectations. CNSs were either moderately or very satisfied with their present positions. They were self-confident and assured in the role. They continuously felt challenged by clinical problems confronted; changes in technology; new projects within the institution; and greater involvement in professional activities, research, and publishing.

CNSs in the *frozen phase* reported major conflicts between their goals and those of the organization. Although these CNSs were confident, self-assured, and at an advanced level of practice, administrative support for programs or goals valued by the CNS was generally lacking. These CNSs believed that they were not achieving their maximum potential and were in a frozen state because of factors beyond themselves and the CNS role. Feelings of anger and frustration were apparent. Reassessment and renegotiation of both the role and position within the organization are necessary to resolve conflicts and further role development.

The *reorganization phase* is typically experienced by CNSs in organizations that are involved with major changes in nursing or hospital administration and financial constraints. These changes often require reorganization in CNS practice that is incongruent with the CNSs concept of role and goals. If the role change is expected to be permanent, the CNS must decide whether this new role is adaptable or whether it can be renegotiated to incorporate elements that preserve the integrity of the CNS role, allow for job satisfaction, and meet the new needs of the organization. For example, in some hospitals CNSs are focusing on new patient care delivery systems such as case management. If no compromise can be found, the CNS may choose to leave the organization.

Hamric and Taylor (1989) found a small number of CNSs in a *complacent phase*. They were settled and comfortable with varying degrees of job satisfaction. Although these CNSs were not necessarily negative, the authors of the study question the extent to which complacent CNSs influence clinical practice. CNSs in this phase for long periods are not seen as change agents but have constructed their practice to meet selected, narrowly focused needs. For example, the CNS who does all of the preoperative education instead of empowering and developing the staff nurses to do this activity is not moving forward. CNSs in this phase need to be reenergized by changing some aspect of their practice or focus on a new population or new institutional need. The CNS role must change to allow for growth.

Role Development Issues

Movement of the CNS through any of these developmental phases is dynamic, occurs at varying rates, and is impossible to predict. The dynamics of role transition are affected by role ambiguity, lack of authority, resistance from staff nurses, lack of support, lack of role models, and role competition.

Role ambiguity occurs when there is a lack of consistency in describing the role and responsibilities of the CNS. Clearly defined goals, role responsibility, and mutual agreement about role expectations are essential. Role ambiguity may be positive in that it provides an opportunity to be creative.

Lack of authority for the CNS is an area of concern. The CNS role has historically been envisioned as purely clinical without administrative responsibilities. The CNS is expected to be the change agent by virtue of advanced knowledge, clinical skills, and expertise. As a result, the CNS is usually assigned a staff position without direct authority. The power base of the CNS is expert power, meaning that, based on the CNS's knowledge and skill, he or she has the ability to affect the behavior and actions of others. The CNS must be highly skilled in interpersonal relationships and in developing and maintaining channels of communication to influence clinical practice.

Resistance from the nursing staff and the nurse manger occurs when they are told by administration that the CNS is needed to improve patient care and patient outcomes. The CNS must establish credibility by focusing on the role of expert practitioner and acting as a role model and patient advocate during the early phases of CNS role development.

Lack of authority may be amplified by lack of visible administrative support for the CNS role. Lack of recognition such as no involvement in the development of clinical standards, no appointment to clinical practice councils, or no recognition of CNS contributions to quality patient care could significantly limit the CNS range of influence and potential.

Lack of role models for the CNS can limit job satisfaction and role development. Peer support can provide a mechanism to exchange ideas, share experiences, and give feedback.

Practice Implications

Although exact time periods cannot be attached to each phase of CNS role development, Benner's framework can be used to describe CNS role development and strategies that can facilitate successful role implementation incorporating the seven CNS competencies.

Novice CNS

The first year of practice as a CNS is crucial in establishing credibility and laying the foundation for future development. Developmental tasks include learning the formal and informal organization, establishing relationships, building a power base, identifying influential individuals in the organization, and clarifying the CNS role to self and others. Role conflict can occur if the CNS's preconceived role expectations do not conform to how the role is expected to be enacted. To learn this new role the CNS must relinquish previous roles such as student and staff nurse.

Whether a novice or experienced CNS, the newly employed CNS needs a thorough orientation. A comprehensive, structured, competency-based orientation and job description must define specific skills to help promote job integration. A competency-based orientation focuses on the integration of knowledge, skills, and attitudes necessary for the role of the CNS. It provides the CNS a method to demonstrate the proficiencies that are of central importance to the CNS role. The CNS job description should be developed on the basis of the competencies required to implement the role, including clinical practice, coaching, consultation, research, leadership, collaboration, and ethical decision-making skills.

The CNS needs time to become familiar with the organizational structure, philosophy, goals, policies, and procedures of the institution and the critical care unit. At the institutional level the CNS supervisor identifies key individuals for the CNS to meet, shares departmental objectives, and helps the CNS identify skill deficits that need attention. Role expectations and goals are discussed and mutually agreed on. The goals should pertain to the enhancement of the individual CNS performance, as well as to program objectives of the institution. For example, if the CNS supervisor wanted to develop nursing research in the critical care unit, one goal for a novice CNS could be to communicate to the critical care nursing staff monthly the findings of one published research study.

The CNS goals should be shared with others whose roles interface with the CNS to ensure that they know what to expect and what not to expect from the CNS. Goals can be shared at staff meetings and/or posted in the critical care unit. This clarification of priorities can help prevent misunderstandings and conflicts.

The novice CNS needs feedback frequently during the first year. For example, the supervisor and the CNS may meet monthly to provide feedback and encouragement to the CNS. The CNS may need assistance in setting limits, addressing a problem situation, or maintaining a sense of perspective. A more experienced CNS should be assigned as a preceptor to act as a role model and advocate for the novice CNS. In addition, meeting and networking with other CNSs in the institution is helpful in learning how the CNS role is implemented. If there are no other CNSs or if all the CNSs are novices, the new CNS can be encouraged to meet with other CNSs in other institutions in the community.

Within the critical care unit, it is imperative that the new CNS demonstrate clinical competence. During the first 6 months, the CNSs clinical knowledge and skills are constantly being tested by the staff. The CNS cannot affect change unless critical care expertise is established. This expertise can be demonstrated through consistent involvement in direct patient care in the critical care unit for which the CNS is responsible. Time scheduled for direct patient care should never be cancelled (Page & Arena, 1991). During this time the CNS can demonstrate clinical skills, clinical competence, and assess the skills and educational needs of the staff. The CNS can start role modeling direct patient care. In addition, the CNS can become familiar with the culture of the unit, as well as the protocols, standards, and levels of practice. Part of the assessment includes identifying the perceived nursing leaders in the critical care unit, the method of staff orientation, the relationship between the nursing staff and physicians, and the leadership style of the nurse manager. In addition, the CNS can spend time in other clinical areas to learn more about the patient population cared for in the critical care unit. For example, it would be beneficial for a new CNS in the cardiac critical care unit to spend time in the cardiac catheterization area. This experience promotes collaboration with the physicians and other clinical areas.

The novice CNS may further substantiate the clinical role by wearing attire similar to the staff nurses and by exhibiting flexibility in scheduling. Working off shifts increases CNS visibility and promotes acceptance by the staff. Off shifts may be scheduled in 1-week blocks or 10- to 12-hour shifts in an effort to overlap shifts. After the initial orientation period the CNS should maintain a flexible schedule to come in early or stay late to maintain contact and enhance use by the evening, night, and weekend nursing staff. Although this type of flexibility may not be required by other management roles, flexibility and clinical visibility are essential to CNS role success.

The CNS must identify and clarify the role to self and others, especially if the role is newly created. Appointments with nursing administrators and physicians are scheduled to introduce the role and discuss implementation. Attending staff meetings on all shifts to discuss the CNS role and placing the CNS job description in visible locations in the critical care unit enhances communication of the role. Integration into the system is further enhanced by being accessible to the nursing staff by pager and distributing business cards to professional contacts.

During this stage information should be absorbed, and judgment on issues reserved until the CNS role is accepted. Keeping a log or a list of needs or ideas for future projects is helpful. Opinions of the CNS will be valued at a later time when the CNS is more knowledgeable and entrenched in the daily operations of the organization.

Once baseline assessment of the critical care unit and the institutional system is completed, the CNS can formulate specific goals and action plans. This process is helpful in providing structure and direction, both of which are important for performance evaluation and a sense of accomplishment. During this phase the CNS must begin to internalize self-worth in the role (Hamric & Taylor, 1989).

Advanced Beginner CNS

The focus of activities during this stage is establishing and implementing the CNS role. The CNS increases visibility and credibility by focusing on clinical practice, role modeling, and being a patient advocate. For example, the CNS can serve as a patient and family advocate by increasing nursing staff awareness about the experience of families with a loved one in the critical care unit. The CNS can ask a family member to write what she perceives as concerns in meeting the needs of her critically ill mother. By sharing this list with the nursing staff and promoting discussion, a better understanding of the critical care unit experience by the nursing staff may be achieved. Establishing these components of the CNS role is important as the CNS begins to implement change and promote education.

The CNS develops the consultant role by implementing walking rounds to increase visibility and develop patient referral patterns. Walking rounds provide the opportunity to identify patient care problems, suggest problem-solving strategies, and assist the staff in providing patient care, all of which help to increase CNS credibility and enhance staff nurse acceptance. Walking rounds are best done with the nurse manager at a time of day that is selected by the nurse manager, CNS, and critical care unit staff. Nursing staff should be encouraged to participate so that it does not appear that the CNS is "policing" care. Participation in multidisciplinary patient care conferences provides an opportunity for the CNS to function as a role model, coach, clinical expert, and an advocate of the nursing staff. The interaction with other team members also helps establish role identity and patient referrals.

Strategies that promote education of the nursing staff, patients, and families are best implemented at this time. Copies of relevant and interesting articles or research can be made available through the patient chart or bulletin board. The CNS should sign his or her name with a "for your information" notice to promote the role of the CNS as a resource person. Providing opportunities for the nursing staff to identify topics is one strategy that can be used in developing staff education programs, including inservices and patient care conferences. The CNS can also serve as a consultant to the nursing staff in developing patient education materials.

The critical care unit nursing staff may not be effectively providing family support because of patient acuity and time constraints on the nursing staff. The CNS can then serve as a liaison for the family. For example, family members arriving from out of town to be with a critically ill loved one may have many questions and concerns. The staff nurse may not able to spend the amount of time with the family that both the family and the nurse desire. The CNS can be with the family initially to address their concerns and communicate back to the bedside nurse. The CNS can also promote staff nurse involvement with families by offering to "cover" the staff nurse's patient assignment so the staff nurse can participate in family conferences. However, if the CNS has a relationship with the family, the CNS may also need to attend the family conference.

During this period of role development, the CNS typically is performing tasks that are requested from a variety of different sources. Directors may request management coverage on units without nurse managers. Nurse managers may solicit assistance for units inadequately staffed, and staff nurses may request patient assignment coverage for a variety of reasons. These requests place the CNS in a difficult situation in which requests for involvement are being initiated but are often inappropriate for the CNS role. The CNS must decide how to handle this dilemma without alienating management and staff. For example, if inadequate staffing is an issue, the CNS can facilitate care by assisting in direct patient care 1 day per week and creating or supporting efforts to create long-term solutions to these staffing challenges. This strategy reconfirms the clinical expertise of the CNS, enhances role modeling and leadership to promote change, and reestablishes clinical credibility in a CNS who has been in the position for years.

Because of the need to establish clinical credibility and concentrate on direct care activities in this stage, clinical research activities are directed at implementing research findings of others into practice through staff education and incorporation into standards of care. Presenting or publishing one's graduate research or project is a useful starting point. Identifying potential research problems can serve as the basis for future research.

Providing concrete examples of when to call the CNS will enhance role acceptance and use. For example, in one community hospital a CNS consultation is automatic if the patient is in the critical care unit for more than 3 days.

A crucial task during this stage is to develop a support system to network with other CNSs. This provides a mechanism for communication, collaboration, and feedback necessary for effective CNS role development. In addition, the CNS

develops a realistic perspective of the work setting in which short-term goals and projects can be implemented and that can provide tangible results and personal gratification.

Competent CNS
By this stage a successful CNS should have established a strong power base and be ready to focus on the role of change agent as a clinical and professional leader. Planned change involves competence in the skills of problem solving, decision making, and interpersonal relationships. If the CNS does not have the administrative authority to implement change, credibility becomes a key element. The CNS can best implement change in clinical practice through collaboration with the nurse manager and nursing staff. This involvement may take the form of committee work with a focus on quality improvement. Beginning steps include identifying the problem, collecting relevant data, and formulating a written proposal for accomplishing the desired outcome. Inclusion of the nurse manager and staff in the process fosters the feelings of involvement and commitment to the planned change.

An increase in the number of patient consultations from nurses and physicians often occurs in this stage. Because of the rapidly changing population and physiological changes in patients that occur in the critical care unit, the competent CNS demonstrates flexibility in responding to priorities. If a crisis occurs, the competent CNS responds appropriately, whether it be to serve as a resource to the staff, work directly with the staff, solve problems, or direct resources.

The CNS is now able to identify educational programs that are consistent with staff needs based on walking rounds, communication with other health team members, and identified problem areas. The CNS is involved with program development and coordination and expanding personal development beyond the critical care unit. The credibility and expertise of the CNS have usually expanded beyond the institution, and there may be requests to present programs locally and regionally. The CNS should consider publication in professional journals.

Working relationships with colleagues and professional networking are usually well established. The CNS is able to participate in more leadership activities in the hospital (e.g., chairperson of a committee) and the community (e.g., AACN chapter officer). Serving as a preceptor for graduate students provided the CNS with an opportunity to contribute to the professional growth and development of others. By working with graduate students, the CNS is able to role model the integration of practical and scientific knowledge into expert clinical practice. These experiences, although satisfying, also stimulate self-evaluation and reassessment of the role. The CNS also serves as a mentor to the nursing staff.

Research efforts during this stage focus on identified clinical issues. The CNS may coordinate a small study or assist the staff in a research project. The formation of a journal club to disseminate research findings that impact practice in the critical care unit helps promote evidenced-based practice.

Proficient CNS

Consultation is the major focus of the CNS in the proficient stage. Time is spent on consultation beyond the critical care unit. The CNS must ensure that the nursing staff has been developed to address clinical issues that the CNS once addressed to successfully move beyond the critical care unit. Consultations may occur outside the hospital as a member or chairperson of a multidisciplinary committee or involvement in projects that impact clinical practice in the critical care unit. However, the opportunity to provide direct patient care and function as a role model and coach for the nursing staff must still be integrated. This ensures that clinical expertise and credibility are maintained and enhanced, communication with the staff maintained, staff learning needs identified, and resource utilization evaluated. In addition, direct care requirements for recertification can be met.

The CNS with more than 5 years' experience has demonstrated competence and problem-solving ability so that he or she is able to serve as a consultant at all levels. Nursing administration may seek advice about handling difficult situations or personalities, program development, or strategies to improve existing services as the CNS has become the management link to the bedside. Staff nurses may consult the CNS in the development of patient education materials, in the revision of patient care forms, or in patient-focused projects. Physicians may consult the CNS for system- or patient-related concerns. The CNS serves as an organizational specialist and change agent as coaching and guidance skills are further developed. A CNS may initiate the plan, mobilize the resources, defuse the politics, and facilitate resolution (Sparacino, 2005).

Presenting at national meetings is an appropriate goal. Collaboration with an experienced researcher or with other CNSs is realistic and rewarding. Serving as a mentor and preceptor to new CNSs continues to expand the expert coaching and guidance skills.

The demands for CNS expertise and guidance outside the institution may be more than the CNS can fulfill. When considering an opportunity, the CNS must examine the focus, the number of people who will be reached, internal or external visibility, and potential cost savings or revenue for the institution. The CNS must carefully balance obligations within the institution with opportunities outside the practice setting.

Many CNSs perceive themselves at this stage to be autonomous, highly motivated, self-directed professionals. The CNS is trusted and perceived as an integral member of the team. Continued role development may become frozen if the goals of the institution or supervisor are seen as restrictive or incompatible or if conflicting or competing demands occur with the CNS's time or attention. When such circumstances occur, support and advice from an objective mentor can be helpful.

Expert CNS

The expert CNS is an individual who has achieved a level of role maturity. CNSs are perceived as dependable, goal directed, organized, and "doers" within the institution. They are viewed as team players, possess strong interpersonal skills, and help others grow through mentorship and empowerment (Boyle, 1997). Role advancement is not perceived as vertical growth into administration but as horizontal growth in which their clinical outcomes move beyond the institution or health care system when they are able to impact nursing curriculum; impact nursing agendas at the local, regional, and national levels; and mentor novice CNSs (Bingle, 2001). Hamric and Taylor (1989) describe factors that enhance continued role evolution for experienced CNSs, including availability of continuous feedback to validate role performance, freedom to develop the CNS role without unnecessary restriction, encouragement and support for broadening their sphere of influence, recognition of the contributions the CNS makes to patients and the institution, and congruent goals and philosophy between the CNS and the employing institution. Examples of support for the expert CNS include involving the CNS in planned change projects, expanding CNS involvement in activities outside their immediate sphere of influence, and facilitating relationships with those who can be a constructive counsel and trusted mentor (Boyle, 1997).

CNS career goals can be addressed within the institution. Hamric and Taylor (1989) discuss a clinical ladder for advanced practice to facilitate ongoing growth and recognition of exemplary CNS practice. Oda, Sparacino, and Boyd (1988) recommend offering sabbaticals for self-renewal, monetary recognition for clinical excellence and entrepreneurship, and facilitating opportunities for creativity and professional growth within the institution. Hazelton, Boyum, and Frost (1993) suggest offering educational programs on marketing strategies, financial management, business law, and organizational structure to advance clinical knowledge.

Expert CNSs can help institutions move from a quality focus to a quality-cost balance by using and moving the CNS from a patient/nurse focus to a systems focus (Wolf, 1990). Examples of this "second-generation" CNS include identifying and correcting system-wide factors contributing to poor patient outcomes such as length of stay or hospital-acquired complications, identifying and correcting system-wide factors contributing to inefficient and ineffective nursing practice, developing strategies to modify nursing practice while maintaining quality outcomes, evaluating new technologies and equipment for cost-effectiveness, developing innovative approaches to care delivery that positively affect quality-cost balance, and evaluating care through research.

An additional strategy that may further challenge the CNS is formalizing a mechanism for offering services and expertise to others (e.g., forming a small company that offers educational programs). Continuing to publish clinical research, developing new research studies based on previous work, and seeking external funding for research offer new challenges. Doctoral study may be considered.

Strategies to Successful Role Development

Additional strategies that can enhance CNS role development are goal setting and mentoring.

Goal Setting

Goals provide a purpose, direction, and focus. The setting of goals between the CNS and supervisor provides a framework for measuring CNS effectiveness, decreases role ambiguity, fosters purposeful activity, and ensures CNS development. Through goal setting dialogue, the institution (represented by the supervisor) and the CNS find the mutuality of purpose that binds them together (Brown, 1989).

In setting a 5-year goal of professional critical care CNS practice, it is useful to list qualities that exemplify that practice, followed by activities that foster those qualities. For example, nursing research is one of the core competencies of CNS practice. If the nursing staff has been exposed to limited nursing research, it is unrealistic to expect the CNS to conduct a research study in the first year. However, rather than let the research component lie dormant, the CNS may develop strategies to expose the staff to nursing research, including posting pertinent studies in the unit, sharing with the staff the research basis for proposed practice innovations, or critiquing a sample study to assist staff in recognizing its merits. Once potential strategies are listed, arrange them along a loose timeline based on the unique needs of the unit. This process is then repeated for other problem areas or aspects of clinical practice that the CNS identifies, such as accountability or continuity (e.g., evaluation of documentation) and communication skills (e.g., assertiveness, conflict management skills, improved family support). After the list is completed, all aspects are arranged along a 5-year steplike timeline. The yearly deadlines may be fluid since some projects are complex and cannot be accomplished by a fixed date.

By creating this timeline, the CNS can stay focused on goals. In daily practice the CNS mentally asks, "Does this activity relate to my goals?" Setting priorities and decisions about time allocation become easier. The resulting flexibility allows the CNS to respond to crises such as staffing shortages and sudden rises in patient acuity without losing sight of progress toward the goal.

Mentoring

Mentoring is defined as the personal and professional nurturing of a less experienced person (Vance & Olson, 1998). The mentor serves as a guide, role model, counselor, teacher, and sponsor for a newer, less experienced person (protégé). Mentoring promotes professional development, career satisfaction, and success. The mentoring relationship occurs along a continuum, ranging from passive role modeling to active precepting of a novice CNS.

Mentoring can be used effectively in the development of the novice CNS. A CNS mentor can assist the novice CNS; clarify the CNS role in the institution; and decrease confusion, frustration, and anxiety. In addition, the CNS mentor can enhance the skills and interpersonal behaviors of the novice CNS through encouragement, guidance, sharing, and caring. The novice CNS may bring new knowledge and an unbiased perception of the CNS role. Through mutual sharing of experience and knowledge, both the mentor and novice may benefit by enhanced self-esteem, professional productivity, and value to the institution.

Selecting a mentor requires careful matching of mentors and protégés. Not all experienced CNSs are appropriate mentors. The first step in seeking a mentor is to identify what one needs assistance with and who can specifically help. For a novice CNS the logical choice is a more experienced CNS. However, the choice should also be based on admiration, respect, and trust and should outweigh feelings of envy or being threatened. Mentoring relationships take time to develop; therefore, as the novice CNS is learning the role and seeking advice and guidance, potential mentors can be evaluated. A novice CNS benefits from someone who can communicate knowledge and skills effectively, is creative, collaborates, and demonstrates entrepreneurship. In addition, someone who is effective with conflict resolution, is assertive, empowers, and is respected may be a potential mentor. Once a potential mentor is identified, the protégé should start sharing ideas to see if the individuals are compatible. Another way to select a mentor is to ask for help so one can tap that source and begin to establish a relationship. As a mentoring relationship develops, both the mentor and protégé gain from ongoing reciprocal communication. For example, a newer CNS may approach a more experienced CNS regarding a clinical issue that the newer CNS has been unable to resolve. The ensuing discussions may bring into focus the newer CNS's inability to work effectively with the nurse manager. The more experienced CNS, through expert guidance, coaching, and role modeling, can demonstrate more effective behaviors to assist in enhancing the CNS/nurse manager relationship.

To facilitate an effective mentoring relationship, congruence must exist between the perception that the mentor and protégé have of the mentoring relationship. The most effective relationships occur when the mentor demonstrates empathy and is genuine, concrete, and provides self-disclosure while the protégé seeks to understand himself or herself and the role of the CNS. Mentors must be willing to help a protégé face the realities of the CNS role and simultaneously help him or her achieve the highest level of functioning possible.

CONCLUSION

The critical care CNS has many unique challenges in role development. Although significant barriers may exist such as limited administrative support and guidance, limited understanding of critical care CNS role, resistance to change, and unrealistic expectations, the critical care CNS can be successful in the role and improve patient outcomes. Considerable responsibility is placed on the CNS to sell the role; and, with an understanding of the CNS competencies, role development phases, and strategies for implementing the role, this can be achieved.

References

American Association of Colleges of Nursing. (1996). *The essentials of masters education for advanced practice nursing.* Washington D.C.: Author.

American Association of Critical-Care Nurses. (2002). *Scope and standards of professional performance for the acute and critical care clinical nurse specialist.* Aliso Viejo, CA: Author.

American Nurses Association. (1995). *Nursing's social policy statement.* Washington D.C.: Author.

American Nurses Association. (2003). *Nursing's social policy statement 2003 draft.* Washington D.C.: Author.

Baker, V.E. (1979). Retrospective exploration in role development. In G.V. Padilla (Ed.). *The clinical nurse specialist and improvement in nursing practice.* Wakefield, MA: Nursing Resources.

Benner, P. (1984). *From novice to expert: Excellence and power in clinical nursing practice.* Reading, MA: Addison-Wesley Publishing.

Benner, P., Tanner, C., & Chesla, C. (1992). From beginner to expert: Gaining a differential clinical world in critical care nursing. *Advanced Nursing Science, 14,* 13.

Biddle, B.J., & Thomas, E.J. (1979). *Role theory: Concepts and research.* Huntington, NY: Robert E. Krieger Publishing.

Bingle, J.M. (2001). A career ladder for the clinical nurse specialist. "To be or not to be." *Clinical Nurse Specialist, 15,* 167.

Boyle, D.M. (1997). Lessons learned from clinical nurse specialist longevity. *Journal of Advanced Nursing, 26,* 1168.

Brown, S.J. (1989). Supportive supervision of the CNS. In A.B. Hamric & J.A. Spross (Eds.). *The clinical nurse specialist in theory and practice.* Philadelphia: Saunders.

Brykczynski, K.A. (2005). Role development of the advanced practice nurse. In A.B. Hamric, J.A. Spross, & C.M. Hanson (Eds). *Advanced practice nursing: An integrative approach* (3rd ed.). Philadelphia: Elsevier Saunders.

Clark, A.P., & Taxis, J.C. (2003). Developing ethical competence in nursing personnel. *Clinical Nurse Specialist, 17,* 236.

Curley, M.A. (1998). Patient-nurse synergy: optimizing patient outcomes. *American Journal of Critical Care, 7,* 72.

Davies, B., & Hughes, A.M. (1995). Clarification of advanced practice nursing: Characteristics and competencies. *Clinical Nurse Specialist, 9,* 156.

Dreyfus, H.L., & Dreyfus, S.E. (1986). *Mind over machine: The power of human intuition and expertise in the era of the computer.* New York: Free Press.

Dreyfus, H.L., & Dreyfus, S.E. (1996). The relationship of theory and practice in the acquisition of skill. In P. Benner, C.A. Tanner, & C.A. Chesla (Eds.). *Expertise in nursing practice: Caring, clinical judgment, and ethics.* New York: Springer-Verlag.

Hamric, A.B. & Taylor, J.W. (1989). Role development of the CNS. In A.B. Hamric & J.A. Spross (Eds.). *The clinical nurse specialist in theory and practice.* Philadelphia: Saunders.

Hamric, A.B. & Hanson, C.M. (2003). Educating advanced practice nurses for practice reality. *Journal of Professional Nursing, 19,* 262.

Hamric, A.B. (2005). A definition of advanced practice nursing. In A.B. Hamric, J.A. Spross, & C.M. Hanson (Eds.). *Advanced practice nursing: An integrative approach,* (3rd ed.). Philadelphia: Elsevier Saunders.

Hanson, C.M., & Spross, J.A. (2005). Collaboration. In A.B. Hamric, J.A. Spross, & C.M. Hanson (Eds.). *Advanced practice nursing: An integrative approach,* (3rd ed.). Philadelphia: Elsevier Saunders.

Hazelton, J.H., Boyum, C.M., & Frost, M.H. (1993). CNS subroles: Foundation for entrepreneurship. *Clinical Nurse Specialist, 7*, 40.

Lyon, B.L. (2004). The CNS regulatory quagmire—we need clarity about advanced nursing practice. *Clinical Nurse Specialist, 18*, 9.

National Association of Clinical Nurse Specialists (2004). *Statement of clinical nurse specialist practice and education*. Harrisburg, PA: Author.

National Council of State Boards of Nursing. (2002a). *Regulation of advanced practice nursing: 2002 National council of state boards of nursing position paper*. Retrieved January 28, 2005 from http://www.ncsbn.org/public/regulation/res/APRN_Position_Paper2002pdf.

National Council of State Boards of Nursing. (2002b). *Requirements for accrediting agencies and criteria for APRN certification programs*. Retrieved January 28, 2005 from http://www.ncsbnorg/pdfs/APRN_approved_criteria_requirements_04.pdf.

Oda, D., Sparacino, P.S.A., & Boyd, P. (1988). Role advancement for the experienced clinical nurse specialist. *Clinical Nurse Specialist, 2*, 167.

Page, N.E., & Arena, D.M. (1991). Practical strategies for CNS role implementation. *Clinical Nurse Specialist, 5*, 43.

Scanlon, C. (1994). Models of discernment: Developing ethical competence in nursing practice. *American Nurses Association Center for Ethics and Human Rights Communiqué, 3*, 1.

Sparacino, P.S.A. (2005). The clinical nurse specialist. In A.B. Hamric, J.A. Spross, & C.M. Hanson (Eds.). *Advanced practice nursing: An integrative approach* (ed. 3). Philadelphia: Elsevier Saunders.

Spross, J.A., & Baggerly, J. (1989). Models of advanced practice. In A.B. Hamric, & J.A. Spross (Eds.). *The clinical nurse specialist in theory and practice*. Philadelphia: Saunders.

Spross, J.A. (2005). Expert coaching and guidance. In A.B. Hamric, J.A. Spross, & C.M. Hanson (Eds.). *Advanced practice nursing: An integrative approach* (3rd ed.). Philadelphia: Elsevier Saunders.

Stark, S.W. (2000). Point of view: The case for combined education for the NP and CNS. *Journal of the American Academy of Nurse Practitioners, 12*, 85.

Tucker, S., & Rhudy, L. (2003). Preparing CNS's for prescriptive authority. *Clinical Nurse Specialist, 17*, 194.

Vance, C., & Olson, R.K. (Eds). (1989). *The mentor connection in nursing*. New York: Springer-Verlag.

Wolf, B.A. (1990). Clinical nurse specialists: The second generation. *Journal of Nursing Administration, 5*, 7.

Synergy Model

Guiding the Practice of the CNS in Acute and Critical Care

Roberta Kaplow

BACKGROUND

Over a decade ago, the Certification Corporation of the American Association of Critical-Care Nurses (AACN) envisioned a new model for clinical practice. In 1993 the Corporation assembled a group of critical care nurses to develop a conceptual framework for certified practice. This group believed that certified practice was more than tasks and should be grounded in nurses meeting the needs of patients and influencing optimal outcomes (Hardin, 2004a).

During the 1994 National Teaching Institute, the Board of Directors of the Certification Corporation expressed the importance of linking certified practice with patient outcomes. Of great importance was the ability to articulate nurses' unique contribution in caring for critically ill patients and their families (Hardin, 2004a).

In 1995, the Certification Corporation Board of Directors appointed a group of subject matter experts to refine the conceptual model and to be involved with a study of practice. The experts concluded that each patient consistently brings a unique set of characteristics to the health care situation (Hardin, 2004a).

THE SYNERGY MODEL

The AACN Synergy Model for Patient Care is based on five assumptions: (1) patients are biological, social, and spiritual entities who present at a particular developmental stage. The whole patient (body, mind, and spirit) must be considered; (2) the patient, family, and community all contribute to providing a context for the nurse-patient relationship; (3) patients can be described by a number of characteristics; all characteristics are connected and contribute to one another; characteristics cannot be looked at in isolation; (4) nurses can be described on a number of dimensions; the interrelated dimensions paint a profile of the nurse; and (5) a goal of nursing is to restore a patient to an optimal level of wellness as defined by the patient; death can be an acceptable outcome in which the goal of nursing care is to move a patient toward a peaceful death (AACN, 2000, p. 55).

The core concept of the Synergy Model is that the needs or characteristics of patients and families influence and drive the characteristics or competencies of nurses (Curley, 1998). Synergy results when the needs and characteristics of a patient, clinical unit, or system are matched with a nurse's competencies. Further, when patient characteristics and nurse competencies match, patient outcomes are optimized (www. aacn.org/certcorp.org).

Outcomes are considered patient conditions measured along a continuum. The group of experts articulated three derivations of outcomes: from the patient, nurse, and health care system. Examples of patient outcomes include changes in functional status, behavioral changes, trust, satisfaction, comfort, and quality of life. Nursing outcomes include changes in physiological status, presence or absence of complications, and the degree to which treatment objectives were attained. Health care system outcomes include recidivism, length of stay, and health care costs (Curley, 1998).

PATIENT CHARACTERISTICS

The eight patient characteristics identified are present in varying levels when patients are admitted for care (wherever care is rendered to acute and critically ill patients):

1. Resiliency
2. Vulnerability
3. Stability
4. Complexity
5. Resource availability
6. Participation in care
7. Participation in decision making
8. Predictability

Each characteristic exists on a continuum from low (level 1) to high (level 5). The patient characteristics are defined in Table 3-1. The continuum of how these characteristics present at the varying stages of illness appears in Table 3-2.

The Synergy Model definition of *resiliency* is "the patient's capacity to return to a restorative level of functioning by using compensatory and coping mechanisms" (Curley, 1998; www.aacn. org/certcorp.org). Some people have the ability to bounce back, regardless of how difficult a situation is (Lauer, 2002). If a patient is resilient, it is implied that adaptation to other stressors has taken place in the past (Kaplow, 2004a). Resiliency has been further defined as the ability to achieve, retain, or regain a level of physical or emotional health after a devastating illness or loss (Felten & Hall, 2001).

TABLE 3-1
Patient Characteristics of the Synergy Model

Patient Characteristic	Definition
Resiliency	The patient's capacity to return to a restorative level of functioning by using compensatory and coping mechanisms
Vulnerability	The susceptibility to actual or potential stressors that may adversely affect patient outcomes
Stability	The ability to maintain a steady-state equilibrium
Complexity	The intricate entanglement of two or more systems (e.g., body, family, therapies)
Resource availability	The extent of resources (e.g., personal, financial, social, psychological, technical) the patient, family, and community bring to the current situation
Participation in care	The extent to which the patient and family engage in care
Participation in decision making	The extent to which the patient and family engage in decision making in aspect of care
Predictability	A summative characteristic that allows one to expect a certain trajectory

Source: www.aacn.org/certcorp.org.

TABLE 3-2

Patient Characteristics on a Clinical Continuum

Patient Characteristic	Explanation of Continuum
Resiliency	Level 1: Minimally resilient—Unable to mount a response; failure of compensatory/coping mechanisms; minimal reserves; brittle
	Level 3: Moderately resilient—Able to mount a moderate response; able to initiate some degree of compensation; moderate reserves
	Level 5: Highly resilient—Able to mount and maintain a response; intact compensatory/coping mechanisms; strong reserves; endurance
Vulnerability	Level 1: Highly vulnerable—Susceptible; unprotected, fragile
	Level 3: Moderately vulnerable—Somewhat susceptible; somewhat protected
	Level 5: Minimally vulnerable—Safe; out of the woods; protected, not fragile
Stability	Level 1: Minimally stable—Labile; unstable; unresponsive to therapies; high risk of death
	Level 3: Moderately stable—Able to maintain steady state for limited period of time; some responsiveness to therapies
	Level 5: Highly stable—Constant; responsive to therapies; low risk of death
Complexity	Level 1: Highly complex—Intricate; complex patient/family dynamics; ambiguous/vague; atypical presentation
	Level 3: Moderately complex—Moderately involved patient/family dynamics
	Level 5: Minimally complex—Straightforward; routine patient/family dynamics; simple/clear cut; typical presentation
Resource availability	Level 1: Few resources—Necessary knowledge and skills not available; necessary financial support not available; minimal personal/psychological supportive resources; few social systems resources
	Level 3: Moderate resources—Limited knowledge and skills available; limited financial support available; limited personal/psychological supportive resources; limited social systems resources
	Level 5: Many resources—Extensive knowledge and skills available and accessible; financial resources readily available; strong personal/psychological supportive resources; strong social systems resources
Participation in care	Level 1: No participation—Patient and family unable or unwilling to participate in care
	Level 3: Moderate level of participation—Patient and family need assistance in care
	Level 5: Full participation—Patient and family fully able to participate in care
Participation in decision making	Level 1: No participation—Patient and family have no capacity for decision making; requires surrogacy
	Level 3: Moderate level of participation—Patient and family have limited capacity; seeks input/advice from others in decision making
	Level 5: Full participation—Patient and family have capacity and patient makes decision for self
Predictability	Level 1: Not predictable—Uncertain; uncommon patient population/illness; unusual or unexpected course; does not follow critical pathway or no critical pathway developed
	Level 3: Moderately predictable—Wavering; occasionally noted patient population/illness
	Level 5: Highly predictable—Certain; common patient population/illness; usual and expected course; follows critical pathway

One of the other factors that has been associated with an individual's level of resiliency is the quality of resources the individual has to help with the adjustment to an adverse situation. These may include one's own resources, family, and community. On any given day or time, any or all of these resources can be used to deal with stress (Callahan, 2003).

It is essential to understand what factors promote or enhance a patient's resiliency (Woodgate, 1999). Theories have been suggested regarding the relationship between resiliency and other factors. Relationships have been reported with spirituality and social support (Poblete, 2000). Other significant factors associated with resiliency include faith, hope, having a living relative, and having memories of one's roots (Lothe & Heggen, 2003). Sequela of resiliency has been reported. These include avoidance of distress and successful ability to cope and function (Tusaie-Mumford, 2001).

The Synergy Model definition of *vulnerability* is the susceptibility to actual or potential stressors that may adversely affect patient outcomes (Curley, 1998; Kaplow, 2004b, www.aacn.org/certcorp.org). Vulnerability consists of anxiety, inferiority, insecurity, lack of intimacy, and disconfirmation (Lidell, Fridlund, & Segesten, 1998). A number of situations can make a person vulnerable. The process of caregiving is one of the factors identified that creates a situation of vulnerability. Situations can occur in "anyone who is feeling threatened and uncertain" (Ebersole, 2002). Another situation is admission to an intensive care unit. McKinley, Nagy, Stein-Parbury, Bramwell, & Hudson (2002) performed a qualitative study of seriously ill patients in an intensive care unit (ICU). The data revealed sources of vulnerability in these patients that included extreme physical and emotional dependency, lack of information, and depersonalized care. The researchers concluded that feelings of vulnerability diminished when patients were kept informed of their status, were provided explanations about care they were to receive, when care was individualized based on their respective needs, and when families were present. Other factors related to

patients' levels of vulnerability include their relationship with primary care practitioners (Shi, Forrest, von Schrader, & Ng, 2003), health variability (Karpati, Galea, Awerbuch, & Levins, 2002), and transition in health care delivery with shorter length of hospital stay (Walker, 2001).

The Synergy Model definition of *stability* is the ability to maintain a steady-state equilibrium (Curley, 1998; Kaplow, 2004c; www.aacn.org/certcorp.org). The limited literature addressing the concept of stability comes from very few perspectives. One way it is addressed evaluates resources consumed by critically ill patients to maintain levels of stability. Patients' level of stability during hospitalization has also been used to predict morbidity and mortality rates and hospital recidivism (Kaplow, 2004c).

Complexity is defined as "the intricate entanglement of two or more systems (e.g., body, family, therapies) (Curley, 1998; Kaplow, 2004d, www.aacn.org/certcorp.org). Patient complexity is often reported in the literature in a variety of ways. Information on patient complexity is important as changes in nursing interventions may be indicated on the basis of a patient's clinical status. For example, patients with multiple organ dysfunction syndrome are complex and require high levels of care in the ICU. Depending on the number of organs involved and the degree of involvement, these patients will have varying levels of complexity (Kaplow, 2004d).

Complexity from a psychosocial perspective is also examined in the literature. One of the more challenging circumstances is a family discussion surrounding withdrawal and withholding of therapies in the ICU. Communication approaches and support that is provided to the family during these difficult times should reflect the complexity of the situation (Curtis et al., 2002).

Based on the Synergy Model, *resource availability* is defined as the extent of resources (e.g., personal, financial, social, psychological, technical) the patient, family, and community bring to the current situation (www.aacn.org/certcorp.org; Mullen, 2002). A patient's clinical situation can be impacted on the basis of availability of resources. Limited availability of resources can impede a patient's recovery. One of the frequently evaluated resources that a patient brings to a clinical picture is human resources—family and significant others (Kaplow, 2004e). The family is an essential factor in the course, outcomes, treatment, and care of the health and illness of its members. Human resources are also essential for prevention of problem behaviors and promotion of psychosocial behaviors (Kerr, Beck, Shattuck, Kattar, & Uriburu, 2003).

The Synergy Model definition of *participation in care* is the extent to which the patient and family engage in care (Curley, 1998; Kaplow, 2004f; www.aacn.org/certcorp.org). Decisions related to health care are complex (Kravitz & Melnikov, 2001). Patient participation is considered valuable and beneficial. The expression has been used interchangeably with patient involvement, partnership, and collaboration (Kaplow, 2004f). Given the notion that there needs to be collaboration between the patient and nurse, this presumes that patients need to be central to decisions that affect their health and well-being (Jewell, 1994).

A growing number of patients are participating in their care. Patients are assuming more accountability for prevention and treatment of health problems. This participation augments or replaces care by professionals (Cahill, 1998). The value and importance of family participation in care is well documented (Henderson & Shum, 2003; Kjelin, Malmborg & Hallstrom, 2002; Portillo Vega, Wilson-Bartnett, & Saracibar Razquin, 2002). Given this importance, participation in care has become increasingly accepted in nursing practice (Cahill, 1998).

The Synergy Model definition of *participation in decision making* is the "extent to which the patient and the patient's family engage in decision making in aspect of care" (Curley, 1998; www.aacn.org/certcorp.org). "The traditional concept of the doctor-patient relationship places the patient in a passive, dependent role with nothing to do but seek competent help and cooperate with the physician in order to get well" (Brody, 1980). In the recent past it was

expected that patients would be passive recipients of care (Biley, 1992). Now participation in decision making is considered the foundation of ethical medical practice (Avis, 1994; Gattelari, Voigt, Butow, & Tattersall, 2002, Kaplow, 2004g).

Patients in western cultures have been encouraged to participate in decision making related to health care issues for a number of reasons, including economic, social, ethical, and legal concerns (Henderson & Shum, 2003). In many cases patients prefer to be informed about treatment options and want to participate in decision making when choices exist (Guadagnoli & Ward, 1998 Kaplow, 2004g).

The degree to which patients wish to participate in decision making can range from the physician having full control to the individual having complete control (Biley, 1992; Kaplow, 2004g; Kravitz & Melnikov, 2001). Tendency for participation in decision making varies with cultural background and the clinical situation. However, at the very least, patients want to be informed (Kaplow, 2004g; Kravitz & Melnikov, 2001).

According to the Synergy Model, *predictability* is a summative characteristic that allows one to expect a certain trajectory (Curley, 1998; Kaplow, 2004h; www.aacn.org/certcorp). Health care providers use a variety of instruments or prediction models to help determine a patient's response to treatment. Nurses are frequently asked to anticipate a patient's needs for the remainder of a shift and complete patient acuity information. These data are used to predict nurse staffing needs on the subsequent shift (Kaplow, 2004h).

Given the increased emphasis on patient outcomes, scientists in numerous specialties often conduct investigations to predict outcomes of care. Physiological response is one outcome used in these studies. Other studies have evaluated the ability to predict complications of interventions (Kaplow, 2004h).

NURSE COMPETENCIES

The experts who were gathered by the Certification Corporation further agreed that there were eight nurse competencies that could be considered essential for providing care to acute and critically ill patients and families. These competencies reflect an integration of knowledge, skills, and experience of the nurse. The nurse characteristics of the Synergy Model are:

1. Clinical judgment
2. Advocacy
3. Caring practices
4. Collaboration
5. Systems thinking
6. Response to diversity
7. Clinical inquiry
8. Facilitator of learning (Hardin, 2004a)

The nurse competencies are defined and explained on the basis of the continuum in which they are seen in clinical practice in Tables 3-3 and 3-4, respectively.

Clinical judgment is defined as the use of clinical reasoning, including decision making, critical thinking, and the global grasp of a situation, coupled with nursing skills acquired through a process of integrating education, experimental knowledge, and evidenced-based

TABLE 3-3

Nurse Competencies of the Synergy Model

Nurse Characteristic	Definition
Advocacy and moral agency	Working on another's behalf and representing the concerns of patients, families, and/or nursing staff; serving as a moral agent in identifying and resolving ethical and clinical concerns within or outside the clinical setting
Caring practices	A constellation of nursing activities that creates a compassionate, supportive, and therapeutic environment with patients and staff; the aim is to promote comfort, heal, and prevent unnecessary suffering
Clinical inquiry	The ongoing process of questioning and evaluating practice, providing informed practice, and creating practice changes through research utilization and experiential knowledge
Clinical judgment	Clinical reasoning that includes clinical decision making, critical thinking, and a global grasp of the situation; nursing skills required through a process of integrating formal and experiential knowledge
Collaboration	Working with others, including physicians, families, and other health care providers, in a way that promotes and encourages each person's contributions toward achieving optimal, realistic patient goals; collaboration involves intradisciplinary and interdisciplinary work with colleagues
Facilitator of learning	The ability to help patients, nursing staff, physicians, and other health care disciplines learn both formally and informally
Response to diversity	The sensitivity to recognize, appreciate, and incorporate differences into the provision of care; differences may include but are not limited to individuality, cultural differences, spiritual beliefs, gender, race, ethnicity, disability, family configuration, lifestyle, socioeconomic status, age, values, and alternative medicine involving patients' families and members of the health care team
Systems thinking	A body of knowledge and tools that allows the nurse to manage whatever environmental and system resources exist for the patient, family, and staff within or across health care and nonhealth care systems

Source: www.aacn.org/certcorp.org.

TABLE 3-4

Nurse Competencies on a Clinical Continuum

Nurse Characteristic	Explanation of Continuum
Clinical judgment	*Level 1:* Collects basic-level data; follows algorithms, decision trees, and protocols with all populations and is uncomfortable deviating from them; matches formal knowledge with clinical events to make decisions; questions the limits of one's ability to make clinical decisions and delegates the decision making to other clinicians; includes extraneous detail
	Level 3: Collects and interprets complex patient data; makes clinical judgments based on an immediate grasp of the whole picture for common or routine patient populations; recognizes patterns and trends that may predict the direction of illness; recognizes limits and seeks appropriate help; focuses on key elements of case while shorting out extraneous details
	Level 5: Synthesizes and interprets multiple, sometimes conflicting, sources of data; makes judgment based on an immediate grasp of the whole picture unless working with new patient populations; uses past experiences to anticipate problems; helps patient and family see the "big picture"; recognizes the limits of clinical judgment and seeks multidisciplinary collaboration and consultation with comfort; recognizes and responds to the dynamic situation
Clinical inquiry	*Level 1:* Follows standards and guidelines; implements clinical changes and research-based practices developed by others; recognizes the need for further learning to improve patient care; recognizes obvious changing patient situation (e.g., deterioration, crisis); needs and seeks help to identify patient problem
	Level 3: Questions appropriateness of policies and guidelines; questions current practice; seeks advice, resources, or information to improve patient care; begins to compare and contrast possible alternatives
	Level 5: Improves, deviates from, or individualizes standards and guidelines for particular patient situations or populations; questions and/or evaluates current practice based on patients' responses, review of the literature, research, and education/learning; acquires knowledge and skills needed to address questions arising in practice and improve patient care (The domains of clinical judgment and clinical inquiry converge at the expert level; they cannot be separated.)
Facilitator of learning	*Level 1:* Follows planned educational programs; sees patient/family education as a separate task from delivery of care; provides data without seeking to assess patient's readiness or understanding; has limited knowledge of the totality of the educational needs; focuses on a nurse's perspective; sees the patient as a passive recipient
	Level 3: Adapts planned educational programs; begins to recognize and integrate different ways of teaching into delivery of care; incorporates the patient's understanding into practice; sees the overlapping of educational plans from different health care providers' perspectives; begins to see the patient as having input into goals; begins to see individualism
	Level 5: Creatively modifies or develops patient/family education programs; integrates patient/family education throughout delivery of care; evaluates the patient's understanding by observing behavior changes related to learning; is able to collaborate and incorporate all health care providers' and educational plans into the patient/family educational program; sets patient-driven goals for education; sees the patient/family as having choices and consequences that are negotiated in relation to education

Continued

TABLE 3-4
Nurse Competencies on a Clinical Continuum—cont'd

Nurse Characteristic	Explanation of Continuum
Collaboration	*Level 1:* Willing to be taught, coached and/or mentored; participates in team meetings and discussions regarding patient care and/or practice issues; open to various team members' contributions
	Level 3: Seeks opportunities to be taught, coached, and/or mentored; elicits others' advice and perspectives; initiates and participates in team meetings and discussions regarding patient care and/or practice issues; recognizes and suggests various team members' participation
	Level 5: Seeks opportunities to teach, coach, and mentor and to be taught, coached, and mentored; facilitates active involvement and complementary contributions of others in team meetings and discussions regarding patient care and/or practice issues; involves/recruits diverse resources when appropriate to optimize patient outcomes
Systems thinking	*Level 1:* Uses a limited array of strategies; limited outlook—sees the pieces or components; does not recognize negotiation as an alternative; sees the patient and family within the isolated environment of the unit; sees self as key resource
	Level 3: Develops strategies based on needs and strengths of the patient/family; able to make connections within components; sees the opportunity to negotiate but may not have strategies; developing a view of the patient/family transition process; recognizes how to obtain resources beyond self
	Level 5: Develops, integrates, and applies a variety of strategies that are driven by the needs and strengths of the patient/family; global or holistic outlook—sees the whole rather than the pieces; knows when and how to negotiate and navigate through the system on behalf of patients and families; anticipates needs of patients and families as they move through the health care system; uses untapped and alternative resources as necessary
Advocacy and moral agency	*Level 1:* Works on behalf of the patient; self-assesses personal values; aware of ethical conflicts/issues that may surface in the clinical setting; makes ethical/moral decisions based on rules; represents the patient when the patient cannot represent self; aware of patients' rights
	Level 3: Works on behalf of the patient and family; considers patient values and incorporates in care, even when differing from personal values; supports colleagues in ethical and clinical issues; moral decision making can deviate from rules; demonstrates give and take with patient's family, allowing them to speak/represent themselves when possible; aware of patient and family rights
	Level 5: Works on behalf of patient, family, and community; advocates from patient/family perspective, whether similar to or different from personal values; advocates ethical conflict and issues from patient/family perspective; suspends rules—patient and family drive moral decision making; empowers the patient and family to speak for/represent themselves; achieves mutuality within patient/professional relationships
Caring practices	*Level 1:* Focuses on the usual and customary needs of the patient; no anticipation of future needs; bases care on standards and protocols; maintains a safe physical environment; acknowledges death as a potential outcome

TABLE 3-4	
Nurse Competencies on a Clinical Continuum—cont'd	

Nurse Characteristic	Explanation of Continuum
	Level 3: Responds to subtle patient and family changes; engages with the patient as a unique patient in a compassionate manner; recognizes and tailors caring practices to the individuality of the patient and family; domesticates the patient's and family's environment; recognizes that death may be an acceptable outcome
	Level 5: Has astute awareness and anticipates patient and family changes and needs; fully engaged with and sensing how to stand alongside the patient, family, and community; caring practices follow the patient and family lead; anticipates hazards and avoids them and promotes safety throughout patient's and family's transitions along the health care continuum; orchestrates the process that ensures patient's/family's comfort and concerns surrounding issues of death and dying are met
Response to diversity	*Level 1:* Assesses cultural diversity; provides care based on own belief system; learns the culture of the health care environment
	Level 3: Inquires about cultural differences and considers their impact on care; accommodates personal and professional differences in the plan of care; helps the patient/family understand the culture of the health care system
	Level 5: Responds to, anticipates, and integrates cultural differences into patient/family care; appreciates and incorporates differences, including alternative therapies, into care; tailors health care culture, to the extent possible, to meet the diverse needs and strengths of the patient/family

guidelines (AACN, 2002; Stannard & Hardin, 2004a). It consists of critical thinking and nursing skills that are acquired through a process of integrating formal and experiential knowledge Stannard & Hardin, 2004a).

The Synergy Model definition of *advocacy and moral agency* is working on another's behalf; representing the concerns of patients, families, and/or nursing staff; and serving as a moral agent in identifying and resolving ethical and clinical concerns within or outside the clinical setting (www.aacn.org/certcorp.org). The nurse serves as a moral agent in identifying and helping resolve ethical and clinical concerns within the clinical setting (Stannard & Hardin, 2004b).

The Synergy Model definition of *caring practices* is a constellation of nursing activities that creates a compassionate, supportive, and therapeutic environment with patients and staff. The aim is to promote comfort, heal, and prevent unnecessary suffering. Caring behaviors include compassion, vigilance, engagement, and responsiveness to the patient and family (Hardin 2004b).

Collaboration entails working with others, including physicians, families, and other health care providers, in a way that promotes and encourages each person's contributions toward achieving optimal, realistic patient goals (www.aacn.org/certcorp.org). The patient, family, and members of various health care disciplines work toward promoting the needs and requests of patients (Hardin, 2004c).

Systems thinking entails using a body of knowledge and tools that allows the nurse to manage whatever environmental and system resources exist for the patient, family, and staff within or across health care and nonhealth care systems) (www.aacn.org/certcorp.org). The ability to understand how one decision can impact the whole is integral to systems thinking. The nurse uses a global perspective in clinical decision making and has the ability to negotiate the needs of the patient and family through the health care system (Hardin, 2004d).

Response to diversity is the sensitivity to recognize, appreciate, and incorporate differences into the provision of care. Differences may include but are not limited to individuality, cultural differences, spiritual beliefs, gender, race, ethnicity, disability, family configuration, lifestyle, socioeconomic status, age, values, and alternative medicine involving patients' families and members of the health care team (Hardin, 2004e; www.aacn.org/certcorp.org).

Clinical inquiry is an ongoing process of questioning and evaluating practice, providing informed practice, and creating practice changes through research utilization and experiential knowledge (www.aacn.org/certcorp.org). Nurses need to recognize the individuality of each patient while observing for patterns that respond to interventions (Hardin, 2004f).

Facilitator of learning is the ability to help patients, nursing staff, physicians, and other health care disciplines learn both formally and informally (www.aacn.org/certcorp.org). Education should be provided on the basis of individual strengths and weaknesses of the patient and family. The educational level of the patient should be considered when designing the plan to educate the patient and family to ensure informed decisions. Creative methods should be developed to ensure patient and family comprehension (Hardin, 2004g).

THE CLINICAL NURSE SPECIALIST

Advanced practice nurses provide health care on a continuum, during times of illness, but also, and perhaps more important, during times of health when this state can be promoted and prolonged (Fitzpatrick, 1998). Advanced practice nursing is the "application of an expanded range of practical, theoretical, and research-based therapeutics to phenomena experienced by patients within a specialized clinical area of the larger discipline of nursing" (Hamric, 1996).

"A CNS is a master's-prepared nurse and an expert in clinical nursing with a specialty focus who advances the practice of nursing through innovative, cost-effective nursing interventions that are based on theory and evidence" (Peterson, 2004; www.aacn.nche.edu/Publications/positions/cerreg.htm).

When the aspects of roles of the clinical nurse specialist (CNS) were initially delineated over two decades ago, they were based on job specifications. These roles included direct care and independent practice, researcher, and consultant (Hamric & Spross, 1983). A few years later, the published subroles and competencies were modified to include clinical practice and direct patient care, consultation, education, research, collaboration, and clinical leadership (Hamric & Spross, 1989).

Presently the roles of the CNS are described based on three spheres of influence: (1) patient/family; (2) nurse-nurse; and (3) system (Moloney-Harmon, 1999). The spheres of influence are described in greater detail in Chapter 4 of this text.

An alternative way to describe the multifaceted role of the CNS who cares for the acute and critically ill patients and their families is based on the Synergy Model. CNSs manage, support, and coordinate the care of acutely and critically ill patients with episodic illness or acute exacerbation of chronic illness (www.aacn.org/certcorp.org).

Advocacy and Moral Agency

In its *Standards of Practice and Professional Performance for the Acute and Critical Care Nurse Specialist* document, AACN delineated several activities of the CNS in relation to advocacy and moral agency and the three spheres of influence.

It is essential for the CNS to advocate for the patient and family notwithstanding personal values. The multifaceted role of the CNS allows for several opportunities to demonstrate competency in advocacy and moral agency as they impact the three spheres of influence of practice. Exemplars have been sited in the literature as well as by AACN. Each of these exemplars has the common thread of the CNS working to promote the best interests of the patient. CNSs work to create an environment for patients and families to participate in ethical decision making. They help resolve ethical issues such as do-not-resuscitate status questions and those related to withholding or withdrawal of medical therapies while ensuring that these wishes are consistent with those of the patient and family. The CNS monitors professional staff to be advocates and moral agents and assist staff to support the family and help resolve ethical issues. Further, they assist in facilitating the development of organizational ethics (Kaplow, 2002; Moloney-Harmon, 1999).

CNSs' decisions and actions are made on behalf of patients and their family members, nursing personnel, and organizational systems and are determined in an ethical manner. They foster the establishment of an ethical environment that supports the rights of all participants. CNSs contribute to the resolution of ethical dilemmas by enhancing the responsiveness of individuals and organizational systems, and they serve as mentors and role models by participating in the resolution of ethical and clinical dilemmas (www.aacn.org).

CNSs influence resource utilization to promote safety, effectiveness, and fiscal accountability in the planning and delivery of patient care. They advocate for patients, family members, and nursing personnel and support policy and services that advocate for patient rights and optimal environments of healthcare.

Caring Practices

Caring practices should be a primary attribute of CNS practice. In its *Standards of Practice and Professional Performance for the Acute and Critical Care Nurse Specialist* document, AACN delineated several activities of the CNS in relation to caring practices and the three spheres of influence. CNSs work with patients and families to promote caring and minimize unnecessary suffering.

They help ensure that the physical, emotional, and spiritual needs of patients and families are met and express compassion to patients and families during care delivery. Further, they assist staff to accomplish the latter and facilitate an organizational culture of caring (Kaplow, 2002; Moloney-Harmon, 1999).

Clinical Inquiry

In the *Standards of Practice and Professional Performance for the Acute and Critical Care Nurse Specialist* document, AACN delineated several activities of the CNS in relation to clinical inquiry and the three spheres of influence. Through many of the performance improvement activities, CNSs develop and use valid and reliable data collection tools. They collect data in all three spheres of influence on an ongoing basis that reflect the dynamic nature of patients and systems and prioritize according to immediate conditions and needs. They identify factors that influence outcomes during the data collection process (e.g., financial and regulatory requirements and effectiveness of interdisciplinary collaboration) and classify and synthesize them as facilitators or barriers to proposed changes. CNSs use and design appropriate tools and methodologies to identify the clinical and professional development needs or gaps in knowledge, skills, and competencies of nursing personnel (www.aacn.org).

It is the CNSs who develop and facilitate a plan that prescribes interventions to attain the expected outcomes for patients, family members, nursing personnel, and organizational systems. They identify interventions within the plan of care that reflect current scientific knowledge and practice and promote continuity of care.

CNSs implement interventions identified in the plan(s) for patients/family, nursing personnel, and organizational systems. They perform evidence-based interventions consistent with patient/family needs.

CNSs evaluate progress toward attainment of expected outcomes for patients, family members, nursing personnel, and organizational systems. The evaluation process is based on advanced knowledge, practice, and research. They incorporate the use of quality indicators and benchmarking in evaluating the progress of patients, family members, nursing personnel, and systems toward expected outcomes.

CNSs systematically develop criteria for and evaluate the quality and effectiveness of nursing practice and organizational systems. They assume a leadership role in establishing criteria for and monitoring quality of care initiatives within the three spheres of influence. They assess the need for, plan, and implement quality improvement (QI) programs; evaluate QI; and formulate evidence-based recommendations to improve quality of care and nursing practice.

CNSs use, participate in, and disseminate research to enhance practice. They critically evaluate existing practice based on current research findings and integrate changes into practice. In addition, they select, apply, or withhold interventions in a manner that is substantiated by relevant research and appropriate to the needs of the patient or system. They use the research process to improve patient outcomes and enhance the environment of care.

CNSs evaluate clinical practice on an ongoing basis. They incorporate research findings and evaluate clinical practice to improve patient outcomes. Further, they serve as a mentor for staff by implementing an evidence-based practice model for nursing care. For the system sphere of influence, CNSs create an environment that supports clinical inquiry with the ongoing quest for excellence. They evaluate clinical practices. Innovations for patients, populations, and systems are honed on the basis of experiential knowledge, literature, outcomes, and benchmarking data. Last, CNSs collaborate with multidisciplinary team staff to support research initiatives of the assigned unit or the institution (Kaplow, 2002; Moloney-Harmon, 1999).

Clinical Judgment

As identified in the AACN *Standards of Practice and Professional Performance for the Acute and Critical Care Nurse Specialist* document, the CNS, while engaging in performance improvement activities, includes the patient, family members, and other health care providers in the data collection process to develop a holistic picture of the patient's needs. Further, these specialists analyze assessment data to determine the needs of the patient, family members, nursing personnel, and organizational systems. They formulate differential diagnoses by systematically comparing and contrasting assessment findings; derive diagnoses from the assessment data; discuss, validate, and prioritize diagnoses in collaboration with patients, family members, nursing personnel, and systems; prioritize diagnoses to facilitate development of a plan of care and to achieve expected outcomes, reevaluate and revise diagnoses when additional assessment data are available; and identify and analyze factors that enhance or hinder the achievement of desired outcomes for patients, family members, nursing personnel, and systems (www.aacn.org).

CNSs identify expected outcomes for patients, family members, nursing personnel, and organizational systems. They formulate expected outcomes with patients, family members, and the multidisciplinary health care team that are based on current clinical and scientific knowledge; they identify expected outcomes, considering associated risks, benefits, and costs; and they modify expected outcomes and plans of care based on changes in condition or needs.

These specialists develop and facilitate a plan that prescribes interventions to attain the expected outcomes for patients, family members, nursing personnel, and organizational systems. They accomplish this by developing a plan that is individualized and dynamic and can be applied across the continuum of acute and critical care services; developing the plan in a collaborative manner, promoting each individual's contributions toward achieving the expected outcomes; and by identifying interventions that reflect current scientific knowledge and practice and promote continuity of care.

CNSs implement interventions identified in the plan(s) for patients and family, nursing personnel, and organizational systems. They deliver interventions in a safe and ethical manner that promotes health and stability and that minimizes complications.

CNSs evaluate progress toward attainment of expected outcomes for patients, family members, nursing personnel, and organizational systems. The evaluation process is based on advanced knowledge, practice, and research. They revise the diagnoses, expected outcomes, and plan of care based on information gained in the evaluation process. Further, they establish, monitor, and evaluate the effect of interventions on patient care, organizational and nursing personnel outcomes, and cost.

Clinical judgment is at the core of the role of the CNS. CNSs demonstrate competency in clinical judgment in a number of ways to impact all three spheres of influence. They assess patients and use advanced knowledge to identify problems. They provide clinical expertise and plan, implement, and evaluate patient care interventions based on the intricacies of the clinical problem. CNSs help ensure that the nursing staff is able to move forward with nursing care. For the system, they ensure that staff support is available (e.g., equipment, education, and resources) needed to deliver care. They plan, implement, and evaluate interventions based on resources of the system (Kaplow, 2002; Moloney-Harmon, 1999; Peterson, 2004).

Collaboration

The CNS collaborates with other members of the multidisciplinary team, especially physicians, social workers, pharmacists, and nutritionists. In its *Standards of Practice and Professional Performance for the Acute and Critical Care Nurse Specialist*

document, AACN delineated several activities of the CNS in relation to collaboration and the three spheres of influence. The CNS discusses, validates, and prioritizes diagnoses in collaboration with patients, family members, nursing personnel, and systems (www.aacn.org).

CNSs identify expected outcomes for patients, family members, nursing personnel, and organizational systems. They formulate expected outcomes that are based on current clinical and scientific knowledge with patients, family members, and the multidisciplinary health care team.

It is the CNSs who develop and facilitate a plan that prescribes interventions to attain the expected outcomes for patients, family members, nursing personnel, and organizational systems. They develop this plan in a collaborative manner, promoting each individual's contributions toward achieving the expected outcomes.

CNSs implement interventions identified in the plan(s) for patients and family, nursing personnel, and organizational systems. They promote implementation of the plan of care collaboratively with patients, family members, and the health care team.

These specialists evaluate progress toward attainment of expected outcomes for patients, family members, nursing personnel, and organizational systems. They include interdisciplinary collaboration and multiple sources of data in the evaluation process.

CNSs systematically develop criteria for and evaluate the quality and effectiveness of nursing practice and organizational systems. They participate in interdisciplinary efforts to address costs, duplication, and barriers to goal attainment based on QI data obtained.

CNSs collaborate with patients, family members, and health care personnel in creating a healing and caring environment. They provide consultation and initiate referrals to other members of the multidisciplinary team to facilitate optimal care. In addition, they provide mentoring to nursing students in the area of CNS preparation in collaboration with schools of nursing and collaborate with other disciplines in teaching, consultation, management, and research activities to improve outcomes in nursing practice and enhance the health care environment.

CNSs use, participate in, and disseminate research to enhance practice. This is accomplished by collaborating with senior investigators and/or members of the interdisciplinary team in conducting research relevant to practice.

CNSs collaborate with patients and families on a regular basis. The CNS recognizes the patient and family as equal partners in care; their contribution is integrated into the care plan. CNSs collaborate with the nurse leader, nurse educator, and senior nursing staff to perform an ongoing staff assessment. They collaborate with members of the multidisciplinary team to support unit initiatives such as new policies, procedures, or standards of care. CNSs further work with members of the multidisciplinary team to implement the most effective interventions and facilitate best practices based on a global grasp of a patient situation (Kaplow, 2002; Moloney-Harmon, 1999).

Facilitator of Learning

In its *Standards of Practice and Professional Performance for the Acute and Critical Care Nurse Specialist* document, AACN delineated several activities of the CNS in relation to facilitator of learning and the three spheres of influence. CNSs contribute to the professional development of peers, colleagues, and other members of the health care team. They identify and participate in opportunities to share skills, knowledge, and strategies for patient care and system improvement with colleagues and other health care providers. This can be accomplished in a one-on-one session with a novice nurse by such methods as role modeling patient care or in a group setting such as a classroom or conference room. CNSs promote a learning environment that enables nurses and other members of the health care team to make optimal contributions and systems to function most effectively (www.aacn.org).

The CNS is a facilitator of learning as a patient and family educator as seen in the application of guidelines in counseling patients and families about lifestyle changes to prevent or modify progression of disease (e.g., diabetes, heart disease). CNSs provide patient and family education based on identified needs. They develop education programs with the purpose of optimizing patient outcomes and quality of care. They provide rationales for care to patients, families, and nurse colleagues. CNSs implement educational interventions to nurses based on identified needs. In collaboration with the nurse educator, the CNS works to develop the psychomotor, critical thinking, and clinical decision-making skills of a nurse new to a specialty or unit. They enhance this new nurse's application of content learned in critical care orientation classes and principles of the sciences learned in the nursing school program. CNSs are also facilitators of learning by serving as role models and mentors for clinical competencies. From a systems perspective, the CNS develops educational programs to improve outcomes and quality of care. CNSs participate in the publication process, present information at meetings and conferences, and are actively involved in their professional organizations (e.g., AACN) (Kaplow, 2002; Moloney-Harmon, 1999).

Response to Diversity

In its *Standards of Practice and Professional Performance for the Acute and Critical Care Nurse Specialist* document, AACN delineated several activities of the CNS in relation to response to diversity and the three spheres of influence. For example, during performance improvement activities, the CNS obtains data from multiple sources that reflect sensitivity to ethnic and cultural differences of individuals (e.g., patient, family members, nursing personnel, and systems) (www.aacn.org).

CNSs incorporate patient and family values into the delivery of care. They assist staff to increase their comfort with values that may be different from their own and lead multidisciplinary teams to learn to appreciate the uniqueness of each individual (Moloney-Harmon, 1999).

Systems Thinking

In its *Standards of Practice and Professional Performance for the Acute and Critical Care Nurse Specialist* document, AACN delineated several activities of the CNS in relation to systems thinking and the three spheres of influence. CNSs evaluate progress toward attainment of expected outcomes for patients, family members, nursing personnel, and organizational systems. They base the evaluation process on the analysis of risks, benefits, and cost-effectiveness (www.aacn.org).

CNSs systematically develop criteria for and evaluate the quality and effectiveness of nursing practice and organizational systems. They participate in interdisciplinary efforts to address costs, duplication, and barriers to goal attainment based on QI data obtained.

These specialists contribute to the professional development of peers, colleagues, and other members of the health care team. They participate in professional organizations such as AACN to address issues of concern in meeting patient needs and improving nursing practice and system effectiveness.

CNSs influence resource utilization to promote safety, effectiveness, and fiscal accountability in the planning and delivery of patient care. They evaluate factors related to safety, effectiveness, availability, and cost to design; implement best practices; facilitate access for patients and family members to appropriate health care services; and serve as a resource to various populations for the purpose of influencing the delivery of health care and the formation of health care policy.

CNSs develop organizational strategies that are based on the needs of patients and their families. They guide health care providers in the use of care delivery models and assess,

develop, implement, and evaluate care delivery models (Moloney-Harmon, 1999).

EXEMPLARS

Moloney-Harmon (1999) illustrated use of the Synergy Model in relation to the CNS's role in leading a multidisciplinary team to develop, implement, and evaluate a new conscious sedation program in a health care system. The program included development of a policy, staff education, and measurement of patient outcomes. In this situation the CNS used available evidence-based data, literature, benchmarking data, and other colleagues to develop the program.

An analysis of the system included financial strength and identification of the unique needs of each department that would be impacted by this new program. Once this assessment was complete, the CNS developed education materials for the patient, family, and members of the health care team. This was accomplished by collaborating with each of these stakeholders to identify their respective needs. The Synergy Model was useful in this situation to help develop a program that was based on the needs of all three spheres of influence: patients, families, members of the health care team, as well as the health care system (Moloney-Harmon, 1999). This exemplar illustrated the CNS as a systems thinker, collaborator, and facilitator of learning.

Hardin and Hussey (2003) described the use of the Synergy Model for a patient in a congestive heart failure (CHF) clinic. A case study is presented involving an elderly patient with New York Heart Association class III CHF. The patient is an African-American widow with minimal financial support for health care. Her past medical history includes a stroke, which left her dependent on assistance with ambulation, hypertension, osteoporosis, atrial fibrillation, and type II diabetes mellitus. The patient has had two exacerbations of CHF in the past 18 months that required hospitalization. Despite not having financial support, the patient paid $350 monthly for her prescription medications. On admission for the most recent exacerbation of CHF, the CNS learned that the patient had not taken her medications for the past 3 days and had not been able to eat appropriately due to lack of financial resources.

In this case presentation, Hardin and Hussey described the patient characteristics using the Synergy Model. These included a decreasing level of *stability* as evidenced by the patient's vital signs and presenting systems; an increasing level of *complexity* given her multiple system compromise and lack of resource availability; uncertain *predictability* because of the patient's decreased stability and increasing complexity; good potential for *resiliency* given the patient's willingness and knowledge to adhere to the required treatment regimen; increased *vulnerability* due to limited financial resources; presence of *participation in care and decision making* as evidenced by the patient having no cognitive impairment and the fact that her daughter is supportive in all other ways aside from providing financial support; and *decreased resource availability* as evidenced by the patient's limited financial resources.

Hardin and Hussey also described the nurse competencies that were essential for the CNS to possess in management of this patient. These competencies include *clinical judgment, clinical inquiry, collaboration, systems thinking, and response to diversity.* The CNS used *clinical judgment* by "synthesizing, interpreting, and making decisions on the assessment data of [the patient's] weight gain, lower extremity edema, elevated blood pressure, heart rate, and her current medication regimen" (p. 75). *Clinical inquiry* was demonstrated by the CNS questioning of the patient regarding adherence to the evidence-based plan of care that was developed to meet her individual, specific needs and by evaluating the patient's thinking and values related to her condition and the therapies prescribed. The CNS in this case *collaborated* with other members of the multidisciplinary team to obtain Meals on Wheels to help ensure that the patient had a balanced diet until her Social Security check arrived. The CNS also helped

obtain financial support for the medications. The authors note that "typically, an advanced practice nurse would use *systems thinking* to develop proactive strategies that could ensure improved utilization of services" (p. 76) through use of the clinic that the patient attended. Last, the CNS demonstrated *response to diversity* by developing a plan to allow the patient to maintain her independence and pride by not accepting charity and recognizing the patient's food preferences when arranging for food.

Heath and Balkstra (2004) described the role of the clinical nurse specialist as helping with a new generation of tobacco harm-reduction products known as "potential reduction exposure products (PREPS)" (p. 40). These products are defined by the Institute of Medicine as "any product that lowers total tobacco-related mortality and morbidity even though the use of that product may involve continued exposure to tobacco-related toxicants" (Stratton, Shetty, Wallace, & Bondurant, 2001). While not referring to the Synergy Model specifically, the authors identify ways that the CNS demonstrates competencies of the model in relation to the identified problem and ways he or she can respond to a call for action. Specifically the CNS demonstrates *clinical judgment* by auscultating breath sounds, evaluating abnormalities on chest films, and facilitating smoking cessation clinics. These actions demonstrate that the CNS has a global grasp of the situation and identifies the lethal effects of tobacco. The authors also note that CNSs "have a history of advocacy initiatives and leadership roles that impact patient and organizational outcomes" (p. 40). These activities demonstrate the CNS's competency with *advocacy and moral agency* and *collaboration.* Further, the CNS demonstrates competency in *response to diversity* and *clinical inquiry* when speaking with patients about PREPS. As noted by the authors, CNSs have to debate whether it is better to encourage tobacco abstinence or sustained tobacco use in some manner if less harmful. The authors concluded by appealing to CNSs' competency in *advocacy and moral agency* by "advocating for legislation regulation for tobacco products and nicotine delivery systems" (p. 44).

CONCLUSION

The purposes of nursing are to meet the needs of the patient and family and to provide safe passage through the health care system. The Synergy Model is a conceptual framework for designing practice. The model has far-reaching implications for the practice of nursing and other health care professions (Curley, 1998).

References

American Association of Critical-Care Nurses (2000). *Standards for acute and critical care nursing practice.* Aliso Viejo, CA: Author.

American Association of Critical-Care Nurses (2002). *Competency level descriptors for nurse characteristics.* Aliso Viejo, CA: AACN Certification Corporation.

Avis, M. (1994). Choice cuts: an exploratory study of patients' views about participation in decision making in a day surgery unit. *International Journal of Nursing Studies,* 31(3), 289-298.

Biley, F.C. (1992). Some determinants that effect patient participation in decision-making about nursing care. *Journal of Advanced Nursing,* 17(4), 414-421.

Brody, D.S. (1980). The patient's role in clinical decision-making. *Annals of Internal Medicine,* 93(5), 718-722.

Cahill, J. (1998). Patient participation—a review of literature. *Journal of Clinical Nursing,* 7(2), 119-128.

Callahan, H.E. (2003). Families dealing with advanced heart failure: A challenge and an opportunity. *Critical Care Nursing Quarterly,* 26(3), 2302-43.

Curley, M.A.Q. (1998). Patient-nurse synergy: optimizing patients' outcomes. *American Journal of Critical Care,* 7(1), 64-72.

Curtis, J.R., Engelbug, R.A., Wenvich, M.D., et al. (2002). Studying communication about end-of-life during the ICU family conference: Development of a framework. *Journal of Critical Care,* 17(3), 147-60.

Ebersole, P. (2002). Situational vulnerability. *Geriatric Nursing,* 23(1), 4-5.

Felten, B.S., & Hall, J.M. (2001). Conceptualizing resilience in women older than 85: overcoming adversity from illness or loss. *Journal of Gerontological Nursing,* 27(11), 46-53.

Fitzpatrick, E.R. (1998). Analysis and synthesis of the role of the advanced practice nurse. *Clinical Nurse Specialist,* 12, 106-110.

Gattelari, M., Voigt, K.J., Butow, P.N., & Tattersall, M.H.N. (2002). When the treatment goal is not cure: Are cancer patients equipped to make informed decisions? *Journal of Clinical Oncology,* 20(2), 503-513.

Guadagnoli, E., & Ward, P. (1998). Patient participation in decision-making. *Social Science and Medicine,* 47(3), 329-39.

Hamric, A.B. (1996). A definition of advanced nursing practice. In A.B. Hamric, J.A. Spross, & C.M. Hanson (Eds.). *Advanced nursing practice: An integrative approach.* Philadelphia: Saunders

Hamric, A.B., & Spross, J.A. (Eds.). (1989). *The clinical nurse specialist in theory and practice* (2nd ed.). Philadelphia: Saunders.

Hamric, A.B., & Spross, J.A. (Eds.). (1983). *The clinical nurse specialist in theory and practice.* Orlando: Grune & Stratton.

Hardin, S. (2004a). Introduction. In S.R. Hardin & R. Kaplow (Eds.). *The Synergy Model: Implications for certified practice in optimizing patient outcomes.* Boston: Jones & Bartlett.

Hardin, S. (2004b). Caring practices. In S.R. Hardin, & R. Kaplow (Eds.). *The Synergy Model: Implications for certified practice in optimizing patient outcomes.* Boston: Jones & Bartlett.

Hardin, S. (2004c). Collaboration. In S.R. Hardin, & R. Kaplow (Eds.). *The Synergy Model: Implications for certified practice in optimizing patient outcomes.* Boston: Jones & Bartlett.

Hardin, S. (2004d). Systems thinking. In S.R. Hardin, & R. Kaplow (Eds.). *The Synergy Model: Implications for certified practice in optimizing patient outcomes.* Boston: Jones & Bartlett.

Hardin, S. (2004e). Response to diversity. In S.R. Hardin, & R. Kaplow (Eds.). *The Synergy Model: Implications for certified practice in optimizing patient outcomes.* Boston: Jones & Bartlett.

Hardin, S. (2004f). Clinical inquiry. In S.R. Hardin, & R. Kaplow (Eds.). *The Synergy Model: Implications for certified practice in optimizing patient outcomes.* Boston: Jones & Bartlett.

Hardin, S. (2004g). Facilitator of Learning. In S.R. Hardin, & R. Kaplow (Eds.). *The Synergy Model: Implications for certified practice in optimizing patient outcomes.* Boston: Jones & Bartlett.

Heath, J., & Balkstra, C.R. (2004). Potential reduction exposure products and FDA tobacco regulation: A CNS call to action. *Clinical Nurse Specialist,* 18(1), 40-48.

Henderson, A., & Shum, D. (2003). Decision making preferences towards surgical intervention in a Hong Kong Chinese population. *International Nursing Review,* 50(2), 95-100.

Jewell, S.E. (1994). Patient participation: What does it mean to nurses? *Journal of Advanced Nursing*, 19, 433-438.

Kaplow, R. (2004a). Resiliency. In S.R. Hardin, & R. Kaplow (Eds.). *The Synergy Model: Implications for certified practice in optimizing patient outcomes*. Boston: Jones & Bartlett.

Kaplow, R. (2004b). Vulnerability. In S.R. Hardin, & R. Kaplow (Eds.). *The Synergy Model: Implications for certified practice in optimizing patient outcomes*. Boston: Jones & Bartlett.

Kaplow, R. (2004c). Stability. In S.R. Hardin, & R. Kaplow (Eds.). *The Synergy Model: Implications for certified practice in optimizing patient outcomes*. Boston: Jones & Bartlett.

Kaplow, R. (2004d). Complexity. In S.R. Hardin, & R. Kaplow (Eds.). *The Synergy Model: Implications for certified practice in optimizing patient outcomes*. Boston: Jones & Bartlett.

Kaplow, R. (2004e). Resource availability. In S.R. Hardin, & R. Kaplow (Eds.). *The Synergy Model: Implications for certified practice in optimizing patient outcomes*. Boston: Jones & Bartlett.

Kaplow, R. (2004f). Participation in care. In S.R. Hardin, & R. Kaplow (Eds.). *The Synergy Model: Implications for certified practice in optimizing patient outcomes*. Boston: Jones & Bartlett.

Kaplow, R. (2004g). Participation in decision making. In S.R., Hardin & R. Kaplow (Eds.). *The Synergy Model: Implications for certified practice in optimizing patient outcomes*. Boston: Jones & Bartlett.

Kaplow, R. (2004h). Predictability. In S.R. Hardin, & R. Kaplow (Eds.). *The Synergy Model: Implications for certified practice in optimizing patient outcomes*. Boston: Jones & Bartlett.

Kaplow, R. (2002). The Synergy Model in practice. Applying the Synergy Model to nursing education. *Critical Care Nurse*, 22(3), 77-81.

Karpati, A., Galea, S., Awerbuch, T., & Levins, R. (2002). Variability, vulnerability at the ecological level: Implications for understanding the social determinants of health. *American Journal of Public Health*, 92(11), 1768-1772.

Kerr, M.H., Beck, K., Shattuck, T.D., Kattar, C., & Uriburu, D. (2003). Family involvement, problem and prosocial behavior outcomes of Latino youth. *American Journal of Health Behavior*, 27(Suppl. 1), S55-S65.

Kjelin, A., Malmborg, M., & Hallstrom, I. (2002). Increased parental participation in care of boys undergoing surgery for hypospadias repair—parents' views. *Vard il Norden. Nursing Science and Research in the Nordic Countries*, 22(2), 38-42.

Kravitz, R.L., & Melnikov, J. (2001). Engaging patients in medical decision making. *British Medical Journal*, 323(7313), 584-585.

Lauer, C.S. (2002). The relevance of resilience. *Modern Healthcare*, 32(33), 29.

Lidell, R., Fridlund, B., & Segesten, K. (1998). Vulnerability factors from a pre- and post-MI perspective: A qualitative analysis. *Coronary Health Care* 2(2), 72-80.

Lothe, E.A., & Heggen, K. (2003). A study of resilience in young Ethiopian famine survivors. *Journal of Transcultural Nursing*, 14(4), 313-320.

McKinley, S., Nagy, S., Stein-Parbury, J., Bramwell, M., & Hudson, J. (2002). Vulnerability and security in seriously ill patients in intensive care. *Intensive and Critical Care*, 18(1), 27-36.

Moloney-Harmon, P.A. (1999). The Synergy Model: Contemporary practice of the clinical nurse specialist. *Critical Care Nurse*, 19(2), 101-104.

Mullen, J. (2002). The Synergy Model as a framework for nursing rounds. *Critical Care Nurse*, 22(6), 66-68.

Peterson, K. (2004). CNS and NP: To blend or not to blend. *AACN News*, 21(4), 5.

Poblete, S.A. (2000). Relationship of spirituality, social support, reciprocity, and conflict to resilience in individuals diagnosed with HIV. Rutgers The State University of New Jersey, Newark. Ph.D. thesis.

Portillo Vega, M.C., Wilson-Bartnett, J., & Saracibar Razquin, M.I. (2002). Study of patients' and families' perception of lay caregiver participation in care of stroke patients: methodology and preliminary results. *Enfermeria Clinica*, 12(3), 94-103.

Shi, L., Forrest, C.B., von Schrader, S., & Ng, J. (2003). Vulnerability and the patient-practitioner relationship: The roles of gatekeeping and primary care performance. *American Journal of Public Health*, 93(1), 138-144.

Stannard, D., & Hardin, S. (2004a). Clinical judgment. In S.R. Hardin & R. Kaplow (Eds.). *The Synergy Model: Implications for certified practice in optimizing patient outcomes*. Boston: Jones & Bartlett.

Stannard, D., & Hardin, S. (2004b). Advocacy and moral agency. In S.R. Hardin, & R. Kaplow (Eds.). *The Synergy Model: Implications for certified practice in optimizing patient outcomes*. Boston: Jones & Bartlett.

Stratton, K., Shetty, P., Wallace, R., & Bondurant, S. (Eds.). (2001). *Clearing the smoke: Assessing the science base for tobacco harm reduction*. Washington, D.C.: National Academy Press.

Tusaie-Mumford, K.R. (2001). Psychosocial resilience in rural adolescents: Optimism, perceived social support and gender differences. University of Pittsburgh, Ph.D. thesis.

Walker, A. (2001). Trajectory, transition, and vulnerability in adult medical-surgical patients: A framework for understanding in-hospital convalescence. *Contemporary Nurse*, 11(2/3), 206-216.

Woodgate, R.L. (1999). A review of literature on resilience in the adolescent with cancer: Part II. *Journal of Pediatric Oncology Nursing*, 16(2), 78-89.

Internet References

The AACN Synergy Model for Patient Care. Available at www.aacn.org/certcorp.org. Accessed April, 2004.

American Association of Colleges of Nursing. Available at www.aacn.nche.edu/Publications/positions. Accessed April, 2004.

Assumptions guiding the AACN Synergy Model for Patient Care. Available at www.aacn.org/certcorp.org. Accessed April, 2004.

Basic information about the AACN Synergy Model for Patient Care. Available at www.aacn.org/certcorp.org. Accessed April, 2004.

Certification and Regulation of Advanced Practice Nursing. Available at http://www.aacn.nche.edu/Publications/positions/cerreg.htm. Accessed April, 2004.

Characteristics of patients, clinical units and systems of concern to nurses. Available at www.aacn.org/certcorp.org. Accessed April, 2004.

Nurse competencies of concern to patients, clinical units, and systems. Available at www.aacn.org/certcorp.org. Accessed April, 2004.

Standards of Practice and Professional Performance for the Acute and Critical Care Clinical Nurse Specialist. Available at www.aacn.org. Accessed April, 2004.

4

Spheres of Influence

Defining the Impact of the CNS

Kathleen Vollman
Brenda Lyons

SPHERES OF INFLUENCE FOR THE CNS

Clinical nurse specialist (CNS) practice has evolved over the past 50 years into highly specialized and complex work in over 40 specialty areas. One of the largest specialty areas is in acute and critical care. The practice area for acute and critical care is defined not by the physical location but rather by the dynamic interaction between acute and critically ill patients and family, the caregiver, and the health care environment. A master's degree has always been the recognized educational entry level requirement for CNS practice; however, only since the late 1990s have core (across specialties) competencies of CNS practice and the standards of acute and critical care CNS practice been articulated.

This chapter presents a brief history of the transition from "subroles" to "spheres of influence" as domains to portray the essence of CNS practice, a description of each sphere, and a CNS exemplar to depict the work of a critical care CNS in creating cost-effective quality patient outcomes through three spheres of influence. The exemplar is a representation of an actual CNS practice scenario.

History of Transition from CNS Subroles to CNS Spheres of Influence

Since the inception of the CNS role, it has been a challenge to adequately capture the richness and complexity of CNS practice in role descriptions. For many years CNS practice was defined by subrole, including expert practitioner, educator, researcher, change agent, administrator, and consultant (ANA, 1980; Hamric, 1989; Hamric & Spross, 1989; Sparacino, 2000). Subrole delineations were used to help differentiate the CNS from other clinically expert nurses. Although the partitioning of CNS practice into subrole silos had some heuristic desirability, artificially segmenting practice activities that in real life are highly integrated made it difficult to evaluate or account for CNS practice. Commonly, attempts to measure or account for CNS practice were made using "time in activity" by subroles as a metric. The "time in activity" metric never became the standard measure because day-to-day CNS practice does not occur in subrole silos and therefore cleanly teasing out subrole times of activity becomes an impossibility (Dayhoff and Lyon, 2001). In addition, the subrole titles, particularly those of educator and researcher, inferred academic preparation and role responsibilities beyond the master's degree.

In an attempt to more realistically capture CNS practice, the National Association of Clinical Nurse Specialists (NACNS) conducted a content review of over 70 CNS job descriptions from a variety of health care agencies with geographic representation. The content review confirmed that CNS practice is highly complex and consistently targeted toward achieving quality, cost-effective outcomes through direct patient care and indirect care activities through advancing the practice of nursing and championing system changes that facilitate or improve patient care. The target focus areas or domains of CNS practice were thus delineated as *patient/client, nursing personnel, and system/network organization.* Although the knowledge and skill competencies required to practice effectively in each of the domains built on each other, they were different from one another. The decision was made to identify core competencies by domain. It was also decided to call these three domains "spheres of influence" since the vast majority of effective CNS work is accomplished through *influence* rather than position authority (NACNS, 1998).

Different Professional Group Perspectives

Core competencies required in the three spheres of influence were drafted and underwent extensive review in the mid 1990s by more than 60 external reviewers, including practicing CNSs, leaders in nursing service, CNS educators, and leaders in the discipline. The core competencies of CNS practice and core CNS-related outcomes across specialties were published in the first edition of the *Statement on Clinical Nurse Specialist Practice and Education* (NACNS, 1998). Recently the statement was updated (NACNS, 2004) to reflect new developments in evidence-based practice, nurse-sensitive outcomes, patient safety issues, special needs of older adults, end-of-life care, and increased emphasis on quality clinical environments. The current edition of the document was also extensively reviewed by practicing CNSs, nurse leaders, and national nursing organizations.

The American Nurses Association (ANA) and the American Association of Critical-Care Nurses (AACN) adopted the three "spheres of influence" framework to describe the scope of CNS practice in their respective documents (ANA, 2004; AACN, 2002). Both ANA and AACN use the nursing process (i.e., assessment, diagnosis, planning, implementation, evaluation) framework to delineate standards of practice (competencies). The standards are described in a generic sense within each component of the nursing process to be applicable to each sphere of influence. The ANA's *Nursing: Scope and Standards of Practice* (2004) is structured to clearly build on the registered nurse (RN) scope of practice. AACN's *Scope of Practice and Standards of Professional Performance for the Acute and Critical Care Clinical Nurse Specialist* (2002) includes strategies for implementing the standards (competencies) and also incorporates the AACN Synergy Model for Nursing Care (Curley, 1998). The NACNS's *Statement on Clinical Nurse Specialist Practice and Education* (1998, 2004) also uses components of the nursing process to identify competencies, but does so for each sphere of influence separately. Although the structure of each of the association's (NACNS, ANA, AACN) documents describing CNS practice is somewhat different, there is a high degree of correspondence between them to describe the scope of CNS practice using three spheres of influence as a foundation.

Each of the three spheres of influence of CNS practice is summarized below. Since the NACNS *Statement* identifies competencies specific to each sphere of influence, it will be used to capture the skills needed by acute and critical care CNSs to accomplish desired outcomes. Desired outcomes* of CNS practice are summarized for each sphere, as well as the competencies required for effective practice in each sphere. Each sphere

---

*"The results of deliberative CNS action within each sphere of influence and may include the initiation and facilitation of change or transformation actions. ... The outcomes ... are unlikely to occur without the deliberative actions which requires expert problem identification and problem solving by the CNS." (NACNS, 2004, p. 65)

incorporates problem-solving processes inherent in the nursing process and demonstrates the integration of the subroles. Following the description of the spheres of influence is a presentation of a critical dare CNS exemplar that demonstrates practice through all of the spheres.

Patient/Client Sphere
"Clinical expertise, embedded in the patient/ client sphere of influence, is the foundation of CNS practice in the other two spheres." (NACNS, 2004, p. 18) The overall goal of care within this sphere is to directly affect the accomplishment of cost-effective quality patient and family outcomes.

Patient/Client Sphere Outcomes. Outcomes of properly collaborative CNS practice in the patient/client sphere of influence encompass:

- Accurate diagnoses based on multiple sources of valid data as appropriate.
- Appropriate plans of care tailored to the preferences of patient and family.
- Measurable desired outcomes of interventions.
- Interventions targeting specific etiologies developed in the context of appropriate collaboration with other health care disciplines.
- Prevention, alleviation, and/or reduction of symptoms, functional problems, and risk behaviors.
- Prevention of unintended consequences or errors.
- Measurement of nurse-sensitive patient outcomes.
- Evidence-based programs of care of developed for specific patient populations.
- Full integration of strategies that facilitate the transition of patients across the continuum of care to decrease fragmentation.
- Development, implementation, and evaluation of innovative educational programs for patients, families, and groups.
- Dissemination of knowledge of new phenomena and/or interventions through presentations and publications.

- Best practice guidelines and policies developed based on evidence of demonstrated effectiveness. (Adapted from NACNS, 2004.)

Patient/Client Sphere Competencies. To accomplish the above outcomes, CNSs must have expert knowledge and skill in the assessment, differential diagnosis, and treatment of illness. The meaning of illness here is not synonymous with disease. Rather it is defined as the experience of somatic discomfort (i.e., physical and/or emotional) and declines or impairment in functional ability below capability level (Lyon, 1990; NACNS Statement, 2004). Consistent with the observations of Nightingale (1859;1969), illness and disease are distinctly different phenomena. Illness can have both disease/pathology–based (including iatrogenic effects of medical therapeutics) and nondisease-based etiologies (including person and environmental factors). A common example is pain. Incisional pain is a disease/pathology–based etiology, whereas muscle strain from coughing or misalignment and tissue stretching are nondisease-based etiologies requiring nursing therapeutics. Disease/ pathology etiologies require "medical" interventions, which may encompass surgery (breaking of the skin), prescriptive medications, complex mechanical (e.g., traction) or electrical (defibrillation) interventions. Nondisease-based etiologies require nonpharmacological or nursing interventions/therapeutics such as proper positioning (includes appropriate prone positioning), and warming or cooling (NACNS, 2004).

CNSs must be experts in both disease phenomena and person/environment phenomena that can cause or exacerbate symptoms and functional problems that require "medical" or nursing interventions, as well as the iatrogenic affects of treatments. It is this knowledge that helps to guide the CNS's comprehensive assessment and accurate differential diagnosis. Therefore CNSs must be excellent in differentially determining which etiologies are contributing to patient/ client illness experiences (symptoms and functional problems) that are resulting in a delay in achieving desirable outcomes or have the potential to result in undesirable outcomes, including but not limited to complications and extended stays. Accurate diagnosis based on valid information from multiple sources is essential to selecting or designing appropriately targeted and effective interventions (NACNS, 2004).

CNSs must be able to conduct clinical inquiries to identify patient population needs/problems that form the design and implementation of population-based programs of care to address common problems either through preventive or treatment efforts. Prevention and treatment programs are designed by CNSs and implemented as appropriate with other health care team members to create synergistic outcomes. The evaluation of nursing practice is critical, and thus the CNS measures nurse sensitive outcomes (NACNS, 2004).

Nurses and Nursing Practice Sphere
CNSs work to advance the practice of nursing and improve patient outcomes through updating standards of care and developing best practice models of care that direct the actions of nurses and nursing practice. CNSs provide leadership and consultation expertise to nursing staff and other health professionals in the implementation of evidence-based practice. Of central importance to CNS effectiveness with nursing personnel in bridging the gap between what is known and what is done at the bedside are the personal characteristics of honesty, communication skills (listening, validating, reflecting, caring attitude), positive self-regard/confidence, personal mastery in managing thoughts and emotions, personal commitment to continued learning, and willingness to take risks (NACNS, 2004).

Nurses and Nursing Practice Sphere Outcomes. Outcomes of effective CNS practice in the nursing/nursing practice sphere of influence encompass:

- Identified knowledge and skill development needs of nurses.

- Nursing personnel using evidence-based practices.
- Nursing care innovations that have an evidence base that is accessible and understandable by nursing staff.
- Nurses who can articulate their unique contributions to nurse-sensitive outcomes and other patient care outcomes.
- Nurses who are empowered to solve patient care problems at the point of care.
- Desired patient outcomes that are derived through nurses collaborating with other health care professionals as appropriate.
- Ongoing career enhancement programs for nurses.
- Nurses experiencing job satisfaction.
- Nurses providing care in a cost-conscious manner.
- Nurses engaging in learning experiences to maintain or enhance competence.
- Educational programs that advance the practice of nursing.
- Nurses exercising an effective voice in decisions affecting patient care. (Adapted from NACNS, 2004.)

Nurses and nursing practice sphere competencies. CNSs conduct assessments to identify and define problems and opportunities within the nursing/nursing practice sphere. Specifically CNSs use valid assessment methods to identify the knowledge and skill competencies of nursing personnel and patterns of outcomes of nursing practice within and across units of care.

To facilitate the practice of nursing, CNSs work in collaboration with nursing personnel and other health care providers to identify needed changes in equipment or other products to enhance clinical outcomes and cost-effectiveness. It is also essential that CNSs assess barriers and facilitators to implementing needed changes in nursing practices (NACNS, 2004).

The diagnoses of what is needed and what is contributing to the needs to change nursing practice are based on valid evidence and anticipation of both intended and unintended consequences. CNSs specify the measurable desired outcomes of practice changes and plans for achieving the outcomes that incorporate facilitators and strategies to overcome barriers. Plans for changing practice are sensitive to cost and resource considerations (NACNS, 2004).

CNSs must be skilled in mentoring staff in the use of evidence-based information and in collaboratively working with nursing personnel to implement innovative interventions that improve outcomes. In addition, CNSs assist nurses in developing innovative programs of care for patients who are sensitive to the complexity of patient care problems and resources of the system (NACNS, 2004).

CNSs are skilled in creating an environment that stimulates self-learning and enables nurses to articulate their unique contributions to patient care, be inquisitive about that care, develop and evaluate innovations in practice focused on improving care and/or cost-effectiveness, and evaluate the outcomes of care. In the spirit of personal growth and advancement, CNSs also mentor nurses to advance their careers in nursing (NACNS, 2004).

Organization/System Sphere

Today's complex health care systems require that CNSs be skilled in affecting system changes to remove barriers to and to enhance facilitators of nursing practice and patient care. CNSs influence the trajectory of care for populations of patients in a system from admission through discharge to facilitate the achievement of desired outcomes and to minimize recidivism and readmission.

Organization/System Sphere Outcomes. The outcomes of CNS work in the organization/system sphere of influence encompass:

- Articulation of clinical problems within the context of the organization/system structure, mission, culture, policies and resources.

- Patient care processes that reflect continuous improvements that benefit the system.
- Change strategies that are integrated throughout the system.
- Policies that enhance the practice of nurses within the context of multidisciplinary teams.
- Innovative models of care that are incorporated across the continuum of care.
- Evidence-based best practice models that are developed for the system.
- Articulation of nursing's unique contribution to patient care outcomes at the system's decision-making levels.
- Informed decision makers at the system level regarding practice problems, factors contributing to the problems, and significance of the problems in terms of outcomes and costs.
- Patient care programs that are aligned with systems mission, goals, and priorities.
- Nursing staff compliance with regulatory requirements. (Adapted from NACNS, 2004.)

Organization/System Sphere Competencies. The CNSs' concern about and accountability for continuous improvement are also evident in their work at the organization/system level. CNSs are skilled in assessing organizational processes, including interdepartmental relationships/functioning, professional climate, multidisciplinary collaboration, external relationships and regulations, and health policy to identify facilitators and barriers to effective patient care. On the basis of valid assessments, CNSs are able to clearly define and articulate system problems that are having deleterious effects on patient outcomes and/or cost-effectiveness of care within the context of the organization's mission, culture, policies, and resources. CNSs work to ensure a common vision of patient care within a multidisciplinary context and develop patient care programs that are consistent with the organization's mission, values, and goals. It is essential that CNSs help to ensure the provision of patient care services consistent with statutory/ regulatory requirements and standards. CNSs must be able to facilitate multidisciplinary collaboration and lead nursing and multidisciplinary teams in developing, implementing, and evaluating innovative patient care programs. The measurable outcomes of system-wide changes to stakeholders are communicated clearly, along with strategies to sustain and diffuse programs of care throughout the system as appropriate (NACNS, 2004).

The ability to continuously evaluate and adapt is essential for the CNS. CNSs document and evaluate the impact of their work on the organization. Deliberative CNS practice within a collaborative multidisciplinary environment helps to ensure that desired patient/client outcomes are attained and sustained.

Critical Care Clinical Nurse Specialist Exemplar

Using a patient case example, the three spheres of influence within CNS practice are highlighted. Within each sphere (patient/client, nurses/nursing practice, and organization/ system) evidence of CNS skill sets and competencies are outlined. The example details how assessments from a single patient encounter can lead to planning and implementation of individual patient management, population-based care changes, education and professional development of the RN, and long-term clinical and financial impact to the health system in which care is provided. Fundamental to influencing the spheres are key characteristics of the CNS that include clinical expertise in a specialty, leadership skills, collaboration skills, consultation skills, professional attributes, ethical conduct, and professional citizenship beyond the specialty and within the profession of nursing. Therefore demonstration of these characteristics is included within this case exemplar.

Case Example

A 40-year-old male was admitted to a medical intensive care unit (MICU) with a diagnosis of community-acquired pneumonia. There was no significant past medical history. He presented to the emergency department with complaints of shortness of breath and a low-grade fever for 2 days. His vitals signs revealed borderline hypotension responsive to fluid administration. The patient's oxygen saturation was 76% on a nonrebreather with a respiratory rate of 40 breaths per minute. He was oriented to self and place. The patient was intubated, placed on antibiotics, and transferred to the MICU. His wife, who was 7 months' pregnant with their first child, accompanied him.

On admission the patient was placed on the ventilator management program. This *population-based initiative* was designed earlier by a multidisciplinary team co-led by the medical director and the CNS to ensure, through standing orders, that all ventilator patients receive consistent evidence-based care. The care included enteral feeding within 24 hours of intubation as part of peptic ulcer disease prophylaxis; deep vein thrombosis prophylaxis; head of the bed at 30 degrees; spontaneous breathing trials for weaning when physiologically ready; every 2- to 4-hour oral care and placement on a protocol for management of pain, anxiety, and/or delirium. On the basis of the evidence, when these components are consistently performed on ventilator patients, they result in shorter time on the ventilator, shorter stay in the ICU, and a reduced incidence of ventilator-induced pneumonia. As a part of the initiative, process and outcome data on the population of ventilator patients are collected on a monthly basis. The CNS coordinates this activity with the unit practice committee and manager, and the results are presented at the collaborative practice meeting to identify areas for process improvement and shared with the hospital's executive management team. (**Sphere:** Patient/client: population-based care; nurses/nursing practice: evidence-based best practice guideline and education. **CNS characteristics:** Clinical expertise in a specialty, leadership skills, collaboration.)

On the third day after admission the patient's RN called the CNS to the bedside. She expressed some concerns with regard to the patient's current physiological condition.

The bedside nurse had spoken with the resident and had received initial orders for culturing and fluid resuscitation. An initial assessment was performed by the CNS identifying the immediate clinical concerns, and a discussion of care strategies with the nurse and medical staff occurred. At a later time, a more thorough assessment of both the disease-and nondisease-based etiologies to guide the complete plan of care was developed in conjunction with the patient's nurse (Table 4-1). The CNS determined that the patient demonstrated clinical signs of severe sepsis and met the clinical definition for adult respiratory distress syndrome (ARDS). As part of the development of the bedside nurse, the CNS used this as an opportunity to assist the bedside nurse in reaching the same conclusion about the patient's condition through a series of questions to stimulate critical thinking. (**Sphere:** Patient/client: Direct assessment and collaboration with the team for appropriate medical and nursing management of the patient; nurses/nursing practice: deductive reasoning and education of clinical criteria to identify severe sepsis and ARDS. **CNS Characteristics:** Clinical expertise in a specialty, consultation, collaboration.)

Immediate Strategies. Early effective fluid resuscitation secondary to third spacing is important to improve oxygen delivery and prevent end-organ dysfunction. The initial orders

received included two 250-ml boluses and instruction to increase the IV fluid to 150 ml/hr. Together with the bedside nurse, the CNS approached the medical team to discuss whether the fluid order was sufficient for an effective resuscitation in a patient with severe sepsis. The CNS facilitated this communication based on the knowledge of recent studies and articles supporting early goal-directed fluid therapy. After the team reviewed the data, an order was given to resuscitate to evidence-driven clinical parameters. In addition, an order for drotrecogin alfa (Xigris) administration was received. The CNS assessed the RN's familiarity with the use of drogrecogin alfa because it was a fairly new medication. The RN caring for the patient shared that this was the first time she had administered the medication. She had received an in-service several months ago. A short in-service was provided at the bedside to ensure safe and appropriate administration of the medication to reduce any potential errors. This encounter sparked a concern that other nurses may also have the same educational deficit. Therefore the CNS assessed the staff's knowledge level and ultimately planned for re-in-servicing and placement of an information fact sheet in a support materials binder at the bedside. **Sphere:** Patient/client: Direct assessment and collaboration with the team for appropriate medical and nursing management of the patient; nurses/nursing practice: education about a new medication immediately to provide safe and appropriate administration and the development of an educational plan and support material for the unit. **CNS Characteristics:** Clinical expertise in a specialty, collaboration, professional attributes.)

The patient was placed on low tidal volume ventilation to reduce ventilator injury. As part of a protocol written by the nursing team during a project to improve mobility, the patient was placed on continuous lateral rotation therapy to help mobilize secretions, improve ventilation and perfusion matching, and reduce the incidence of pneumonia and atelectasis. Part of the role of the CNS was to ensure that the staff were

TABLE 4-1	
CNS Assessment of Patient Problems by Category	
Disease-Based	**Nondiseased-Based**
Community-acquired pneumonia	Early recognition of instability
Hypotension	Impaired coping/family
Severe sepsis	Immobility/deconditioning
Acute respiratory distress syndrome	Powerlessness
Bloodstream infection	Potential for skin injury
Failure to wean	Failure to wean

knowledgeable about the therapy and monitor its use for appropriateness to cost-justify the benefits. The patient continued to require significant support by the ventilator with high levels of oxygen (FiO_2 90%) and positive end-expiratory pressure (PEEP) (18 cm H_2O) with a PaO_2 of 58 mm Hg and a saturation of 87%.

Recently the CNS had attended a national conference where there were many sessions on the benefits of a prone position maneuver for patients with ARDS. With limited knowledge about the topic, the CNS contacted a colleague who was considered to be knowledgeable about the use of prone positioning and received the necessary resources to consider trying this maneuver with the patient. The CNS then suggested considering the use of the prone position to the team. Aware that the hospital did not have a policy and procedure for prone positioning, the CNS accessed the Internet and available professional resources and identified several examples from which to develop a protocol for the future but for the present was able to download one and provide a safer strategy for the positioning technique. The staff was educated and started prone positioning on a 6-hour schedule, which helped to reduce the support needed on the ventilator and resulted in improved patient oxygenation. Subsequently a policy and procedure was developed, and staffs within all the ICUs were educated. (**Sphere:** Patient/client: Direct assessment and collaboration with the team for appropriate medical and nursing management of the patient; nurses/nursing practice: education of a new positioning technique; organization/system: writing a policy, a method to measure appropriate use of a therapy to demonstrate its cost effectiveness. **CNS Characteristics:** Clinical expertise in a specialty, collaboration, leadership, professional attributes.)

The patient's wife was 7 months' pregnant with their first child, exhausted, and frightened. The staff nurse was able to support the family when at the bedside but requested additional intervention by the CNS. Providing *direct patient care*, the CNS assessed the social support structure (i.e., tangible factors that were increasing

the stress level and current coping strategies). The need for information about and access to her husband were key to reducing her stress levels. Resistance to opening the visiting hours was a continuing challenge within the unit. The CNS helped to develop a contract, taking into account the needs of the patient, family, and staff. To ensure consistency in practice with regard to visiting, the CNS was critical in helping the practice committee examine the evidence-based concept of open visiting. Access is a key family need when a loved one is in the ICU. After guided review of the literature by the practice committee, the visiting policies were rewritten, and open visiting occurred. Challenges continue to occur with this policy, and those issues are brought forth to the committee for review and problem solving. Patient/family satisfaction data as a nurse-sensitive outcome is collected monthly and shared with the staff to celebrate and discuss opportunities for improvement.

In addition, the CNS's assessment also revealed that the patient lived in a neighboring city about 1 hour away from the hospital. Assistance for arrangements to stay at the hospitality rooms provided by the hospital helped ensure her proper rest while remaining close to her husband. A lounge chair was placed in the room for increased comfort and to facilitate napping while remaining close. A discussion with family members and friends occurred to discuss strategies to support the patient and his wife by rotating time spent with the patient. The CNS arranged a family meeting with the lead intensivist at weekly intervals to keep them accurately informed about the patient's progress. (**Sphere:** Patient/client: Direct assessment and collaboration with family and team for care interventions; nurses/nursing practice: involved staff in development of the visiting policy, assisted in developing their skills of critiquing research; organization/system: measurement of patient and family satisfaction, sharing that data and intervention strategies at a system level. **CNS Characteristics:** Clinical expertise in a specialty, collaboration, leadership, professional attributes, ethical conduct.)

The patient began to turn the corner and was showing significant signs of improvement. Vasoactive medications were weaned off; ventilator support was at FiO_2 of 50% with 8 cm of PEEP. On ICU day 10 the patient's condition worsened. He was showing signs of sepsis again. Cultures revealed a bloodstream infection caused by the central venous catheter. The catheter was removed, and the patient was started on the appropriate antibiotics by the medical team. Because of the prolonged ICU stay, the patient was weakened and challenged with successful liberation from the ventilator. The CNS was again consulted by the nursing team. A progressive mobility program was designed in concert with physical therapy, respiratory therapy, medical and nursing staff, and family. In addition, the CNS diagnosed powerlessness and worked with the patient, family, and nursing staff to develop a daily schedule to reinsert control into the patient's choices of daily activities. The patient was successfully weaned and transferred to a facility for rehabilitation. (**Sphere:** Patient/client: Direct assessment and collaboration with the team for appropriate management of the patient, development of a progressive mobility plan; nurses/nursing practice: role modeling, education on strategies to reduce powerlessness; organization/system: writing a policy, reducing and measuring ventilator patient's length of stay. **CNS Characteristics:** Clinical expertise in a specialty, collaboration, leadership).

Impacting Practice at a Larger Scale

From this type of patient encounter, direct patient care outcomes, and nursing personnel development to advanced practice were realized through mentoring and application of evidence-based practice, development and education about nursing practice protocols, and assisting with individual and long-range strategies for helping families cope. In addition to direct care and nursing personnel outcomes, the CNS was able to formulate one systems initiative, a reduction in bloodstream infections (BSIs), and two patient population—specific programs to include early recognition and

rescue of physiologically unstable patients and the design and development of a progressive mobility program for mechanically ventilated patients (Table 4-2).

Systems Initiative: Reducing Bloodstream Infections. During the second consultation, the CNS heard the information that the infection was from the central line. Knowing the unit's current BSI rate was above the national average, the CNS saw an opportunity to improve on this outcome for other patients that enter the unit. A multidisciplinary quality improvement team was formulated; the CNS served as co-chair.

Assessment of the current process for line insertion occurs. Monthly evaluation of the BSI rate per 1000 catheter days was tabulated and compared to the national benchmark. Staff nurses from the unit were included in the development of the data collection tools and the process for collection. The national evidence-based guidelines from the Centers for Disease Control and Prevention (CDC) were used to rewrite a unit policy for central line management. The policy was taken through an approval structure, including a unit practice council and collaborative practice group. An implementation plan was created with the team.

The goal of the new evidence-based policy was to improve on the insertion process/sterile field, dressing care, and length of time the line is in placed. The implementation involved an educational plan designed by the CNS outlining the science and presenting baseline data to the staff. Before implementing the policy, the team reviewed all educational materials. In addition, a number of environmental changes addressing barriers and facilitators to support appropriate practices were addressed. This included invasive line carts stocked with the necessary supplies to create an appropriate field. The CNS and nursing staff conducted a transparent dressing product evaluation. The goal was to obtain a dressing that had the highest moisture vapor permeability rate and occlusiveness. In addition, the bedside RN was given the power to stop a line procedure if the sterile field was inappropriate. Significant role modeling by

TABLE 4-2

Examples of Influence Care Activities of the Sphere within the Case

Patient/Client	Nurses/Nursing Practice	Organization/System
Ventilator management program	Oral care policy	Reduction of bloodstream infections
Antibiotics		
Rapid fluid resuscitation/early goal directed therapy	Early recognition of trouble/ prevent complications Critical thinking skills	Early recognition and response to patients in trouble and measurement of outcomes
Drotrecogin alfa (Xigris) administration	Education/staff information sheet	
Low tidal volume ventilation		
Continuous lateral rotation therapy (CLRT)/prone positioning	CLRT policy written and monitored Networking prone positioning policy and education	
Progressive mobility plan for the patient and then developed for the mechanically ventilated patient	Team development Literature review skills Critique research articles	Measurement of outcomes
Reversal of powerlessness through development of a daily schedule	Role model behavior	
Contract visiting with family	Open family visiting policy	Measurement of patient/family and staff satisfaction
Arrangements for wife to stay near by		
Weekly meetings with care staff for consistent information updates		

the CNS and nurse manager were required to make the program successful. The process was incorporated into monthly physician meetings and new nurse orientation.

The results of implementing the new policy demonstrated a reduction of the BSI rate from 6.8 per 1000 catheter days to 2.9 per 1000 catheter days. The project was presented as an abstract at the American Thoracic Society meeting. The cost-benefit analysis revealed a reduced mortality and avoidance of 27 BSIs with a financial savings close to 1 million dollars a year. The evaluation and reporting of these data became a standard report at the monthly collaborative practice and unit practice meetings.

Congratulation/good job signs were posted in the bathroom as well. Creating the need for a larger system change, the CNS and the medical director reported data at a hospital-wide critical care committee, and the CNS co-chaired the development of a hospital-wide policy and procedure based on the new guidelines from the CDC released in 2002. Product changes occurred to combat some of the challenges identified within the unit before moving the policy housewide. BSI rates and reporting occurred at a unit level and a system level, and process improvement continues toward a zero target rate. (**Sphere:** Nursing personnel: Support the nurses patient advocacy role, involve staff in ownership of the care process; systems: measurement of BSI rates, process measurements, product evaluation, sharing data and intervention strategies at a system level, presentation to nursing groups of strategies to reduce BSIs regionally and nationally. **CNS Characteristics:** Clinical expertise in a specialty, collaboration, leadership, professional attributes, professional citizenship.)

Population-Based Initiative/Systems Initiative: Early Recognition and Response. The patient demonstrated signs of deterioration on day 3 in the ICU. Early recognition of patients who are in trouble with a developing sepsis or cardiac difficulty is essential to improve survival, whether the patient is in an ICU, the emergency department, a medical-surgical floor, or the postanesthesia care unit. To prevent avoidable delays, it is imperative that nurses be skilled at recognizing the clinical signs of patients in trouble and be able to initiate a system that will bring immediate assessment and initial resuscitation. The CNS was aware of the national statistics on in-house survival of cardiopulmonary resuscitation and through evaluation of the literature had evidence of documented improvement in outcome for patients in trouble if they were recognized early.

The CNS approached the code blue team for a discussion of the opportunity to reduce code blues by focusing on early recognition, alerting, and immediate resuscitation. The code blue team believed that it went beyond the scope of their charge and requested that this issue be discussed at the hospital-wide critical care committee. Networking to gather support, the CNS approached the chair of the critical care committee to discuss the idea. Support was obtained, and a physician champion was designated to co-chair the program or concept development and create a presentation of the literature for the full committee. The presentation was an overwhelming success; and a task force, including frontline practitioners of respiratory, nursing, medicine, and pharmacy and an operations administrator, was designated to design a process for the hospital for

early recognition and response for patients in trouble.

An extensive literature review was done, and two site visits of facilities that had implemented a similar process occurred. The process was tested in a surgical and medical floor and triage in the ER. Process and outcome measures were designed. Request for a data manager for the improvement process was approved after multiple attempts. The pilots were successful. Minor changes where made in the process, and a full-scale implementation would occur over the next several months. If predicted outcome measures of reduced in-house cardiac arrest, improved rescue rates, and improved mortality occur, plans to publish and present have been discussed. (**Sphere:** Nursing personnel: Support the nurse's patient advocacy role, involve staff in ownership of the care process; systems: develop a system-wide process to promote early recognition and resuscitation of patients wherever they are, outcome measures designed, cost-benefit analysis performed, plans to publish and present to a variety of audiences, including administrators, nurses, and doctors. **CNS Characteristics:** Clinical expertise in a specialty, collaboration, leadership, professional attributes, professional citizenship).

Population-Based Initiative/Progressive Mobility for Mechanically Ventilated Patients. The CNS was consulted again later in the patient's hospital stay because of difficulty weaning from the breathing machine. The assessment clearly demonstrated that significant deconditioning had occurred from prolonged bed rest, which was confirmed by a myelogram. The CNS saw this as an opportunity to look at the problem of deconditioning on a broader scope with all patients on a mechanical ventilator for longer than 3 days. The practice issue was introduced at the monthly nursing practice committee meeting. A discussion occurred, and several staff nurses expressed interest in looking at this issue. They appeared to be the nurses who consistently are assigned to the "chronic vents" and wanted to see if there was anything they could do to improve patient outcomes and get patients off the ventilator sooner. The task force co-chaired by the CNS and a clinical nurse III set up the initial meeting. It was decided to include a physical therapist because of their expertise in mobility/tolerance.

The CNS used the first meeting as an opportunity to educate the nurses about how to do a literature search and how to critique research articles. A tool for scoring a research article was created to help with consistency. The literature review was completed, and the articles divided among the task force members. After 2 weeks the group met and discussed the findings. An initial progressive mobility protocol was created and piloted on two patients. Results of the pilot were shared with the group, and necessary changes were made. Once completed, the protocol was taken to the unit-based collaborative practice meeting for approval. The protocol was accepted with minor changes, and an education and implementation plan was designed. Outcome measures of length of time on the ventilator, stay in the ICU, and long-range mobility goals after hospitalization are measured. (**Sphere:** Patient/client: Development of a progressive mobility protocol for patients on a ventilator for longer than 3 days; nursing/nursing practice: involved staff in ownership of the care process, education on how to do a literature review and critique a research article, team participation skills; organization/systems: process and outcome measurements that can result in cost avoidance or revenue generation. **CNS Characteristics:** Clinical expertise in a specialty, collaboration, leadership)

CONCLUSION

The three spheres of influence serve as a foundational dynamic working diagram to guide CNS practice. The case example demonstrates that CNS practice begins with an expert clinician who skillfully assesses, diagnosis, plans, and intervenes using evidence to influence patient management, the nurse/nursing practice, and the system to impact cost-effective quality outcomes. The CNS must develop and possess the key quality characteristics of collaboration, leadership, consultation skills, and professional attributes within an ethical framework that encompasses active citizenship for the continued growth and development of the profession of nursing.

References

American Association of Critical-Care Nurses (2002). *Nursing: Scope of practice and standards of professional performance for the acute and critical care clinical nurse specialist.* Aliso Viejo, CA: Author.

American Nurses Association (1980). *Nursing's social policy statement.* Kansas City, MO: Author.

American Nurses Association (2004). *Standards of clinical nursing practice.* Washington, D.C.: Author.

Curley, M.A. (1998). Patient-nurse synergy: Optimizing patients' outcomes. *American Journal of Critical Care,* 7:64-72.

Dayhoff, N., and Lyon, B.L. (2001). Assessing outcomes of clinical nurse specialist practice. In Kleinpell, R. (Ed.). *Outcome assessment in advanced practice nursing.* New York: Springer Publishing.

Hamric, A.B. (1989). History and overview of the CNS role. In A.B. Hamric & J.A. Spross (Eds.). *The clinical nurse specialists in theory and practice* (2nd ed.). Philadelphia: Saunders.

Hamric, A.B., & Spross, J.A. (Eds.). *The clinical nurse specialist in theory and practice* (2nd ed.). Philadelphia: Saunders.

Lyon, B.L. (1990). Getting back on track: Nursing's autonomous scope of practice. In N.L. Chaska (Ed.). *The nursing profession: Turning points.* St. Louis: Mosby.

National Association of Clinical Nurse Specialists (1998). *Statement on clinical nurse specialist practice and education.* Glenview, IL: Author.

National Association of Clinical Nurse Specialists (2004). *Statement on clinical nurse specialist practice and education.* Harrisburg, PA: Author.

Nightingale, F. (1859/1969). *Notes on nursing.* New York: Dover.

Sparacino, P.S.A. (2000). The clinical nurse specialist. In A.B. Hamric, J.A. Spross, & C.M. Hanson (Eds.). *Advanced practice nursing: An integrative approach* (2nd ed.). Philadelphia: Saunders.

PART II
Dimensions of Practice for the CNS in Acute
and Critical Care: Synergy in Motion

CHAPTER

5

Clinical Judgment*

Marla J. De Jong

INTRODUCTION

Clinical Nurse Specialists (CNSs) manage a vast amount of patient care data and make decisions that directly impact patients and families. Changes in the workplace environment have complicated decision-making processes. For example, patients live longer and present with complex medical problems, electronic patient care resources are more readily available, regulatory requirements abound, insurance payers aim to control health care costs, and nurse shortages persist. One hallmark of CNSs is their use of clinical judgment to achieve positive outcomes for those within the sphere of influence: patients and their families, nurses and other health care providers, and the organizational system. Furthermore, CNSs are responsible to help clinical nurses develop clinical judgment expertise.

The purpose of this chapter is to describe clinical judgment and discuss how CNSs apply clinical judgment to their practice. The content of this chapter is organized in a way that reflects *Scope of Practice and Standards of Professional Performance for the Acute and Critical Care Clinical Nurse Specialist* (Bell, 2002).

---

*The opinions or assertions contained herein are the private views of the author and are not to be construed as official or as reflecting the views of the Department of the Air Force or the Department of Defense.

DEFINITION OF CLINICAL JUDGMENT

Clinical judgment is the use of clinical reasoning, including clinical decision making, critical thinking, and global perspectives, coupled with nursing skills acquired through a process of integrating education, experiential knowledge, and evidence-based guidelines (American Association of Critical-Care Nurses Certification Corporation, 2005; Curley, 1998). Clinical judgment is anchored in extensive clinical expertise, experience, and available data. Intrinsic to judgment is the need to relate something to something else or to conclude something about the disparity between the current state and a fixed standard (Busch & Schmidt-Hellerau, 2004). Thus, to form a clinical judgment, CNSs compare patient assessment data with normative assessment data and conditions within the organizational system with established criterion. Clinical judgment is intrinsic to nursing practice and is vital in acute and critical care environments where CNSs and clinical nurses practice with a high degree of autonomy.

However, the concept of clinical judgment is difficult to articulate. Acute and critical care clinical nurses and CNSs care for critically ill and unstable patients in diverse and complex settings and must often initiate complicated, highly specialized, and time-sensitive interventions amid uncertainty. In addition, health care organizations routinely rely on CNSs to develop evidence-based and system-wide policies,

BOX 5-1	
Definitions	
Concept	**Definition**
Critical thinking	"The process of purposeful thinking and reflective reasoning where practitioners examine ideas, assumptions, principles, conclusions, beliefs, and actions in the context of nursing practice. . . . This process is associated with a spirit of inquiry, discrimination, logical reasoning, and applications of standards" (Brunt, 2005, p. 61).
Clinical reasoning	The cognitive process of thinking, connecting, and forming judgments about information (Johnson & Webber, 2005)—the overall process of figuring things out (Paul, 1993).
Clinical judgment	The use of clinical reasoning, including clinical decision making, critical thinking, and global perspectives, coupled with nursing skills acquired through a process of integrating education, experiential knowledge, and evidence-based guidelines (American Association of Critical-Care Nurses Certification Corporation, 2005; Curley, 1998).

promote efficient practice, analyze clinical data, create centers of excellence, achieve relevant performance measures, and execute regulations, all with the goal of providing optimal patient care. Particularly in situations in which answers are often not obvious or in which information is incomplete, CNSs rely on clinical judgment to guide practice.

Although some use the terms *critical thinking, clinical reasoning,* and *clinical judgment* interchangeably, these are not synonymous concepts (Box 5-1). Clinicians use critical thinking and clinical reasoning to make clinical judgments (Alfaro-LeFevre, 1999). In other words, clinical judgment is the outcome of critical thinking and clinical reasoning.

Aspects of Clinical Judgment

Six aspects of clinical judgment have been described (Benner, Hooper-Kyriakidis, & Stannard, 1999). First, *reasoning-in-transition* refers to practical reasoning during clinical situations that are evolving or changeable. CNSs use reasoning to resolve contradictions or confusion, form conclusions, and prioritize work. For example, a CNS guides a novice nurse to apply clinical reasoning skills and correctly

conclude that a patient's emergency is aortic dissection, not acute myocardial infarction.

Second, *skilled know-how* is knowing when and how to intervene. Astute assessment skills are an essential part of skilled know-how. Skilled know-how is evident, for instance, when a CNS observes unsafe patient transports between the emergency and radiology departments and then adeptly develops protocols to promote patient well-being. Skilled know-how is not limited to direct patient care but also pertains to other areas such as clinical leadership, communication, and care of families.

Third, *response-based practice* involves a flexible response to the patient's changing situation and needs. Clinicians must "know the patient" and have an immediate understanding or clinical grasp of the situation before they can rapidly respond to a changing situation. Clinicians with a good grasp of the situation do not rigidly adhere to strict protocols but rather understand the unique characteristics of each patient, see the big picture, and individualize care based on the patient's responses. For example, CNSs may adjust visiting hours to meet individual patient or family needs.

Fourth, *agency* refers not only to the ability to act on or influence a situation but also to appreciating how one impacts patients and contributes to the health care team (Benner, Tanner, & Chesla, 1996). Imbedded in this aspect are experiential learning, high-quality practice, independent thinking, confident decision making, self respect, advocacy, and capability to respond to changing circumstances (Benner, Hooper-Kyriakidis & Stannard, 1999; Benner, Tanner & Chesla, 1996). For instance, a CNS arranges a multidisciplinary care meeting for a patient who must decide whether to begin chronic dialysis.

Fifth, *perceptual acuity* is the ability to recognize important clinical problems. Coupled with perceptual acuity is the *skill of involvement* that refers to interpersonal connections between the clinician and patient and/or family. CNSs who engage with the patient and family learn the particulars about the patient's chief complaint, medical and sociocultural history, preferences, values, and response patterns and are positioned to make sound clinical judgments regarding, for example, end-of-life care.

Sixth, *links between clinical and ethical reasoning* refers to the fact that clinical judgment has both clinical and ethical components. The CNS applies experiential learning, practical wisdom, and reflection to make clinical judgments that are in the best interests of patients, families, nurses, and organizational systems. For example, CNSs may consult the hospital ethics committee when a patient's daughter glibly remarks that she signed "do not resuscitate" paperwork for her mother and hopes to soon acquire her mother's life insurance money.

CNS Level of Expertise

The CNS's clinical judgment improves and matures with time and experience. As with clinical nurses, a CNS's level of expertise ranges from competent to expert. Table 5-1 contains descriptions and examples of CNS activities for the novice, competent, and expert CNS, thereby illustrating the role development of the CNS.

A CNS who is new to the role makes it a priority to learn the responsibilities and expectations of the position. In doing so, the CNS develops relationships with other clinicians and leaders, learns about the patient population, gains familiarity with policies and procedures, and assesses the care environment within the unit and organization. These activities are important because inexperienced CNSs may feel unsettled, uninformed about specific responsibilities, and unsure about interactions with other members of the health care team.

New CNSs may be anxious and question their ability to make clinical judgments regarding nursing practice, unit or organizational policies, patient or nurse education, clinical outcomes, resource allocation, or research findings. In these cases, inexperienced CNSs may be paralyzed with inaction or be tempted to revert to a previous and more comfortable role. For example, the CNS may spend too much time performing direct patient care while neglecting responsibilities to develop an evidence-based protocol for care of potential organ donors. For some, transition to the CNS level is difficult, and even skills that previously seemed easy seem awkward. Nonetheless, it is essential that new CNSs demonstrate sound clinical judgment and clinical competence.

The novice yet prudent CNS enhances clinical judgment by using resources both within and outside the institution. For example, when appropriate, the CNS avoids "reinventing the wheel" but uses existing standards or practice guidelines to guide clinical judgment. The CNS seeks nonthreatening avenues by which to hone clinical judgment and consults experts for advice or direction regarding particular subjects.

Novice CNSs often exercise clinical judgment in their immediate area of responsibility (e.g., in the neonatal intensive care unit [NICU]). With time and practice, however, NICU CNSs broaden their focus to collaborate with and influence relevant areas such as referring organizations, neonatal transport team members, and obstetrical clinics.

With experience, the CNS becomes more at ease in making clinical judgments. Competent CNSs are less intimidated by complex situations and

TABLE 5-1

Descriptions and Examples of Clinical Nurse Specialist (CNS) Activities for the Novice, Competent, and Expert CNS

Level of Expertise	Description of Selected CNS Activities	Example of Selected CNS Activity
Level 1 novice	Collects basic information: patient/family assessment data, outcomes data, clinician competency data, availability and adequacy of unit policies and procedures	Demonstrates a comprehensive patient assessment to new critical care nurses and determines that 65% of the unit's nurses are competent in continuous renal replacement therapy
	Uses existing algorithms, decision trees, and protocols when making clinical judgments and is uncomfortable deviating from them	Implements AACN's end-tidal carbon dioxide protocol as written
	Matches formal knowledge with clinical events to make decisions	Applies advanced knowledge of hemodynamic monitoring to detect cardiac tamponade in a patient whose condition is rapidly deteriorating and directs team to prepare for emergency pericardiocentesis
	Questions ability to make clinical judgments and seeks input from CNS colleagues, unit leaders, and/or health care professionals when making decisions	Before implementing a sedation break protocol, posts a message on the Advanced Nursing Practice in Acute and Critical Care (ANPACC) list serve or another CNS list serve to learn whether other organizations use a similar protocol
Level 3 competent	Collects and interprets complex patient/family, clinician, and unit data	Identifies different standards of practice regarding tracheostomy care among the medical, surgical, and progressive care units
	Makes clinical judgments based on an immediate grasp of the whole situation for routine patient populations	Collaborates with other health care professionals to design a product line for high-risk obstetrical patients
	Recognizes patterns and trends that may predict patient outcomes	Recognizes a sharp decline in the number of levels III and IV nurses on the night shift schedule and collaborates with the unit manager to ensure an appropriate skill mix on all shifts
	Recognizes personal expertise and limits; seeks assistance as needed	Applies diabetes management expertise, as validated by Advanced Diabetes Management Certification, as chairperson of a multidisciplinary group charged with forming policies about tight glycemic control

TABLE 5-1

Descriptions and Examples of Clinical Nurse Specialist (CNS) Activities for the Novice, Competent, and Expert CNS—cont'd

Level of Expertise	Description of Selected CNS Activities	Example of Selected CNS Activity
Level 5 expert	Synthesizes and interprets multiple, sometimes conflicting, sources of data	Critiques research data, clinical papers, and existing practice guidelines when updating policy about pediatric extracorporeal membrane oxygenation therapy
	Makes judgment based on an immediate grasp of the whole picture picture unless working with new patient populations	Immediately activates and directs the unit's emergency response plan when the organization receives 193 patients from a train crash
	Uses past experiences to anticipate problems	Implements AACN's Essentials of Critical Care Orientation course when the education department cut the number of critical care courses by 50%
	Helps patients, families, nurses, and the health care system see the big picture	Recommends central line dressing that costs $15 more per patient but which is associated with a 13% decrease in costly bloodstream infections
	Recognizes the limits of clinical judgment and seeks multidisciplinary collaboration and consultation with comfort	Conducts a site visit to a reputable health care organization and consults with experts when asked to open a bone marrow transport center

adeptly make clinical judgments based on an immediate grasp of the whole situation. Unlike novice CNSs, competent CNSs do not feel bound to existing protocols or standards, understanding that there is not always one correct answer and that certain circumstances call for different clinical judgments. For instance, when a physician refuses to resuscitate a patient with end-stage liver failure who refused to sign do not resuscitate orders, the CNS directs the resuscitation team to follow her orders instead of the physician's orders.

As competent CNSs witness favorable outcomes from previous clinical judgments, they become more confident about their abilities. Consequently they generally function independently but understand when to confer with experts.

Expert CNSs possesses an exceptional grasp of the total situation and quickly make clinical judgments with aplomb. Expert CNSs welcome multifaceted situations that require extraordinary clinical judgment and are invigorated by such challenges. Circumstances that seem overwhelming to novice CNSs are straightforward to expert CNSs. CCNS certification is one way that expert and competent CNSs can validate their clinical judgment.

Expert CNSs are well positioned to exert clinical judgment well beyond the boundaries of their organization. They can mentor and teach relevant aspects of clinical judgment to graduate students and inexperienced CNSs. Expert CNSs also share their clinical judgment expertise as they publish clinical and research papers, present at local and national meetings, participate in professional organizational activities, and conduct research.

IMPLEMENTATION WITHIN THE DIMENSION OF PRACTICE

The art and science of nursing practice requires clinical judgment. Clinical judgment is an essential competency for CNSs who orchestrate and deliver care for acutely and critically ill patients. CNSs base clinical judgments on experience and advanced knowledge of clinical and research literature, realizing that their decisions have important consequences for patients' future well-being. If clear scientific evidence is unavailable, CNSs are able to "make the leap between the best available evidence and the realities of practice to develop sound and pragmatic guidelines for the bedside clinician" (Beecroft, 2001, p. 191).

CNSs use intentional and multidimensional thought processes when making clinical judgments. According to Pesut, "Mental fluency to reason "forward" from problems and "backwards" from outcomes to make clinical judgments supports thinking success in nursing practice" (Pesut, 2001, p. 215). On the one hand, CNSs can make clinical judgments using backward reasoning. This means that CNSs first identify the optimal outcome and then reason backwards to form a plan of care (Pesut, 2001). For example, CNSs judge which interventions will prevent unplanned extubation, which orientation program will meet learning objectives of new graduates, and which proposed progressive care unit (PCU) design will promote efficient and safe patient care. On the other hand, CNSs may use forward reasoning to make a clinical judgment. In this case, CNSs assess the patient or situation, identify the problem, and use forward reasoning to make practice decisions.

The nursing process is a forward-reasoning model. The sequential steps of the nursing process (i.e., assessment, diagnosis, outcome identification, planning, implementation, and evaluation) can facilitate clinical judgment.

Although some argue that the nursing process is overly restrictive and does not fully and accurately capture the thought processes of nurses (Benner, Hooper-Kyriakidis & Stannard, 1999; Tanner, 2000), it is a systematic and widely accepted approach for organizing professional nursing practice (Alfaro-LeFevre, 2006; American Nurses Association, 2004; Bell, 2002).

Assessment

CNSs model their inherent clinical judgment skills as they assess patients. The aspects of clinical judgment that directly pertain to patient assessment include reasoning-in-transition, skilled know-how, response-based practice, perceptual acuity, and skill of involvement. For purposes of this chapter it is assumed that CNSs demonstrate expert clinical judgment. Therefore the focus of this chapter is how CNSs assess the clinical judgment of clinical nurses. For example, CNSs consider how nurses reason, comprehend patient problems and concerns, execute the nursing process, respond to changes in the patient's condition, respond to salient information, and initiate interventions.

It is difficult to measure complex concepts such as clinical judgment. The *Clinical Decision Making in Nursing Scale* (Jenkins, 2001) has been used to measure clinical judgment (Bowles, 2000); however, CNSs and nurse educators more commonly assess critical thinking, a component of clinical judgment. Box 5-2 lists formal instruments that CNSs can use to assess critical thinking of clinical nurses. Of concern though is that most are not specific to nursing, their validity has been questioned, and some investigators have not found consistent relationships between measures of critical thinking and clinical judgment (Brunt, 2005; Follman, 2003; Hicks, Merrit, & Elstein, 2003; Kakai, 2003; Staib, 2003). In addition, budget constraints may prevent CNSs from using formal instruments.

CNSs also assess critical thinking and the six aspects of clinical judgment as they interact with clinical nurses, present case studies, and conduct patient care conferences (Oermann, 1998).

BOX 5-2

Formal Instruments Used to Assess Critical Thinking

California Critical Thinking Dispositions Inventory (Facione, Facione & Giancarlo, 1994)
California Critical Thinking Skills Test (Facione, Facione, Blohm, & Giancarlo, 2002)
Critical Thinking in Clinical Nursing Practice for RNs (National League for Nursing, 2002)
Minnesota Test of Critical Thinking (Edman, Bart, Robey, & Silverman, 2004)
Watson-Glaser Critical Thinking Appraisal (Watson & Glaser, 1994)

During everyday discussions with clinical nurses, CNSs ask clinical nurses open-ended questions about care of a particular patient (Oermann, 1998). Examples of questions include:

- What patient assessment findings concern you?
- What data did you use when deciding how to intervene?
- Which data did you consider most important and why?
- What other assessment or treatment options could you consider?
- How confident are you that you made the correct care decision?
- What research evidence supports your decision?
- What ethical principles, if any, are relevant to your patient?
- How will you know whether you made an incorrect decision and how will you alter your interventions?
- How is this patient similar to or different from the last patient you cared for with this diagnosis?

CNSs can assess critical thinking and clinical judgment by having clinical nurses discuss case studies during orientation, competency verification sessions, patient care conferences, small group meetings, or other professional development forums (Oermann, 1998). Case studies may be based on previous or current patients, published clinical exemplars, sentinel or near-miss events, a new patient population, or high-volume, high-risk, high-cost, or problem-prone situations. CNSs should avoid straightforward case studies that clinical nurses can solve with a pat memorized answer. The best case studies are complex and characterized by puzzling or conflicting assessment data, making it difficult for nurses to rapidly diagnose the problem and allowing for several possible approaches to treatment. Such case studies require clinical nurses to explain how concepts, theories, assessment data, previous experience, and research pertain to the situation.

As they lead patient care conferences, CNSs can assess critical thinking and clinical judgment. Patient care conferences are usually characterized by their multidisciplinary focus. By using questioning and active listening, CNSs ascertain how clinical nurses think and reason when collaborating with other health care professionals. Through patient care conferences, interactions with clinical nurses, and case studies, CNSs gain insight about nurses' assumptions, thought processes, nursing knowledge, reasoning, and decision-making processes.

Diagnosis

Although CNSs do not usually generate traditional nursing diagnoses, CNSs will find it useful to use a framework or model to help validate and organize assessment data. According to one such model, the AACN Synergy Model for Patient Care, when patient characteristics drive nurse competencies, patients and families experience optimal outcomes (Bell, 2002). The model stresses knowing and understanding the patient and family; therefore clinical judgment is paramount. Sometimes, CNSs consult nurse managers, nurse practitioners, physicians, or other health care clinicians to authenticate their understanding of given situations and promote collaborative relationships.

Outcome Identification

CNSs must clearly delineate desired outcomes, considering assessment data and the characteristics and goals of patients, families, clinicians, and the organizational system. CNSs rely on available resources such as colleagues, nursing and medical literature, clinical practice guidelines, research and benchmarking data, and the organization's mission and vision to identify outcomes. CNSs should not identify goals in isolation but rather obtain "buy-in" from those who have a vested interest in quality outcomes.

Planning and Implementation

As with outcome identification, planning and implementation requires input from the health care team, patients, families, and the organizational system. CNSs use clinical judgment as they resolve differences of opinion, outline a unified approach, and commence appropriate interventions. CNSs champion for a healthy work environment in which clinicians are encouraged to use their clinical judgment. Examples of planning and implementation are described in the remainder of this chapter.

Evaluation

The nursing process is not complete until identified problems are resolved. Thus evaluation is a continuous process that feeds back to reassessment, additional planning, further interventions, and reevaluation.

INTEGRATION OF THE STANDARDS OF PROFESSIONAL PERFORMANCE

Quality Care

Historically, health care consumers assumed that health care professionals provided quality care and that most health care systems were equivalent in terms of quality. However, during the past 15 years the health care environment has changed dramatically. Today health care is a complex, costly, competitive, and highly regulated industry. As a result, health care organizations are keenly aware of their accountability to consumers, emphasizing access to care, optimal health outcomes, patient autonomy, cost-effectiveness, and patient satisfaction.

Health care organizations face tremendous pressure to prove that they provide high quality and economical care. Quality of care is paramount to the success of health care organizations. Third-party payers channel their patients toward health care organizations with a track record of consistently delivering high-quality care. Consumers also demand quality care; and many are quick to complain, report, or sue if their expectations are unmet. As consumers "shop" for health care, they can readily compare quality reports or "report cards" from various health care organizations and thus determine which will best meet their needs. Table 5-2 lists selected Internet sites where consumers can review quality measures for health care organizations.

Good clinical judgment necessarily contributes to quality care. CNSs are challenged to demonstrate how nursing care positively impacts patient outcomes and to initiate practice improvements that promote the highest possible level of safe, quality, cost-effective, and patient-centered care. In addition to nurse-sensitive indicators (e.g., medication errors, needlestick injuries, and patient satisfaction), CNSs are interested in multidisciplinary quality indicators (e.g., pain level and hospital-acquired pneumonia rates) because these pertain to all legitimate stakeholders within the organizational system. CNSs often collect data, generate reports, interpret results, and communicate summary information to supervisors, administrators, and managers throughout the organization. For example, CNSs may collect data regarding peripheral intravenous line infiltrations, pressure ulcers, and nursing care hours in accordance with the National Database of Nursing

TABLE 5-2	
Selected Internet Sites of Quality Measures for Health Care Organizations	
Quality Report	**Uniform Resource Locator (URL)**
Joint Commission on Accreditation of Health Care Organizations Quality Check	http://www.jcaho.org/quality+check/index.htm
Consumers' CHECKBOOK Guide to Hospitals	http://www.checkbook.org/
Health Grades, Inc.	http://www.healthgrades.com/
U.S. Department of Health & Human Services Hospital Compare	http://www.hospitalcompare.hhs.gov/hospital/home2.asp
U.S. News & World Report Best Health	http://www.usnews.com/usnews/health/best-hospitals/tophosp.htm

Quality Indicators (NDNQI) specifications. CNSs can use the NDNQI quarterly reports for quality improvement purposes.

A major challenge for the CNS is to facilitate clinical judgment of the health care team through teaching, role modeling, coaching, and/or mentoring. As summarized in Table 5-3, numerous methods have been used to cultivate critical thinking and clinical judgment (Benner, Hooper-Kyriakidis, & Stannard, 1999; Marshall, Jones, & Snyder, 2001; Staib, 2003). CNSs can also simply point out patient responses, patterns, trends, or distinctions to less experienced clinicians because this type of teaching stimulates open dialogue and discernment as clinicians consider how to intervene in a specific situation (Benner, Hooper-Kyriakidis, & Stannard, 1999). Novice nurses learn best by applying theoretical knowledge and participating in rule-based activities. For example, based on the patient's diagnosis, they should recognize relevant rules, identify worrisome signs and symptoms, and name potential interventions. More experienced nurses strive to individualize care, interpret the patient's concerns, orchestrate care in accordance with patient preferences and coping style, and recognize how the patient is similar to or different from comparable patients (Benner, Tanner & Chesla, 1996).

Individual Practice Evaluation

CNSs are vital clinical leaders; thus it is important that they continually sharpen their clinical judgment through nursing care, reflection, and self-evaluation. Although CNSs practice in diverse settings, by nature of their clinical expertise and role, they are expected to make and facilitate sound clinical judgments. Self-evaluation enables CNSs to pause and critically contemplate their effectiveness in managing, supporting, and coordinating care for acutely and critically ill patients.

CNSs may evaluate their practice using various approaches. First, CNSs can compare their performance with existing national standards. For example, *Scope of Practice and Standards of Professional Performance for the Acute and Critical Care Clinical Nurse Specialist* (Bell, 2002) describes competent CNS practice and articulates the roles and behaviors expected of CNSs. Second, CNSs evaluate their clinical judgment according to individual position descriptions, performance criteria, and expectations within the organizational system. The prudent CNS helps write performance standards that reflect solid clinical judgment. Third, CNSs seek feedback from others about their ability to render clinical judgment. CNSs serve as liaisons among nurses, physicians, other health care specialists,

TABLE 5-3

Selected Methods Used to Cultivate Critical Thinking and Clinical Judgment

Method	Description	Example of Implementation
Simulation	Demonstration of psychomotor and cognitive skills using a human patient simulator that is programmed to mimic real lifelike clinical situations	Demonstrate use of a transthoracic pacemaker
Journaling	Reflective process of writing free text or prompted notes about experiences, thought processes, and decision making related to patient care activities	Review ethical dilemmas encountered during nursing practice
Concept mapping	Drawing a hierarchical diagram or map that depicts relationships among related concepts and ideas, thus displaying one's knowledge or understanding of a situation	Assess understanding of the physiological derangements associated with decompensated heart failure
Role playing	Pretend and risk-free opportunities to practice clinical, communication, and leadership skills	Communicate a patient death to family members
Clinical questioning	Open-ended questions about assessment data, assumptions, differential diagnoses, thought processes, rationale for decisions, and preparedness to manage patient care situations	Question approach to resuscitating a patient with ventricular fibrillation
Games	Playful learning activity that features rules, competition, collaborative teamwork, rewards, and relevant learning	Determine knowledge of continuous renal replacement therapy
Interactive computer-based instruction	Computerized scenarios containing patient data and varied options for further assessment, interventions, and evaluation	Evaluate ability to assess, manage, and evaluate postoperative pain
Clinical narrative	Reflective process of writing a first-person story about a memorable clinical situation that stands out as significant or meaningful	Record circumstances of evacuating critically ill patients after a hurricane rendered the hospital inoperable

and patients; thus peer review can be an especially effective approach to practice evaluation. Finally, outcome data and other quality reports may reveal lapses in the clinical judgment of clinicians. For example, a CNS may suspect poor clinical judgment when noting a higher trend of reintubations for patients who were recently extubated.

It is important that CNSs devote adequate time and energy to self-evaluation. Although formal self-evaluation should occur at least annually, CNSs' self-evaluation is an ongoing process. An open-minded approach is needed to ascertain whether the clinical judgment skills of oneself and others truly foster first-rate, patient-centered care. If CNSs identify deficiencies in their clinical judgment, they should initiate a self-improvement plan. Although it is easier to maintain the status quo, expert CNSs look for new or different approaches that may revolutionize the delivery of health care.

Last, it is crucial that CNSs document their impact on clinical judgment. Examples of noteworthy documentation include decreased length of stay, decreased nosocomial infection rates, improved patient/family satisfaction, decreased prevalence of pressure ulcers, or earlier identification of potential organ donors. In this way CNSs attest their worth to the organization.

Education

Education is a lifelong endeavor. CNSs are responsible for maintaining current knowledge and competency within the three spheres of their influence. Novice CNSs should seek out and participate in experiences that will advance their personal knowledge and capacity to make intelligent clinical judgments. For example, a cardiac CNS who has little experience with ventricular assist devices (VADs) may quickly learn about these devices if he or she temporarily works with an expert clinical nurse, attends industry-sponsored hands-on training or a continuing education program, completes computer-based modules, and/or interacts with patients with a VAD.

More experienced CNSs may learn to render broader clinical judgments that have system-wide impact. For example, consider an organization that plans to build a new NICU. The CNS may review the literature to learn the advantages of various NICU designs, meet with architects to review floor plan options, negotiate with suppliers for state-of-the-art equipment, and visit several existing NICUs to ask health care personnel, families, and administrators which environmental features best promote functionality and safe care while meeting the expectations of staff and parents.

CNSs are also responsible for promoting the clinical judgment and professional development of other health care personnel. For instance, to enhance clinical judgment, CNSs might teach a class about critical thinking or clinical reasoning, conduct grand rounds conferences, moderate a clinically focused debate, or reward or praise nurses who demonstrate improved clinical judgment. CNSs may also invite a well-known expert in clinical judgment to speak at an education program or facilitate small discussion groups.

Collegiality

Collegial relationships are characterized by mutual respect and trust, open and honest communication, collaboration, and nurturing interactions. Genuine collegiality is not short-lived or self-serving. Nonetheless, CNSs can use collegial relationships to foster the clinical judgment and professional development of others while enhancing their own effectiveness and credibility. Conversely, the lack of collegial relationships contributes to disjointed efforts, feelings of isolation, and risk of confusion and conflict.

As a clinical expert and leader, it is essential that CNSs have healthy and positive collegial relationships with health care professionals. A recently hired CNS, whether a novice or expert, must devote time and energy to building and maintaining collaborative relationships with superiors, peers, and subordinates. A key to success is the ability to communicate effectively. CNSs must be available and willing to listen to new ideas and should avoid condescending language or behaviors.

The goal of the CNS is for clinicians to make sound clinical judgments. Consequently, CNSs want clinical nurses to feel safe and comfortable sharing their concerns and needs. When CNSs practice collegiality, clinical nurses are more likely to consult with them or confide in them; thus the value of a collegial relationship cannot be overemphasized. For example, consider an orientee who is struggling to learn interpretation of cardiac rhythms. The orientee feels intimidated by his or her preceptor but develops a collegial relationship with the CNS. Thus he or she easily discusses concerns with the CNS, who works with him to help him learn the skill. Similarly, when patient care problems arise, managers may be confident that a CNS known for collegiality will be able to investigate and solve the problem with ease.

Ethics

As previously mentioned, clinical judgment has an ethical component. CNSs make clinical judgments in an ethical manner that is sensitive to the best interests of patients and families, nurses, and organizational systems. First, CNSs' chief commitment is to patients and families; therefore the patients' rights always receive primary consideration in all decisions regarding their care (American Nurses Association, 2001). To make patient-centered clinical judgments, CNSs attempt to understand patients' values and beliefs. CNSs are accountable for quality patient care and must maintain and promote standards of excellence. CNSs are obligated to maintain their personal clinical competence and exhibit clinical judgment while simultaneously promoting the same for clinical nurses. To protect patients, it may be necessary for a CNS to temporarily or permanently bar an incompetent clinical nurse from providing patient care. For example, nurses may be unable to perform required skills or may have attempted to make clinical judgments outside their scope of practice. Finally, CNSs may desire to use interesting or unusual patient situations as case studies to highlight real-world successes or lessons learned from others' experience. When using case studies, CNSs take measures to safeguard the confidentiality and dignity of the involved patients and clinical nurses.

Second, CNSs are ethically responsible to the clinical nurses and other health care professionals. CNSs educate clinical nurses, role model

high quality care, and advance the nursing profession as they develop, maintain, and implement professional standards of practice. Although CNSs must interact with other health care professionals in a respectful, nonjudgmental, honest, and fair manner, they should point out and correct or report errors in clinical judgment. Given the authority of their position, CNSs must avoid inappropriate coercion that may adversely affect the clinical judgment of other clinicians.

Third, CNSs have a duty to make clinical judgments that contribute to the mission and well-being of the organizational system. CNSs avoid clinical judgments that promote a self-serving agenda, misrepresent the organization to the public, or otherwise reflect poorly on the organizational system. In addition, CNSs' clinical judgment must not be clouded by individual economic interests or financial incentives.

Collaboration

CNSs collaborate with patients, families, and health care personnel to create a healing and caring environment. A collaborative environment is characterized by open dialogue, creativity, supportive behaviors, connectivity, and shared credit.

As mentioned, clinical judgment is especially necessary in situations in which answers are unclear. Collaborative practice can facilitate optimal care and outcomes because clinicians pool their knowledge, data, experience, problem-solving abilities, values, and goals to produce prudent clinical judgments that are often better than judgments made by one person.

It is important that novice CNSs establish themselves as an integral member of the multidisciplinary health care team. Initially clinicians will test the clinical judgment of a novice CNS. However, as CNSs demonstrate expertise, other clinicians will seek and value the CNS's input when clinical judgments need to be made. CNSs from other departments, physicians, and hospital administrators are more likely to consult and collaborate with CNSs who have a reputation for clinical expertise, level headedness, collegiality, follow-through, leadership ability, and teamwork. For example, an administrator may rely on and value CNSs with proficiency in case management and discharge planning. Finally, as an active member of a multidisciplinary group, CNSs have already formed professional relationships with colleagues who can help solve a practice dilemma, negotiate change, or amend organizational policy.

Research

Research improves practice because it tests and generates theory, answers clinical questions, and extends knowledge. Clinicians constantly make important clinical judgments and decisions and should base these on the best available scientific evidence. Practice based on evidence promotes high-quality, consistent, and cost-effective care and ultimately optimal patient outcomes. Regrettably, many practicing clinicians either seem uninterested in research or find it difficult to comprehend individual research reports and "make sense" of the growing body of research literature. As a result, they fail to consider research evidence as they make clinical judgments in daily practice.

Research is futile unless clinicians incorporate findings into practice. By virtue of their graduate education and clinical expertise, CNSs are well prepared to create an organizational climate that values evidence and to infuse evidence into nursing practice. The CNS's goal is to model evidence-based practice and help clinicians integrate research evidence with clinical judgment and patient preferences so that patients receive the best care possible.

Although it is beyond the scope of this chapter to describe the evidence-based practice process in detail, unit-based or product line CNSs first should assess current nursing practice and identify which practices should be modified. Of those, CNSs place highest priority on those practices that are associated with high morbidity, mortality, and/or cost or those of special importance to the organizational system. It is important that CNSs use clinical judgment to carefully decide which practices to modify because clinical nurses cannot be expected to make numerous changes during a short time frame.

CNSs often lead multidisciplinary groups of colleagues who are committed to evidence-based practice. CNSs and other team members use critical thinking and clinical judgment as they identify and recruit group members, find and synthesize available evidence, collect baseline data, design and implement the evidence-based practice guideline, and evaluate outcomes. Critical thinking and clinical judgment are important for several reasons. First, some studies are poorly designed so their findings may be of little value. Second, data that the group needs to answer its questions may not exist. Third, findings and conclusions of similar studies may contradict each other. Fourth, investigators or team members may advance or hold firm to preconceived ideas due to conflicts of interest. Fifth, the necessary components of evidence-based practice guidelines may not be obvious or clear-cut. Finally, the group may need to decide which outcome data are most important or whether results from a study conducted with a narrowly defined population can be generalized to their particular patients. Before the group adopts or adapts existing evidence-based practice guidelines (see Table 9-2), they should review the work to ensure that the guidelines are current and free of error or undue bias.

Critics of evidence-based practice argue that its "cookbook" approach ignores ubiquitous patient variability and the patient's cultural, religious, and personal preferences, limiting the clinician's ability to individualize patient care. Conversely, proponents of evidence-based practice remind clinicians that guidelines are not intended to replace the clinical judgment of those who best know the patient's unique circumstances. No evidence-based practice guideline is applicable to every patient or practice setting.

CNSs often discover areas in which there is insufficient research to make practice decisions. Many CNSs identify research questions and conduct research to generate the necessary knowledge. CNSs use clinical judgment to prioritize needed research and usually consult with experienced researchers to design and conduct a research study.

Resource Utilization

Two major goals of health care organizations are to provide high quality and cost-effective care. Today the economic environment of health care is highly competitive and regulated. Hospital administrators expect CNSs to use clinical judgment when designing practice protocols and allocating resources and will not support practices that adversely affect an institution's economic health. CNSs continuously balance responsibility for high-quality care with demands for cost effectiveness.

The use of evidence-based practice guidelines often produces cost savings. For example, a CNS who introduces interventions to reduce ventilator-associated pneumonia may be able to document decreased pneumonia rates, decreased ventilator days, and decreased ICU length of stay.

CNSs have the necessary skill sets and clinical judgment to systematically evaluate programs to improve efficiency and/or reduce costs. For example, CNSs have used the American Association of Critical-Care Nurses' Essentials of Critical Care Orientation (ECCO) to improve the efficiency of orientation. As they complete the ECCO modules, newly hired nurses learn the fundamentals of critical care nursing at a pace conducive to their learning and without having to wait for the next formal class. The use of ECCO also has the potential to reduce the length of orientation and thereby reduce costs.

Effective resource utilization may mean that CNSs need to eliminate or reduce work that does not add value or redistribute work to other team members. For example, CNSs may streamline a change-of-shift report, advocate for a computerized documentation system, or propose an electronic supply system that prevents supply shortages.

CNSs also use clinical judgment as they evaluate equipment and supplies. They consider whether supplies referred to in evidence-based practice guidelines are readily and consistently available to clinicians. When making decisions about equipment or supplies, CNSs and clinicians use clinical judgment as they conduct and evaluate trials of similar products. CNSs also collaborate with supply custodians to ensure that the correct equipment and supplies are purchased for the best possible price.

More broadly, CNSs advise administrators of organizational systems about how to provide high-quality and cost-effective care. For example, based on their knowledge of patient care standards and clinical judgment, CNSs partner with administrators, clinicians, and others to determine admission criteria for a new PCU. The appropriate use of PCU beds can free up more costly ICU beds and minimize situations in which the hospital goes on divert status.

CONCLUSION

Clinical judgment is a central component of nursing competence, especially given the demands of the health care environment. CNSs are equipped with the knowledge, skills, and experience needed to not only demonstrate sound clinical judgment but also foster the clinical judgment of other clinicians. This chapter provided concrete examples of how CNSs apply clinical judgment in their practice and thus contribute to positive outcomes for patients and their families, nurses and other health care providers, and the organizational system.

DISCUSSION QUESTIONS

1. Describe how clinical judgment and critical thinking differ.
2. List and describe the six aspects of clinical judgment.
3. Discuss how the CNS's clinical judgment improves and matures with time and experience.
4. Describe ways that CNSs foster the clinical judgment of clinical nurses.

References

Alfaro-LeFevre, R. (1999). *Critical thinking in nursing: A practical approach* (2nd ed.). Philadelphia: Saunders.

Alfaro-LeFevre, R. (2006). *Applying nursing process: A tool for critical thinking* (6th ed.). Philadelphia: Lippincott Williams & Wilkins.

American Association of Critical-Care Nurses Certification Corporation. (2005). *The AACN Synergy Model for patient care*. Retrieved October 19, 2005, from http://www.aacn.org/certcorp/certcorp.nsf/vwdoc/SynModel?opendocument.

American Nurses Association. (2001). *Code of ethics for nurses with interpretive statements*. Retrieved January 16, 2006, from http://www.nursingworld.org/ethics/code/protected_nwcoe303.htm.

American Nurses Association. (2004). *Nursing: Scope and standards of practice*. Washington, D.C.: Author.

Beecroft, P.C. (2001). Clinical judgment in evidence-based practice. *Clinical Nurse Specialist, 15,* 191-192.

Bell, L. (Ed.). (2002). *Scope of practice and standards of professional performance for the acute and critical care clinical nurse specialist*. Aliso Viejo, CA: American Association of Critical-Care Nurses.

Benner, P., Hooper-Kyriakidis, P., & Stannard, D. (1999). *Clinical wisdom and interventions in critical care: A thinking-in-action approach*. Philadelphia: Saunders.

Benner, P.A., Tanner, C.A., & Chesla, C.A. (1996). *Expertise in nursing practice: Caring, clinical judgment, and ethics*. New York: Springer.

Bowles, K. (2000). The relationship of critical-thinking skills and the clinical-judgment skills of baccalaureate nursing students. *Journal of Nursing Education, 39,* 373-376.

Brunt, B.A. (2005). Critical thinking in nursing: An integrated review. *Journal of Continuing Education of Nurses, 36,* 60-67.

Busch, F., & Schmidt-Hellerau, C. (2004). How can we know what we need to know? Reflections on clinical judgment formation. *Journal of the American Psychoanalytic Association, 52,* 689-707.

Curley, M.A. (1998). Patient-nurse synergy: Optimizing patients' outcomes. *American Journal of Critical Care, 7,* 64-72.

Edman, L.R., Bart, W.M., Robey, J., & Silverman, J. (2004). Psychometric analysis of the Minnesota test of critical thinking. *Psychology Report, 95,* 3-9.

Facione, P., Facione, N., & Giancarlo, C. (1994). *The California critical thinking dispositions inventory manual*. Millbrae, CA: California Academic Press.

Facione, P.A., Facione, N.C., Blohm, S.W., & Giancarlo, C.A. (2002). *The California critical thinking skills test manual: Form A, Form B, Form 2000*. Millbrae, CA: California Academic Press.

Follman, J. (2003). Research on nurses' critical thinking: Cul de sac? *Nurse Education, 28,* 255-256.

Hicks, F.D., Merritt, S.L., & Elstein, A.S. (2003). Critical thinking and clinical decision making in critical care nursing: A pilot study. *Heart and Lung, 32,* 169-180.

Jenkins, H.M. (2001). Clinical decision making in nursing scale. In C.F. Waltz & L.S. Jenkins (Eds.). *Measurement of nursing outcomes* (2nd ed., pp. 33-40). New York: Springer.

Johnson, B. M., & Webber, P. B. (2005). *An introduction to theory and reasoning in nursing* (2nd ed.). Philadelphia: Lippincott Williams & Wilkins.

Kakai, H. (2003). Re-examining the factor structure of the California critical thinking disposition inventory. *Perception of Motor Skills, 96,* 435-438.

Marshall, B.L., Jones, S.H., & Snyder, G. (2001). A program design to promote clinical judgment. *Journal of Nursing Staff Development, 17,* 78-84.

National League for Nursing. (2002). *Critical thinking in clinical nursing practice for RNs*. Retrieved February 6, 2006, from http://www.nln.org/testprods/pdf/97-7002p.pdf.

Oermann, M.H. (1998). How to assess critical thinking in clinical practice. *Dimens Crit Care Nurs, 17,* 322-327.

Paul, R.W. (1993). *Critical thinking: What every person needs to survive in a rapidly changing world*. Santa Rosa, CA: Foundation for Critical Thinking.

Pesut, D.J. (2001). Clinical judgment: foreground/background. *Journal of Professional Nursing, 17,* 215.

Staib, S. (2003). Teaching and measuring critical thinking. *Journal of Nursing Education, 42,* 498-508.

Tanner, C.A. (2000). Critical thinking: Beyond nursing process. *Journal of Nursing Education, 39,* 338-339.

Watson, G., & Glaser, E. M. (1994). *Watson-Glaser critical thinking appraisal—short form manual*. San Antonio: Harcourt Assessment.

Clinical Inquiry

6

Christine Schulman

INTRODUCTION

When bedside clinicians routinely question practice using the AACN Synergy Model for Patient Care, individual patient needs are met, nursing competencies are established and updated, and the health care system provides evidence-based, cost-effective patient care (Hardin & Hussey, 2001). In short, an active environment of clinical inquiry (CI) optimizes patient outcomes (Bostrom & Suter, 1993; Heater, Becker, & Olson, 1988). In addition to this, there are numerous professional benefits to having staff nurses actively involved in CI, such as increased recruitment and retention, enhanced professional image, and opportunities for continuing education (Campbell & Chulay, 1990). Successful CI depends on a culture willing to question routine, intuitive, and ritualistic practices and explore different options to delivering care.

Creating and fostering such an environment is fundamental to clinical nurse specialist (CNS) practice. Although the CNS role has traditionally included research activities, the need to increase participation is especially critical now because of the increasing emphasis on quality of care, financial considerations, evaluation of technology, and analysis of nursing practice (Fitzgerald, Milberger, Peden-McAlpine, Meiers, & Sherman, 2003). This chapter reviews strategies the CNS can use to create an environment of clinical inquiry.

BACKGROUND

CI has its foundation in evidence-based practice (EBP), now the cornerstone of both nursing and medical practice, and is frequently mandated by governmental policies, accrediting agencies, consumer demands, and professional organizations. EBP is the "ongoing process of questioning and evaluating practice, providing informed practice based on available data, and innovating care standards through research and experiential learning" (Curley, 1998). It means that the current, best evidence is used to make decisions about the care of individual patients, integrating clinical expertise with systematic research (Sackett, Rosenberg, Gray, & Haynes, 1996).

As a fundamental component of evidence-based nursing (EBN), CI uses scientific knowledge together with experiential knowledge, reviews existing information, and promotes research to answer clinical questions. EBN has a broad influence and means more than simple integration of research into practice. It is an entire process that results in improved patient outcomes. First there is the identification of a question concerning a specific patient or system issue. Then there is the review of the literature that addresses the clinical question. This information is evaluated for its validity, relevance, and applicability. A plan is developed to integrate new information into practice, and finally the practice change is evaluated in terms of the desired outcomes (Ciliska, Pinelli, DiCenso, & Callum, 2001). The CNS is the main driver of this process.

TABLE 6-1

Levels of Nursing Experience When Considering Clinical Questions

The new staff nurse in the unit asks a simple question: How can I suction this patient more effectively?
She gets four different answers from the individuals she approaches:

Experience Level	Characteristics of Answer
Novice nurse	"I was told by my preceptor (who showed me in the procedure book) that we can use normal saline to make the patient cough and loosen secretions better. That's how I'll do it every time I suction a patient."
Competent	"You can use normal saline to illicit a stronger cough, but it's so uncomfortable for the patient that I rarely use it. I sure wouldn't want someone to do that to me!"
Expert	"I know saline has been used, but I also know that there are studies that suggest using it may actually cause harm to the patients. Are there other strategies that might be more comfortable *and* more effective? Which is the best for our patients? How do we find this information?"
Clinical nurse specialist	"There are several nursing studies that suggest that using normal saline with endotracheal suctioning does not benefit and may actually harm the patient. Let's do a literature search to see if these studies reflect our concerns, have some discussions with the staff, and update our policies to reflect the best practice for this clinical issue. If the literature doesn't address our specific question, then maybe we should do our own research study."

CI can be found at all levels of nursing practice, from novice to expert. The characteristics of the questions change, but the intent is still the same: to optimize patient recovery (Table 6-1). Bedside nurses are invaluable participants in CI since they are the ones who identify critical questions and evaluate practice changes. Unfortunately staff nurses are frequently uncomfortable and inexperienced with research, delaying its use in everyday practice, a phenomenon known as the "research-practice gap" (Chulay, 1997; Valente, 2003).

Multiple barriers to the use of research findings have been cited in the literature; a critical CNS responsibility is to identify which of these barriers exist and collaborate with administration to provide institutional support for CI (Table 6-2). The three predominant barriers are a lack of knowledge and negative attitudes about nursing research, lack of institutional support, and limited research findings applicable to actual clinical practice (Hodge, Kochie, Larsen, & Santiago, 2003; Nicswiadormy, 1998). Nurses

believe they are unfamiliar with how to search for and evaluate research findings, state that research results are not communicated in understandable ways to the bedside practitioners, and believe findings are often impractical in the clinical setting. They fear criticism should they suggest practice that is different from the status quo. They also quote tremendous workloads, lack of administrative support, and inadequate library resources as contributing to the lack of integrated research (McKibbon, 1999; Melnyk, Fineout-Overholt, Stone, & Ackerman, 2000; Silagy & Haines, 1998). Removing these roadblocks and making reader-friendly research available to nurses, along with clear practice implications, should be a primary responsibility of any CNS.

CREATING AN ENVIRONMENT OF CLINICAL INQUIRY

A strong partnership between the CNS and all levels of nursing administration is fundamental to the success of a practice model based on CI.

TABLE 6-2	
Barriers to Nursing Participation in Clinical Inquiry	
Barrier	**Clinical Nurse Specialist Role**
Lack of knowledge about how to access the literature	• Consult with administration to make sure library facilities are adequate. • Schedule time with hospital librarian to demonstrate literature searches to staff. • Post useful websites in the nursing unit for 24-hour access to information. • Assist nurses with literature searches. • Create worksheets with questions to help nurses critically evaluate articles.
Lack of knowledge to evaluate studies for clinical relevance	• Conduct classes on how to critically evaluate research studies. • Partner with the nurse scientist or faculty from nearby nursing schools to help teach research classes. • Organize and implement journal clubs. • Invite advanced practice nurses from related specialties to lend their expertise to discussion of the study. • Develop a unit-based research group to review recently published studies relevant to specific patient populations; post discussion summaries in unit.
Difficult access to library resources	• Collaborate with unit manager to make sure computer terminals with website access are available at the nurses' station. • Post a map to the hospital library. • Request that unit administration subscribe to key nursing journals, especially those on-line. • Post clinically useful websites in several locations on the nursing unit. • Post key articles in the unit lounge and facilitate formal and informal discussions about the content.

Administration

At the nursing division level, general administrative philosophies should value a climate that fosters inquiry and creativity, promotes innovative change in nursing practice based on CI, and directs financial resources to support research activities. Annual goals related to research should be included in the yearly strategic plans (Campbell & Chulay, 1990). Discussions impacting patient care delivery should always ask for supporting evidence. Annual evaluations should include participation in clinical research projects. To provide research expertise, the division should employ a nurse scientist or develop a formal collaborative relationship with a nearby school of nursing to provide faculty skilled in designing and guiding clinical research.

At the unit level, the nurse manager must clearly communicate that staff are expected to participate in CI activities. To send the clear message that research activity is highly valued, the unit budget must be developed to provide paid time for nurses to attend research classes, professional research conferences, and meetings. There must also be paid administrative time for staff to review literature and do project work. Additional finances must be allotted to cover secretarial support, publication costs, and travel expenses when staff journey to present findings at regional and national conferences (Campbell & Chulay, 1990; Hodge, Kochie, Larsen, & Santiago 2003; Lieske, 1985). Although the resources required are not insignificant, they can be justified because successful CI projects help achieve organizational goals and can be measured by improved patient outcomes, decreased costs, improved staff retention, and increased patient and family satisfaction.

Clinical Nurse Specialist

Continually juggling the multiple responsibilities of the CNS role is challenging at best. Because research projects occur over an extended time period, they are often put on the "back-burner" for issues requiring more immediate attention. However, given the requirement that nursing care must be evidence based, the CNS must be committed to keeping research activities at the top of the priority list. General CNS responsibilities include sharing the philosophies of administration regarding research, fostering good partnerships with nurse managers, developing an operational model for CI, evaluating project outcomes, and mentoring staff throughout the process. Specific responsibilities are identified in Table 6-3.

STRATEGIES FOR CLINICAL INQUIRY

A unit culture that embraces CI will use a variety of strategies to make sure that staff are aware of current information and integrate it into their practice. Some of these strategies include journal clubs, EBP rounds, and clinician-led research.

TABLE 6-3

CNS Roles in Clinical Inquiry

Read key studies and clinical guidelines relevant to unit practice.

Attend critical professional and research conferences.

Conduct literature reviews and access key websites.

Diplomatically challenge current practice routines.

Include research findings into daily patient rounds.

Include current research findings when teaching critical care content.

Post current, clinically relevant research findings in visible places in unit, discuss during rounds and staff meetings, or place in staff mailboxes.

Develop policies and procedures, care standards, and guidelines based on current evidence.

Teach staff to review the literature and critically evaluate research studies.

Collaborate with administration to create structure for nurses to willingly and easily participate in CI.

Facilitate research work groups.

Partner with academic faculty to help with research projects and statistical analysis.

Consult with other advanced practice nurses to lend their clinical expertise to answer clinical questions.

Mentor staff as they write results of research studies, submit abstracts, and present projects to nursing group.

TABLE 6-4

Levels of Evidence

Level	Description
1	Randomized, prospective, controlled investigations; meta-analysis
2	Nonrandomized, concurrent, or historical cohort investigations
3	Theory-based, expert consensus group
4	Peer-reviewed, state-of-the-art articles, review articles
5	Nonpeer reviewed published opinion textbooks, organizational publications, manufacturers' recommendations

Hodge, M., Kochie, LD., Larsen, L., & Santiago, M. (2003). Clinician-implemented research utilization in critical care. *American Journal of Critical Care*, 12(4):361-365.

All include the need to understand the importance of levels of evidence when evaluating research (Table 6-4) and knowing the best websites for information (Table 6-5). These will be discussed in the following paragraphs. along with specific responsibilities for the CNS.

Journal Clubs

Gathering staff members together to discuss current articles is an excellent way to stimulate discussion about areas of interest and help staff feel comfortable in reviewing clinical literature. This first step toward EBP does not require significant financial resources; the biggest challenge to journal clubs is finding a time and place that promotes consistent staff involvement. The CNS will need to partner with the manager and a staff leader to facilitate participation. Meetings held in the unit will likely be well attended, and staff can benefit from the discussion even if attendance is intermittent due to unit acuity. Frequent interruptions are likely and may be disruptive to the flow of the meeting. Journal clubs also take place in individual's homes or in neutral places such as restaurants or coffee shops. The challenge here is simply the added burden of identifying where meetings will be held from one month to the next, distributing directions, and various "catering" issues such as whether there will be refreshments.

The CNS collaborates with the group leader to select and distribute the articles and share meeting minutes with staff unable to attend.

TABLE 6-5

Internet Sources for Evidence-Based Practice

www.guidelines.gov (NIH sponsored site)
www.cdc.gov (Centers for Disease Control and Prevention)
www.nih.gov (NIH site with links to various institutes)
www.cochrane.org (Cochrane Collaboration site)
www.ahrq.gov (Federal agency site for Agency for Healthcare and Quality)
www.ana.org (American Nurses Association)
www.aacn.org (American Association of Critical-Care Nurses)
www.ena.org (Emergency Nurses Association)
www.aorn.org (Association of Operating Room Nurses)
www.ons.org (Oncology Nursing Society)
www.sccm.org (Society of Critical Care Medicine)
www.hirshinstitute.com (Sarah Cole Hirsh Institute for EBN)
www.evidencebasednursing.com (Nursing journal with abstract databases)

The key to success is to select articles of clinical interest that are easily understood (with simple research design and minimal research jargon), and have obvious implications for practice. Articles that do not meet these criteria will not invite participation from the staff. Evidence-based protocols and guidelines can also be discussed. Materials should be posted in the unit, placed in staff mailboxes, or e-mailed within 1 to 2 weeks before the meeting. An additional page with discussion questions should also be included to guide reading. The CNS may want to invite the hospital's nurse scientist or a faculty member from a school of nursing to help discuss study design and statistical analysis. The unit manager must clearly communicate expectations for participation along with plans to cover staff so they can attend meetings and how to pay staff for participating during off-time. The CNS models commitment to the activity through regular participation, asking thoughtful and nonthreatening questions, and facilitating practice changes from any recommendations made by the group.

Evidence-based Practice Rounds

EBP rounds are another easy, nonthreatening way to encourage nurses to become committed to CI. Melnyk (2002) describes a process during which an individual with significant clinical expertise in a particular area researches clinical questions and presents the findings to colleagues during regularly scheduled meetings. Ideally, helping staff nurses give these presentations will promote better participation in EBP at the unit level. Facilitated by the CNS, nurse scientist, or consulting school of nursing faculty, group discussion includes analysis of study design, results of the study, and implications for practice. Strategies for implementation and outcomes of implementing the practice change are also identified (Melnyk, 2002). Summaries of the discussions in the form of Practice Alerts or Fact Sheets should be distributed throughout the unit via posters, e-mail, or the communication book to ensure that all staff members are

aware of pending practice changes. Feedback should be encouraged. The CNS is responsible for organizing the group, participating in the identification of research questions, guiding discussion, and assisting staff members with the literature review and interpretation of the study. The CNS also plays a key role in guiding the staff as they implement practice changes and in evaluating their impact.

Clinician-led Research

Another effective method to help nurses see the value of research in everyday practice is for the CNS to mentor them as they conduct their own research project. Bedside nurses are in an excellent position to identify and answer important practice questions warranting additional study (Burns, 2002). In addition to answering specific clinical questions using scientific methods, nurses who participate in research learn about the research process in a nonthreatening, clinically practical format, and have the opportunity to publish and present their work to professional colleagues. The CNS should take heart: this is not the tedious, intimidating master's thesis project with an endless literature review and close scrutiny of advising professors! Rather, clinician-based research facilitated by the CNS is short and simple and directly answers a specific clinical question with realistic attention to background information. Suggested resources for developing a clinical research program are identified in Box 6-1.

FACILITATING CLINICIAN-LED RESEARCH

Meetings

Many nurses balk at research for reasons described earlier, so the first challenge in developing clinician-led research studies is to generate staff enthusiasm for participating in a research study. Avoiding use of the word "research" may be helpful, and substituting titles such as "Clinical Inquiry" or "Best Practice" may seem more enticing to nurses who wish to enhance

BOX 6-1

Suggested Resources for Developing a Clinical Research Program

Burns, S.M. (2002). Clinical research is part of what we do: The experience of one medical intensive care unit. *Critical Care Nurse*, 22(2): 100-109.

Campbell, G.M. & Chulay, M. (1990). Establishing a clinical nursing research program. In J. Spicer & M.A. Robinson (Eds): *Environmental management in critical care nursing*. Baltimore: Williams & Wilkins.

Granger, B. & Chulay, M. (1999). *Research strategies for clinicians*. Stamford, CT: Appleton & Lange.

their practice. All staff nurses should be invited to participate, but the CNS should also specifically recruit staff with good follow-through, clinical expertise, solid communication skills, and experience in group work. In addition to nursing staff, other health care professionals (e.g., respiratory therapists, pharmacists, physical therapists) can also be included, especially when the topic is within their expertise. Consistent attendance of the unit manager is not required but is strongly encouraged as a show of support to the staff as they undertake a project. Research teams of two to three people are probably too small to feel productive, whereas keeping the team to no more than eight to ten members will help prevent it from becoming so large that it is unproductive (Granger & Chulay, 1999). Team members should be encouraged to take on tasks that they are comfortable with (e.g., writing minutes, copying articles, actively participating in discussion) to avoid overwhelming them in the early stages of the project. Consistent participation from group members is essential to completing any research project, but the logistics of regularly getting staff nurses to meetings is difficult. Nurses can commit to a project even if unit acuity or life circumstances cause them to miss meetings, and they should be encouraged to join the group at any time.

For the project to be successful, all unit staff should receive meeting summaries and be informed of project status even if they are not "official" team members.

As with any new group, ground rules and expectations should be established early. In general, staff are more likely to commit to a project if work is only done during meetings, with minimal or no homework assignments. Meeting times and sites need to be scheduled. Meetings in the report room promote attendance by nurses working that day; meetings in a room off the unit minimize interruptions but may be harder for on-duty staff to attend. One member of the group is established as the leader, with the CNS as coach. The leader should be someone who has good rapport with his or her peers and is detail oriented (Burns, 2002). The group leader can post meeting times, record and distribute minutes, and distribute reading materials to staff before the meeting work. The CNS consults with the unit manager to arrange staff coverage to attend the meeting. The CNS sets meeting agendas, follows up with individuals if assignments are made, and facilitates meetings.

Identifying Clinical Questions

It is difficult for staff nurses to identify research questions off the top of the head; therefore it is important to establish methods that can help them recognize questions in the course of their workday. In their book, *Research Strategies for Clinicians*, Granger and Chulay (1999) describe two methods useful in helping nurses identify meaningful clinical questions. Both methods help staff generate many topics for consideration as research projects.

The "stick method" works on the assumption that nurses come up with excellent questions throughout their shift, but don't have time to write them down or don't consider them appropriate research questions. Post-it notes are placed in highly visible spots in the unit (near a patient's bedside, in the nursing break room, or at the nurses' desk) for staff to write down a question immediately after it arises. The questions are then collected by the CI group for review. Questions are categorized according to one of four pathways for obtaining an answer:

- Staff development: Can the question be easily answered by an in-service, a simple conversation, or looking it up in a reference book? If so, it is referred to the clinical educator or other appropriate person.
- Policy and procedure: Can the question be easily answered by writing a new policy or procedure? Has new evidence become available that now mandates updating an existing policy or procedure? If so, it is referred to the appropriate unit-based or hospital committee.
- Administrative: Can the question be easily resolved by consulting with administration? If so, it is passed on to the unit manager or responsible administrative committee.
- Clinical research: Is the question clinically relevant? Is there existing evidence that addresses the issue? If so, the CI group evaluates the literature and disseminates the information and implications for practice to staff. If not, the question can be considered a potential research project (Granger & Chulay, 1999).

The "focus group" method is another effective strategy used to identify research topics. In addition to helping staff feel more comfortable with asking clinical questions, this method also promotes the opportunity for everyone in the unit to ask questions, resulting in group ownership of the chosen topic. The first step is series of 1-hour meetings with unit staff. A facilitator, usually the CNS, uses a flip chart to lead the staff through a series of questions aimed at identifying questions about their clinical experiences.

- Patient population: Ask the nurses to identify high-volume patient populations and common problems. List main demographics of patients on the unit by age, medical diagnoses, nursing diagnoses, and symptoms.
- Frequent nursing interventions: Ask the nurses to name common nursing interventions they perform for their patients such as endotracheal suctioning, insertion of intravenous catheters, arterial blood-gas sticks, medication administration, and family support.
- Common technologies: Have the nurses list the equipment they use when caring for their patients and describe challenges they experience when using the equipment. These may include infusion pumps, ventriculostomies, suction catheters, pulmonary artery catheters, SvO_2 computers, and point-of-care testing devices such as thermometers, 12-lead ECG machines, and arterial blood-gas analyzers.

After the above discussions, clinicians may identify between 10 and 20 relevant practice questions after only two to three meetings (Granger & Chulay, 1999).

In the second step of the focus group method, the CNS helps the group generate researchable questions from the most clinically important and interesting topics. In the third and final step the CNS helps them prioritize the best research questions appropriate for a group of busy, inexperienced, but enthusiastic clinicians to pursue (Granger & Chulay, 1999).

Selecting Ideal Research Projects

To create an environment in which nurses will be successful with their first project, it is critical for the CNS to help the CI group select good questions to avoid roadblocks commonly experienced by novice researchers. Projects should meet as many as possible of the following criteria:

- Use the clinical expertise of the staff.
- Sustain staff interest throughout a potentially lengthy time period.
- Be politically neutral.

- Stay within nursing domain.
- Be relevant to clinical practice and patient outcomes.
- Recognize institutional priorities.
- Provide potential cost savings to the institution.
- Include large numbers of patients (at least one patient per day).
- Use previously established measurement tools.
- Require minimal or no funding from administration or outside sources.
- Incorporate data collection into unit routines.

Possible research questions are prioritized using the above criteria with an objective scoring system that differentiates feasible projects from those that will be more difficult to complete. Each topic is given a score based on how it meets the criteria; the question with the highest score is chosen as the group's project. An example of an evaluation tool is found in Fig. 6-1. In the event of a tie, nurses can be given no more than two articles on each potential topic to read. They should consider that their project will look very similar to the studies they've just read, which will help them assess feasibility and resources needed for each potential project. The final selection is made when the group votes on the remaining topics. The CNS facilitates this via consensus building, calling for nominations, or passing out ballots (Granger & Chulay, 1999). Once the question has been selected, the group is now ready to begin working on the project itself.

Writing the Protocol

Writing a protocol from scratch is difficult, especially for novice researchers. Two straightforward approaches are to write a replication of a well-designed and practical study or to use a completed protocol as a template, exchanging text as appropriate. A replication study simply duplicates an entire study as written and should look exactly like the original protocol. Using a published article would suffice if the original protocol is unavailable. When using a previous study as a template, the original patient populations, definitions, technology, and even methodology are crossed out; and the new

Scoring System:	0 = not present	+ = present/yes	++ = highly present/strong yes	
Criteria	Topic	Topic	Topic	Topic
Area of staff interest				
Staff have clinical expertise				
Important to clinical practice, patient outcomes				
Large number of pts eligible				
No political landmines				
Potential financial impact				
No additional $ required				
Measurement tools available				
Data collection fits with unit routines				
Data collection could be finished quickly				
Miscellaneous				

FIG 6-1   Example of a rating worksheet to prioritize possible research topics. (From Granger, B. & Chulay, M. [1999]. *Research strategies for clinicians.* Stamford, CT: Appleton & Lange, p. 47.)

content is substituted. All writing is done as a group during the meeting with the CNS leading dialogue and confirming content. A staff nurse may scribe the new content. The CNS takes the reworked material, edits it into a new document, and presents it to the staff for their approval at the next meeting.

Components of a protocol include:

- Cover letter or abstract.
- Statement of the problem and background information. (Of note, in the Granger and Chulay model, the review of the literature [ROL] is not done early in the protocol development phase because staff can become overwhelmed or sidetracked by too much information. Rather, the brief ROL occurs *after* the protocol is completed so that staff can focus on their own design and then merely fine-tune what they've developed.)
- Research question or hypothesis.
- Definition of terms.
- Methodology: study design, sample size, sample patient population, setting, inclusion/exclusion criteria, data collection.
- Data analysis.
- Risks/benefits to patient.
- Costs.
- Consent.
- Confidentiality and ethical considerations (Granger & Chulay, 1999).

The CNS will likely need to consult with the nurse scientist, a statistician, or academic faculty regarding study design, sample size calculation, and statistical analysis to ensure that the protocol is scientifically sound.

Navigating the Approval Process

Before data collection can begin, the Institutional Review Board (IRB) must give the study formal approval (Granger & Chulay, 1999). Every facility has different requirements for their approval process with strict regulations governing consent and confidentiality. Counsel from the nurse scientist or academic faculty are essential at this stage of the research project. Some facilities may require approval from additional committees such as the Nursing Research Committee and the ICU Research Committee to avoid inundating patients with studies and potential conflicts with other ongoing research.

Understanding Data Analysis

Support for statistical analysis must be done before data is collected to ensure that the study design will be strong enough to answer the clinical question (Granger & Chulay, 1999). Again, this is a time when the nurse scientist or academic faculty must be involved. Some institutions can provide statisticians; however, they must be careful to not overwhelm and confuse novice researchers. By remembering that the data will be collected during the course of daily nursing routines, the data tool must be simple, ask only for information critical to the study, and use as few data points as necessary. When the statistics are basic and straightforward, staff will have an easier time understanding the results of their work and discussing them as they share their findings.

Sharing Results of the Study

The first place to start with sharing findings of the study is within the unit itself and then within the institution. This can be done a variety of ways, including e-mail, posters, newsletters, staff meetings, or hospital nursing research meetings. All of these methods help the staff gain experience and increase confidence in talking about their work to other professionals. Another good venue for sharing findings is to present them at local, regional, and national professional meetings. Posters are easy for staff to create and are of minimal cost. Many staff members are interested in public speaking and are willing, with guidance, to present to an audience. Finally the entire CI group should write up their results for publication in specialty-based journals. The CNS mentors staff throughout all of these pathways, from abstract submission to practicing slide presentations or revising written drafts. These professional activities are highly energizing to staff nurses, promoting job satisfaction and retention. In fact, some nurses may consider the value of these activities to be equal in value to the study itself.

Keeping the Unit Informed

Throughout the entire process, from question development to sharing of findings, the CI group must keep the rest of the unit staff informed. By being aware of project status, the remaining staff will be more likely to support the project, help in data collection, cover staff for meetings or group work, and value the effort put into the project. Indeed, many may become intrigued enough to join the group in progress or sign up to participate in the next project. Good communication fosters staff cohesiveness, eliminates the notion of the "privileged few," and allows the entire unit to take pride in the final project.

Overcoming Roadblocks to the Research Process

The CNS faces many challenges when facilitating a clinical research project. Probably the biggest is that of balancing multiple job responsibilities in such a way that priority is given to research activities. Constant reprioritization of responsibilities based on the needs of the unit is a fact of life; thus the CNS must frequently communicate with the unit manager and other nursing administrators to make sure research activities remain at the top of the list. Inevitable time management conflicts will require that the CNS routinely evaluate the importance of immediate clinical issues over the long-term benefits that the research might provide (Fitzgerald, Milberger, Peden-McAlpine, Meiers, & Sherman, 2003).

Another challenge is establishing rapport within the team, some of whom have yet to be convinced of the usefulness of nursing research (Fitzgerald, Milberger, Peden-McAlpine, Meiers, & Sherman, 2003). The CNS must make sure

that progress is seen with every meeting to help staff feel productive and promote commitment to the group. Meeting agendas must be productive, and the CNS should bring updated manuscripts to review at meetings, distribute articles in a timely way, and foster discussion that is nonthreatening and builds on staff expertise. Above all, the group should have fun as they work together; this more than anything else will create group cohesiveness and respect.

For the research team to be successful, good communication pathways are essential within the team itself and with the remaining nursing staff. Getting the rest of the unit to support the project is crucial; thus the team and the CNS must have strategies to keep staff informed of the group's work. Regular updates on the status of the study should be done, along with frequent one-to-one conversations between the CNS and staff members to sustain support for the research project.

Financial concerns are a potential roadblock, but can be easily avoided with careful topic selection and planning. Choosing projects that require no additional funding is important to avoid cost concerns, but some financial aid can be found through nursing endowment funds, institutional quality assurance grants, professional organizations, and technology companies (Burns, 2002). A big issue will be how to pay nurses for participating in the project. While this issue will vary between institutions, the CNS should dialogue with the unit manager to make sure meetings are held when most of the group are already scheduled to work and that they can be covered to be out of patient care so payroll costs are kept to a minimum. Making sure that data collection is done during normal work hours will also control expenses. Costs for poster development and transportation for nurses who travel to professional conferences need to be considered during planning of yearly budgets. Improved recruitment and retention and institutional visibility seen as a result of clinician research may well outweigh the minimal costs associated with the any research project.

MEASURING OUTCOMES OF CI

Determining the impact of CI is important to guarantee its place in daily nursing practice. Some outcomes will be simply observed: nurses will quote relevant literature and ask thought-provoking questions during report, rounds, and staff meetings. They will include new data in in-services and posters they create. They will be familiar with key websites that give the most useful information. Policies and procedures will show the references used to develop the document. Nurses will actively participate in research groups. The CNS measures these by developing a questionnaire asking nurses about their participation in these activities and can intervene as needed. Annual evaluations and clinical ladder applications can also assess staff participation in research activities.

Outcomes can also be measured more formally with audit tools that evaluate prevalence of practice changes and their impact on patient care. Patient care outcomes can include length of intensive care unit stay, length of hospital stay, patient satisfaction, family satisfaction, patient costs, unit costs, and quality of pain control, to name a few. Nursing outcomes can be measured in terms of recruitment and retention data, number of presentations accepted at professional conferences, and number of publications. Over time, as nurses become more confident with their research skills, the number of projects initiated, coordinated, and mentored by bedside clinicians can be measured as a way to assess success of the clinical research model (Granger & Chulay, 1999).

Finally, an excellent way to highlight the work of the CI groups is for the CNS to organize an annual Nursing Research Day, where staff members present their posters to colleagues and hospital administrators. It is empowering to see their work formally considered by influential people within the institution, validating their efforts, and encouraging continued participation. Practice alerts, revised care standards, protocols, and policies and procedures can also be displayed at this venue, further illustrating the infusion of evidence into routine nursing practice.

CONCLUSION

State-of-the-art nursing practice will occur only when the gap between research and the bedside is virtually nonexistent. The CNS plays a pivotal role in not only making sure nurses are aware of current evidence, but that they know how to independently find it, understand it, and integrate it into their practice. The CNS has a fundamental responsibility to create an environment that encourages nurses to actively question their practice. Although there are a number of approaches to increasing nurses' familiarity with research, perhaps the most effective strategy to help them value its role in practice is for the CNS to guide them through their own research projects. Participating and understanding research is a primary competency for the CNS. When the CNS mentors a team of clinicians through all phases of a research study, not only will nursing science be advanced, but nurses will increase their influence on professional colleagues and enhance their own personal professional satisfaction.

DISCUSSION QUESTIONS

1. What strategies for promoting evidence-based nursing are currently in place?
2. Identify current barriers to evidence-based practice in your unit and what you can do to minimize them.
3. What are the best Internet-based resources for your unit's patient population? How would you go about educating the nurses on how to access them?
4. Who would be the "unofficial" unit leaders who could help establish a clinical research project?
5. How would you establish a formal relationship with a nearby school of nursing to support clinical research?
6. How does the CNS mentor staff as they develop and publish a research study?

References

Bostrom, J., & Suter, W.N. (1993). Research utilization: Making the link to practice. *Journal of Nursing Staff Development, 9*, 28-34.

Burns, S. M. (2002). Clinical research is part of what we do: The experience of one medical intensive care unit. *Critical Care Nurse, 22*(2), 100-113.

Campbell, G., & Chulay, M. (1990). Establishing a clinical nursing research program. In J. Spicer, & M.A. Robinson (Eds.). *Environmental management in critical care nursing* (pp. 52-60). Baltimore: Williams & Wilkins.

Chulay, M. (1997). Bridging the research-practice gap. *Critical Care Nurse, 17*(1), 81-85.

Ciliska, D.K., Pinelli, J., DiCenso, A., & Callum, N. (2001). Resources to enhance evidence-based nursing practice. *AACN Clinical Issues, 12*(4), 520-528.

Curley, M.A. (1998). Patient-nurse synergy: Optimizing patients' outcomes. *American Journal of Critical Care, 7*(1), 64-71.

Fitzgerald, J., Milberger, P., Peden-McAlpine, C., Meiers, S. J., & Sherman, S. (2003). Clinical nurse specialist participation on a collaborative research project. *Clinical Nurse Specialist, 17*(1), 44-49.

Granger, B., & Chulay, M. (1999). *Research strategies for clinicians.* Stamford, CT: Appleton & Lange.

Hardin, S., & Hussey, L. (2001). The synergy model in practice. *Critical Care Nurse, 21*(2), 88-91.

Heater, B.S., Becker, A.M., & Olson, R. (1988). Nursing interventions and patient outcomes: a meta-analysis of studies. *Nursing Research, 37*, 303-307.

Hodge, M., Kochie, L.D., Larsen, L., & Santiago, M. (2003). Clinician-implemented research utilization in critical care. *American Journal of Critical Care, 12*(4), 361-365.

Lieske, A.M. (1985). Utilizing clinical research as a human resource management tool. In E.M. Lewis & J. G. Spicer (Eds.). *Human resource management handbook: Contemporary strategies for nursing managers* (p. 77). Rockville: Aspen Publishers.

McKibbon, A. (1999). *PDQ. Evidence-based principles and practice.* Hamilton: B.C. Decker.

Melnyk, B.M. (2002). Strategies for overcoming barriers in implementing evidence-based practice. *Pediatric Nursing, 28*(2), 159-161.

Melnyk, B.M., Fineout-Overholt, E., Stone, P., & Ackerman, M. (2000). Evidence-based practice: The past, the present, and recommendations for the millennium. *Pediatric Nursing, 26*(1), 77-80.

Nicswiadormy, R.M. (1998). Communication and utilization of nursing research., *Foundations of nursing research* (3rd ed., pp. 313-335). Stamford, CT: Appleton & Lange.

Sackett, D.I., Rosenberg, W., Gray, J.A.M., & Haynes, R.B. (1996). Evidence-based medicine: What it is and what it isn't. *British Medical Journal, 312*, 71-72.

Silagy, C., & Haines, A. (1998). *Evidence-based practice in primary care.* London: BMJ Books.

Valente, S.M. (2003). Research dissemination and utilization: Improving care at the bedside. *Journal of Nursing Care Quality, 18*(2), 114-121.

The Clinical Nurse Specialist as Facilitator of Learning

Karen K. Carlson

From their inception in the early 1960s, critical care units have become progressively more sophisticated. The requisite knowledge and skills for the acute and critical care nurse necessary to facilitate successful outcomes for today's critically ill patients are extensive, rich in technology, and at times overwhelming. Although specialty units are still found in major medical centers, as a result of tight economic times, many institutions have combined all specialties into large multispecialty units. This has greatly expanded the knowledge and skills competent critical care nurses must possess. In addition, in light of the current nursing shortage, the hiring of new nursing graduates into the critical and progressive care arenas increases the complexity of the already complicated orientation and educational needs of the critical care staff in the 21st century.

The knowledge and skills once needed only within the walls of a critical care unit are commonplace in other patient care areas, both in and out of the hospital (e.g., need for telemetry monitoring in outpatient clinics). The traditional education department may no longer exist or may consist of one educator focused on general staff orientation, mandatory updates, and regulator

requirements for education (e.g., cardiopulmonary resuscitation, advanced cardiac life support [ACLS]).

In pursuit of positive patient outcomes, critical care clinical nurse specialists (CNSs) are challenged by the reality of their environment in all aspects of their role. One goal of CNSs must be to create a learning environment for their realm of influence. This sets the stage for educational partnerships between the CNS and his or her audience and should be based on adult learning principles. Practical tips for integrating adult learning principles into educational opportunities are presented in Table 7-1.

In early work on the development of competency-based orientation programs, Alspach (1984), defined critical care nursing education as "education that is directed at facilitating the acquisition and application of the knowledge, skills, and attitudes that are required for competent critical care nursing practice." Components of critical care education include knowledge or cognitive skills, psychomotor or technical skills, interpersonal or attitudinal skills, and critical-thinking ability (Alspach, 1982).

The educational role of the CNS is the role of facilitator of educational experiences.

TABLE 7-1

Applying Adult Learning Principles

Content should:
- Be logical and related to the learner's practice.
- Be relevant to the role of the learner.
- Build on previous knowledge and experience.
- Be able to be readily applied to practice.
- Be presented in manageable increments.
- Be presented by a credible presenter.
- Be presented creatively.
- Be presented with opportunity to implement new knowledge or skills.

Adapted from Dickerson, P. (2003). 10 Tips to Help Learning. *J Nurs Staff Dev*, 19(5), 240-246.

By definition, to facilitate is to make easier. Learning is to gain knowledge or understanding of or skill by study, instruction, or experience. Kolb (1984), an early researcher of the psychology of learning states, "Learning is a process by which knowledge is created through the transformation of experience." The acquisition of knowledge alone is not the goal in learning but rather the acquisition of knowledge for the purpose of applying that knowledge to practice in a competent fashion. Competency, as defined by Benner (1982) is "the ability to perform a task with desirable outcomes under the varied circumstances of the real world."

The AACN Synergy Model for Patient Care (Curley, 1998) defines nurse competency in terms of eight essential characteristics. One of those characteristics is possession of the skills and knowledge necessary to be an effective facilitator of learning, which encompasses the ability to facilitate learning for nursing staff, patients, physicians and other health care disciplines, and community. This competency includes both formal and informal learning.

Therefore, simply translated, CNSs are responsible not only to make the acquisition of knowledge easier for their audiences but also to assist the nursing staff in their own development as facilitators of learning for their audiences (primarily other staff, patients, and families).

Each CNS has a learning facilitation component in his or her role and in that role has a diverse audience. CNSs often assume educational responsibilities for a variety of groups, including nursing staff (e.g., registered nurses [RNs], licensed practical nurses [LPNs], nurse technicians or assistants, agency staff, traveling nurses, float pool staff), patients and families, nursing students (e.g., undergraduate from both associate and baccalaureate programs along with graduate students), peers, and other members of the health care team (e.g., physicians, respiratory care). Their focus may be unit based, specialty based, population based, or institution based. Time devoted to educational responsibilities can consume much of a CNS's time and is variable, dependent on institutional expectations and the CNS's personal role development. In a national survey of practicing CNSs, the group ranked their education role as their second highest time consumer (24% to 89% of their time), following expert clinical practice (29% to 91% of their time) (Scott, 1999). This author would suggest that most expert clinical practice time can also be informal education time, reflecting that the great majority of a CNS's time is spent in facilitation of learning through a variety of venues.

CNS LEVEL OF EXPERTISE

The CNS's level of expertise as a facilitator of learning develops over time with experience, personal education, mentoring, and experimentation. The curriculum content in many master's programs is deficient in preparing the CNS for the educational responsibilities of his or her role. Each master's program places a different emphasis on the educational role while educating nurses in their advanced practice roles. An older study showed that, although over half of the master's programs had required education courses, 16.3% of the programs that completed the questionnaire had no courses in nursing education (Oermann & Jamison, 1989). Cox and Galante (2003) have proposed a master's curriculum specifically designed to prepare the new graduate in the CNS role, using the Synergy Model as a foundation. However, some master's programs that focus on educating graduate nurses as CNSs may have education courses available as electives but not as a required course of study. Given that, new CNSs come into their roles with a great variance in their background in formal education and have different learning needs of their own (Bachman, Kitchens, Halley, & Ellison, 1992).

Orientation to the CNS role is crucial. Working with an experienced peer whose role is similar to that of the new CNS is an excellent way to begin a new job as a CNS. Orientation to the role should be individualized to the person, his or her experience, his or her specialty, the institution, and his or her role. Orientation for a new CNS position is different from that for a new person in a position that already existed (i.e., the new person will be picking up the goals/projects already identified by the predecessor). Several authors have suggested use of a competency-based orientation for the CNS. This type of orientation would provide structure and should include orientation to not only the CNS's areas of responsibility but also to the institution (DiMauro & Mack, 1989, Vezina, Chiang, Laufer, Garabedian, Padre, & Sanders, 1996).

IMPLEMENTATION WITHIN THE DIMENSION OF PRACTICE

Assessment

As the CNS conceptualizes the assessment of learning needs for staff, any approach should be with the goal of developing an educational plan framework. Although there is a growing body of evidence to support the positive effect of CNSs on patient outcomes (i.e., length of stay, complications, use of services, mortality rate) (Wheeler, 1999), there is little evidence that demonstrates a connection between continuing education and improved patient care (Tennant & Field, 2004). However, one study of physicians demonstrated a positive relationship between a continuing education intervention that resulted in acquiring new skills and improved patient

outcomes (Wiecha & Barrie, 2002). Similarly, since the primary goal of the CNS is to improve patient care, specifically patient outcomes, an educational plan of excellence should be constructed in a manner that allows the connection between intervention and outcomes to be measured. This approach would involve five steps: (1) defining the level of current of practice, (2) defining the desired level of current of practice, (3) identifying the gaps, (4) determining the intervention, and (5) defining how the completed transition will be evaluated (how will we know when we get to the new level of practice?). This "beginning with the end in mind" mindset provides a firm foundation for the assessment, diagnosis, intervention, and evaluation aspects of the CNS's educational plan (Covey, 1989). Clinical objectives, most often used with new employees or orientees, may be useful in establishing a baseline level of practice and in determining the minimum level at which all staff should function (McKane, 2004). Use of the Benner Model (Benner, 1984) of staff competencies applied to individual staff is another tool that could be helpful in determining what is needed to help staff in their movement from one level of competency to another. Good and Schulman (2000) present the development of a clinical competency pathway for use from hire through orientation, continuing through development over the first few years after hire. It incorporates both clinical and regulatory agency competencies.

As a facilitator of learning, the CNS is constantly assessing learning wants and needs. Consideration must be given to needs on an individual (i.e., nursing, ancillary personnel, patients and their families), unit, department, service line, and organizational basis, using a wide variety of data sources (Table 7-2). As a part of this assessment, evidence of learning from past interventions should be considered. Although assessment can be done formally or informally, use of a combination of formats will provide the CNS with the most accurate portrait of the needs and outcomes in their area of responsibility (Table 7-3).

TABLE 7-2

Learning Needs Assessment Data Sources

Source	Role in Learning Needs Assessment
Individual staff member	In an organizational culture that values employee development, the individual staff member has a right and a responsibility to identify and document his/her learning needs through a formal assessment process.
Workgroup	Groups of employees may identify a common learning need among the work sections or units and jointly submit a completed assessment form that reflects their shared need.
Professional disciplines	Senior and key members of the various disciplines represented among the organization's staff have an awareness of the critical issues confronting the profession/occupation, its customary and changing work requirements and processes, and trends affecting the profession as a whole. These staff personnel can recognize and document learning needs on behalf of agency employees within the profession/occupation.
Department/service	Managers with a department/service-wide perspective have a wealth of information about the learning needs of their employees at both an individual and employee group level. Managers who view staff development and education as important contributors to process and quality improvements within the department may submit several completed assessment forms on behalf of their subordinates.
Committees	In the course of conducting their business, committees are often aware of trends, work processes, and outcomes within the organization that require adjustments or improvements and that may reflect the need for educational interventions within the organization. The committee chairperson, on behalf of the committee, may submit a staff learning needs assessment form identifying the need and anticipated target audience.
Corporate headquarters initiative	All new initiatives need to be examined by administrators, managers, and educators for staff training implications. When learning needs are reflected in new initiatives, educators and others can ensure that these are addressed by submitting completed assessment forms.
Administrators	These key personnel not only hold a comprehensive view of the agency's mission, functions, resources, and performance but also anticipate the future of the organization. Their participation in the identification of employee learning needs, most commonly aimed at group needs, is critical to the development of a facility education plan that is responsive to needs and proactive in preparing its work force for the present *and* the future.
Supervisory observations	Whether observations and recommendations for learning activities reflect the need(s) of one or more employees, few individuals are in a better position than the immediate supervisors to identify staff learning needs and potential remedies because they have an intimate knowledge of what is needed to successfully perform the assigned work.
Results of organizational performance measures/ clinical outcomes	Many factors contribute to stellar or less than excellent results on performance measures or in clinical outcomes. When employee knowledge and skill deficits are determined to contribute to performance or outcomes below what is expected, key personnel have a responsibility to document staff training needs using the learning needs assessment form.

TABLE 7-2	
Learning Needs Assessment Data Sources—cont'd	
Source	**Role in Learning Needs Assessment**
Strategic goals of facility/ corporation	Strategic goals may require updated or new employee knowledge and skills. These should be examined in light of performance or productivity to determine whether employee training is a necessary strategy for goal attainment and, if so, learning needs assessments should be submitted.
Health care literature & trends (clinical, technical, & administrative)	Administrators, managers, educators, and other key personnel have an obligation to be aware of trends in health care, findings of research, and evidence-based practices that will impact service delivery. Such knowledge may serve as the basis for submission of learning needs forms.
Critical incidents/sentinel events	Root cause analyses (RCA) of these events frequently result in recommendations for employee training. Because of the serious nature of these events, all RCA reports should be carefully reviewed by appropriate officials and educators to ensure that learning needs are documented and educational strategies planned.

Informal opportunities for assessment of learning needs are inherent in every CNS interaction. For example, the CNS, as part of shift report, hears that a patient was started on an experimental medication. Immediately the CNS should recognize that both staff and patient would benefit if the staff understood the intricacies of this new medication.

Each time CNSs are consulted for their expertise, apparent learning needs may appear. DeBourgh (2001) describes three different types of consultation: process, resource, and expert. Each type may uncover a learning need. *Process* consultations provide direction in "how to"

TABLE 7-3
Strategies for Assessment of Learning Needs

- Shift report
- Informal consultation
- Other discipline consultation
- Written evaluations (examinations)
- Competence checks (skill validation)
- Q/A critical incidents
- Evaluation of unit/institutional standards
- Survey (one-on-one, small focus groups, written)

situations, such as how to set a patient up with a transcutaneous pacemaker. *Resource* consultation provides direction for "where to find" or "what to use" such as locating a rectal tube for the hyperkalemic patient who needs a sodium polystyrene sulfonate (Kayexalate) enema. *Expert* consultation involves providing advanced levels of knowledge, information, and assistance with direct patient care in a complex situation such as appropriate medication titration in the hypotensive patient with a high systemic vascular resistance. The CNS should try to capture the essence of all consultations and references requested and then group and trend data. Carrying a small notebook to record the nature of consultations as they occur may be helpful. Transferring this information on a regular basis (e.g., daily, weekly) to an Excel spreadsheet and coupling these data with assessment data from another source along with frequency data can help identify and trend needs.

Likewise, opportunities for formal assessment of learning needs are multiple. One option might be to use a written evaluation of knowledge when a new staff member is hired or has finished orientation, or randomly with experienced staff. One such written tool is The Basic Knowledge

TABLE 7-4
Evaluation of Unit or Institution Standards

- Are they present?
- When were they developed?
- By whom were they developed?
- Are they research based?
- Are they reflective of best practice?
- Is their implementation evident at the bedside?

Assessment Tool (Toth, 2003). Some institutions opt to use the examination given at the end of their own critical care orientation programs.

Another means of assessment is an evaluation of current unit or institutional policies and procedures. Table 7-4 lists the questions to be used in this evaluation. It is not uncommon for a unit or institution to have the appropriate standards in writing yet not integrated into practice. The necessary integration into practice is a learning need. Annual competence checks, often referred to as skill validations, may reveal skill and/or knowledge deficiencies. Some institutions actually verify competence in these sessions, whereas others use them more loosely to review content related to their low-volume, high-risk patient populations. In either scenario, learning needs often present themselves in this process.

The term *critical incident* often carries a negative connotation. A critical incident does not need to be a crisis but rather should be viewed as any situation that caused staff to reflect on or question what happened, what was done, or how a situation was handled. Follow-up on critical incidents is useful in determining the source of the incident as well as identifying potential learning needs and research questions (Elliott, 2004). If the negative association can be removed and staff refocused to recognize the importance of reflecting on practice, it may be possible to identify the nature and the sources of critical incidents, giving the CNS opportunities to intervene so future similar issues can be addressed more successfully.

A learning needs survey is often one of the least helpful tools in determining "real" learning needs. Surveys can be administered in a one-on-one format, in focus groups (Bamford & Gibson, 2000), or to a wide audience in a written format. A staff survey may be developed for staff to indicate their perceived needs and wants. Using a survey may also be helpful in eliciting information from patients and their families about their experiences. The wise CNS recognizes that a written survey may often gather more information about learning wants than actual learning needs. Surveys done in a personal manner such as one-on-one or small focus groups are usually more helpful in gathering insightful, qualitative information (Bamford and Gibson, 2000). For example, on a written staff survey, a need repeatedly stated was for treatment of the hypokalemic patient. This finding puzzled the CNS who knew that the staff did an excellent job of treating these patients. When the survey was further discussed in a staff meeting, it was revealed that the staff was frustrated in treating these patients because of the lag time in obtaining potassium supplements from the pharmacy and receiving follow-up by the laboratory in drawing repeat potassium. This was not a learning need but rather a system-wide process issue.

Diagnosis

As assessment data are gathered, they should be analyzed to determine the focus of learning opportunities. It is common for the CNS to be asked to address nearly every issue that arises with an educational intervention; however, all identified needs are not learning needs. Differentiating between the needs best addressed with education and those best addressed in other ways is the most important task of the CNS in the diagnosis phase.

Most issues can be categorized into one of four groups, using the APES approach. Is the issue a problem/deficit in *A*ttitude, *E*ducation, *P*rocess, or the *S*ystem? For example, poor staff compliance with a new standard may be an issue of attitude (they don't like or agree with the new standard), education (they don't know the new standard), process (they can't comply because they are lacking necessary supplies), or system (they are lacking needed support from another department).

The CNS needs to approach diagnosis of the "real" need using the same mindset, determining the real need or needs so that the planned interventions are appropriate.

Case Application
An order is received for a patient from the telemetry unit to be transported to the radiology department for a computed tomography scan. The patient, who was being cardiac monitored, leaves the unit unmonitored, transported by a transport technician. During the CT scan the patient reports that "my heart is racing," becomes diaphoretic and short of breath, and starts to complain of chest pain. The radiology RN, unsure how to respond to the patient, pages the CNS for assistance. After appropriate intervention the patient is transported back to the unit with the CNS assisting. The radiology manager follows up with a request to the CNS for training of the radiology staff on interpreting rhythms and responding to emergencies.

The CNS should explore all available aspects of the situation and attempt to determine if the issues in this situation are attitudinal, educational, process oriented, or system based. Many times, on quick examination the first issue to surface is one that can be addressed with an educational fix. Let's evaluate this example. On the surface, the CNS recognizes that this situation may not have deteriorated if the patient had been monitored and the radiology RN could interpret rhythms and treat them; therefore education must be the answer. However, as he or she thinks more broadly and approaches the situation with APES in mind, the CNS explores other options. He or she looks for attitude. There does not appear to be an attitude problem. What about a process issue? A patient who was monitored on the telemetry unit is transported off the unit without monitoring or without appropriately trained transport personnel.

If a policy was adopted that required monitored patients who travel off the unit to wear a monitor with appropriately trained staff, in this situation the radiology RN would not need education (except on the new policy). Which need causes the patient to be less vulnerable? It's the system. Why is it safe for a monitored patient to travel off unit without appropriate monitoring? If a patient requires continuous monitoring, how does one decide if the patient does not have arrhythmias (with the potential to be symptomatic and require intervention) while he or she is off unit, in an elevator, and in another environment that is not prepared? In this situation the real need was a change in policy, not more education. Some may encourage both change in policy and education of the radiology staff. CAUTION: Remember that educating staff on a skill infrequently used is not ideal. Long-term concerns such as how competency will be maintained must also be addressed before the decision would be made to train the radiology staff.

Outcome Identification

Each educational intervention should be designed with an expected outcome that is based on current clinical/scientific knowledge. The expected outcome would rarely be simply an increase in knowledge. Is the expected outcome a change in practice? Is the need local or system wide? If a change in process is identified, determine how other departments will be affected. Are needs related to a specific unit or more globally, across unit lines or even across health system lines (e.g., multiple hospitals in one system). If the identified issue is one of attitude, no amount of educational intervention will create a change.

Planning

The planning phase is when determination is made of how best to address the need after it has been identified. The CNS facilitates the plan and prescribes intervention, with a focus on outcome, and ensures all of the right players are involved.

All individuals have unique learning styles that develop in childhood, and they tend to teach the way they learn. The CNS should be aware that most audiences are a combination of visual and auditory learners. He or she should also consider the style of the audience or the fact that all styles most likely are represented and learning interventions need to be created that match these styles. For example, when choosing a clinical preceptor, the CNS tries to match the student's and the preceptor's learning styles (Chase, 2001).

Kolb (1984) authored a learning styles inventory that is used to measure an individual's preferred learning style. Although his tool has been widely used since its introduction, the Kolb Learning Styles Inventory (1985) has been met with mixed reviews concerning both its validity and the true impact of its findings on educational program planning (DeCoux, 1990; Thompson and Crutchlow, 1993; Cavanagh, Hogan, & Ramgopal, 1995; Janing, 2001; Armstrong & Parsa-Parsi, 2005). It does seem reasonable to consider using learning styles in planning for different types of educational interventions.

Learning is translated into retained knowledge through the way individuals perceive and then process information. Figure 7-1 illustrates Kolb's four basic learning styles. Sequencing learning experiences so the learner moves from quadrant one through quadrant four is considered the best design for educational planning purposes (Kolb, 1984).

When planning for opportunities to facilitate learning, the CNS needs to consider the Who,

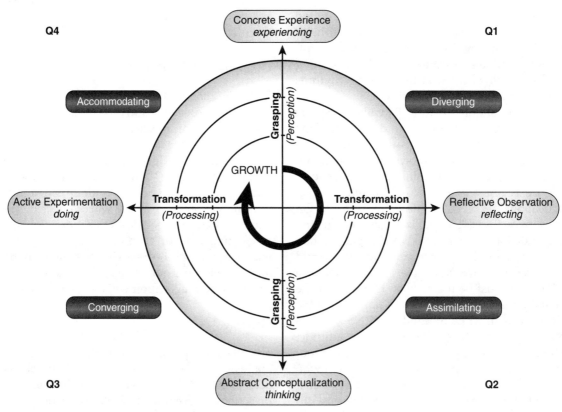

FIG 7-1 The four basic learning styles.

What, When, Where, Why, and How of each intervention. *Who* should participate (e.g., new graduates, experienced staff, other disciplines)? *Who* will prepare or present the content (e.g., CNS, experienced staff nurse, unit physician, other discipline)? *What* will be prepared or presented (content)? *When* (e.g., time of day, available to all shifts, dedicated time off? Is the class mandatory or voluntary?); *Why* (a clear goal in mind to meet a true learning need)? *Where* (e.g., at bedside, conference room, off unit). *How* (What is the best venue? Should it be an in-service, half or full day seminar, part of rounds, informally at the bedside, or self-study module?).

Activities that facilitate learning can be formal (e.g., orientation of new staff [clinically and didactically]), in-service, routine program/repetitive programs (preceptor training, specialty training [IABP, cardiac surgery, cardiac assist devices]) or informal (role modeling in direct patient care by "doing with, not for") staff or impromptu interventions (i.e., bedside education about titrating vasoactive medications). In an ideal situation an education plan would provide a system of learning available to staff at all times and would include not only clinically related topics such as pathophysiology and development of critical thinking and clinical reasoning skills but also professional development and research utilization.

Morton (2005) proposes use of an annual employee education calendar. Using a thorough planning process, a minimum of 3 months is the preparation time recommended in the development of such an undertaking. Ten criteria are suggested for prioritizing education needs (Table 7-5).

Implementation

Although most teaching occurs in classrooms, most learning does not. As a facilitator of learning, the goal of a successful CNS should be to improve patient outcomes. Research has demonstrated that a unit-based expert nurse such as a CNS increases patient-focused care (Hanneman, 1996). All interventions should be evidence based and delivered in a safe and ethical manner and collaboratively as appropriate. One strategy is to involve the more senior staff member in the entire educational process for their area, serving as a mentor.

The necessary sharing of skills and knowledge required to target such a goal encompasses many diverse activities. From orientation (new graduates, experienced medical-surgical nurses, and experienced critical care nurses from other units or institutions) to continuing education and mentoring of experienced staff, implementation of a strong educational plan is vital. Formal classroom teaching (critical care courses, both for the beginner and the experienced provider), in-services, all day programs, self-paced learning modules, and computer-assisted and online learning may all be involved.

Informal learning can be planned or spontaneous. Simply because the CNS is not planning a formal 15-minute in-service does not mean that informal interactions cannot be planned in advance. Perhaps an identified need is for external pacing. The CNS is aware of this need and capitalizes on a clinical situation in which an external pacemaker is applied to involve as many staff as possible. He or she makes more frequent rounds and invites staff into the patient's room where the pacemaker is in use. The CNS uses this as the opportunistic learning moment that it is and involves as many staff as possible.

A wise CNS should capitalize on opportunistic learning moments. The strength of these moments is that the involved staff, student, or patient and family have an immediate need to know. Capturing this need-to-know moment allows for immediate application and, in theory, better retention. One study (Jannings and Artitage, 2001) found that on average a CNS has a minimum of one to three episodes, with an average of five per day, of opportunities to capture an opportunistic learning moment. CNSs facilitate learning without realizing that they are doing it, which may cause them to devalue certain interactions. With the outcome-based nature of many CNS performance

TABLE 7-5

Criteria and Considerations in Setting Priorities of Educational Needs

Criterion	Questions to Consider
Strategic goals and objectives of organization	Does the expected learning outcome contribute to the achievement of one of the organization's strategic goals or objectives?
Compatibility with mission and services	Is achievement of the expected learning outcome mission or service critical? Does it support mission or service(s) of the organization?
Potential for contributing to achievement of performance measures	Is the expected learning outcome a significant factor in maintaining or meeting one or more of the organization's performance measures?
Potential impact on process or quality improvements	Can meeting this learning need have a significant impact on process or quality improvements planned within the organization?
Severity of problem	Does the identified problem reflect a staff training need rather than a need for some other type of remedy within the organization? If so, is the problem significant enough to warrant expenditure of educational resources?
Number/types of patients potentially affected	Would achievement of the learning outcome be expected to improve the quality of care or services to patients or select groups of patients? If so, under what circumstances, to how many, and to what extent?
Potential impact on new programs or services	Will meeting this educational need support the implementation of a planned new program or service? If so, is it critical to successful implementation?
Universality of need among staff	If the learning need is unique to one or a few individual(s), can coaching or other informal processes meet the need? Is the learning need widespread among a group of employees? How important is the expected learning outcome in enhancing the performance of the individual or group?
Application to job/role	Does the expected learning outcome contribute to performance in the current job or role? If not, is there adequate justification to meet the need as preparation for an expanded or different job or role? If the perceived learning need is not directly related to current job or role, would meeting this need contribute to employee satisfaction or retention?
Resources available	Can the learning need be readily met with internal resources? If not, does the benefit to the organization justify the cost of outsourcing? What are the consequences of not meeting the need, and are they acceptable at this time?

evaluations, the need to defend legitimate use of CNS time is at a premium. Being able to demonstrate the link between CNS involvement and positive patient outcomes is powerful.

Less formal interventions such as bedside teaching, precepting, and assisting with patient care are often undervalued as opportunities to facilitate learning. Demonstrating applied clinical expert knowledge and problem-solving skills in real-time, authentic settings greatly impact the development of staff. The CNS should be the leader in efforts to create a practice environment that supports and promotes the diffusion of innovative, creative nursing practice and evidence-based approach to care delivery (DeBourgh, 2001). Use of an evidence-based approach to plan, deliver, and evaluate nursing education requires bridging the gap between theory and science for clinical practice.

Bedside interventions allow for techniques such as Benner's (Benner, Stannard, & Hooper, 1996) "thinking-in-action" approach to teaching clinical judgment to be put into place. Through this approach the CNS can model and help guide staff to identify the relevant clinical problems, focus clinical problem solving on relevant goals, practice reasoning, learn the ethical skill of engaging a problem interpersonally, and take a responsible stand by making clinical judgments, acting on those judgments, and performing as an advocate for patients and their families. This format builds on the staff's ability to think in a critical fashion.

Use of case studies as a learning tool facilitates effective critical-thinking and problem-solving skills and uses adult learning principles. Case study discussion changes the focus from teaching to learning (Tomey, 2003). Similarly, this use of problem-based learning can help the CNS move from being an efficient teacher to being an effective facilitator of learning (Baker, 2000).

Use of technology-based interventions such as AACN's interactive, computer-based critical care orientation program, Essentials of Critical Care Orientation (ECCO), can provide educational access to a large number of participants at a variety of times throughout the day. Another nice feature is that each participant can work at his or her own pace instead of being forced to move forward with a large group in a classroom setting. This may be very useful for learners who are easily intimidated in the classroom because they can review a section as many times as necessary.

One study compared education of staff on performing a 12-lead electrocardiogram using interactive, multimedia CD-ROM versus a self-study module that was accompanied by a brief lecture, skill demonstration, and hands-on practice. Both a pretest and posttest were done with both groups. Both groups were satisfied with their process and had similar capabilities in performing skills (Jeffries, Woolf, & Linde, 2003).

The literature revealed a new, creative venue. An interactive-online educational program was designed for family practice physicians on the care of patients with osteoarthritis (Bellamy, Goldstein, and Tekanoff, 2000). Follow-up data demonstrated improved patient outcomes as a result of this educational intervention. This model could be adapted by the CNS for use on an institution's Intranet to address a variety of educational needs.

Encouraging reflective thinking is another means the CNS can use to provide informal learning opportunities. By using critical incidents (any situation that causes staff to pause and contemplate events that have occurred to give them meaning [Elliott, 2004]) and framing questions to assist with reflective thinking, the CNS can create opportunities for learning.

Performance review via videotape is another strategy that may be used to improve clinical practice (Scherer, Chang, Meredith, and Battistella, 2003). Skill performance is videotaped and played back for review. One study used this method to video and evaluate trauma resuscitation response. Although giving verbal feedback on performance for a 3-month period made no change in practice, practice improved within 1 month of video feedback.

Another means of facilitating learning is through the use of simulations. Life-size manikins that model critical events can be used to educate and evaluate acute care skills (Boulet, Murray, Kras, Woodhouse, McAllister, & Ziv, 2003; Morton, 1997). Simulations have been used effectively to teach resuscitation (Long, 2005) and patient safety (Paparella, Mariani, Layton, Carpenter, 2004).

Interdisciplinary rounds with a focus on improved patient outcomes and increased staff professionalism is another avenue that the CNS may explore in ways to facilitate learning (Halm, Gagner, Goering, Sabo, Smith, & Zaccagnini, 2003). Also, the institution of nursing grand rounds can provide information and education. The CNS can involve members of nursing staff to plan and present interesting cases, along with a review of current literature pertinent to care.

The CNS can assist resources, perhaps by helping with literature review or audiovisual (AV) materials but encouraging staff growth by allowing them to do the actual presentation and lead the discussion. As a double bonus, the literature review may bring to light deficits in care or highlight that current practice is consistent with best practice (Cohen, Crego, Cuming, & Smyth, 2002). Focused rounds, using the topic of need (e.g., weaning from the ventilator, nutrition, arterial blood-gas interpretation, prophylaxis) are other informal learning facilitation strategies.

FORMAL INTERVENTIONS

It is important to remember that not all learning must be facilitated by the CNS. Use other experts (other CNSs, physicians, respiratory therapist, pharmacist, dietician, ACNP) when appropriate.

When asking a group of novice CNSs how they would provide education in their new roles, a frequent response is to do an in-service or lecture. Although experience may help them understand that lecturing should often be a last resort, learning to develop and present a successful lecture is a common need for the new CNS. Even the most experienced CNS most likely remembers his or her first lecture, especially to a large group.

"Lecturing is a skill (learned over time), a strategy (used when large amounts of information need to be covered), and a practice (developing the ability to interpret a learning situation by reading faces, questioning, determining background, and assumptions)" (Young & Diekelmann, 2002). Use of guided reflection in which an experienced CNS works with less experienced CNSs and discusses classroom situations that stand out to them and how they dealt with the situation is helpful in the development of lecturing skills (Young & Diekelmann, 2002).

To develop a lecture, in actuality CNSs are developing three components: student materials, their own materials, and AV materials. Some can do double duty (e.g., some lecturers use their PowerPoint slides as their student handout).

If students have a reference book, CNSs refer to it but don't read it to them. As with other interventions, they start with a clear outcome in mind. For example, if the goal is to change practice in caring for renal failure patients, CNSs think through what is needed to accomplish that goal. They clarify assumptions about prior knowledge. Does the CNS assume that students have an understanding of normal renal physiology? Use of adult learning principles and knowledge of learning styles are reminders to build on previous knowledge. Can the CNS assess knowledge before giving the lecture? Can the CNS give a quiz? This may be better received if it is formally called *an assessment of present knowledge for purposes of building on that knowledge.* (The word quiz is threatening to many.) Can the CNS present a case study to evaluate prior understandings? The ability to clearly describe prior knowledge varies, depending on the audience. If the CNS is preparing a lecture for the unit's staff, one of the above ideas may be used. On the other hand, if the CNS is preparing a lecture for a city-wide critical care course, he or she often does not have that option. Again, dependent on the setting, it perhaps would be best to begin the intervention with assessment and then tailor the lecture (this takes a sophisticated educator) accordingly. Comparisons of unit practice (if this is a local intervention) with literature review of best practice (as defined by outcome) must be included.

The easiest way to begin a new lecture is to use another educator's lecture outline as a template and then personalize it (be sure to give credit!). The CNS starts with a content outline detailing the headings of content to be covered. For example, a lecture on caring for the patient with pancreatitis may need to include a review of gastrointestinal anatomy and physiology. Other topics would include etiologies, assessment, nursing and medical interventions, and expected patient outcomes. Ideally the CNS would set the time frame; in reality, the time frame is often dictated because it fits into a master schedule of some sort. The CNS determines what can be covered in the allotted time frame. Trying to cover too much material in too little time is a common pitfall for the new lecturer. As lecturers become more experienced, they will be able to shrink or stretch lectures as time dictates. The well-prepared lecturer develops the skills to alter their time frames by up to 30 minutes as need dictates.

Adequate preparation time should be allowed. It is foolish to think that a new 1-hour lecture can be written in 1 hour. Often a review of the literature is necessary before the lecturer can even begin. Realistically I plan at least 6 to 8 hours of preparation time for every hour of new lecture content to be delivered, just for preparation of the lecture. Development of AV materials requires additional time.

After the lecture is developed, attention is turned to using AV materials effectively. Given that the lecturer will most likely be addressing both auditory and visual learners, slides or overheads should not contain only words. Well-placed pictures can greatly enhance learning. Imagine the difference between seeing a picture of a heart failure patient in crisis and having it described with words. Remember that learners retain 5% to 15% of what they read or hear, 10% to 20% of what they see, and 40% to 45% of what they do (Jackson, 1993).

In addition, for whatever type of AV materials the CNS chooses, he or she should be prepared to use them and be ready should the equipment fail. Having a backup plan such as overheads or a white board for illustrating points should the LCD crash in the middle of the presentation will add to his or her confidence.

There is no simple answer as to whether or not the CNS must provide a student handout when lecturing or doing any other type of learning facilitation. To promote best learning for auditory or visual learners, some CNSs provide full content outlines, some provide take-home messages (summary of content), and others provide highlights of the content. Some provide nothing. When asked, most students will say that some sort of handout is helpful; I have often heard learners ask for more complete outlines so they can listen and not be focused on note taking. Some CNSs provide students with a copy of the PowerPoint slides as a handout. An important reminder is that students do not want to be read to; thus the actual presentation should not just be reading the handout.

Handouts must follow the lecture, and content must be complete. Checking for missing pages before final copying will prevent student frustration at the time of the lecture. If using PowerPoint slides as a handout, there should be no more than three slides to a page. If there are slides with detailed information (e.g., coagulation cascade), they should be single full-scale pages, or they may be unreadable.

FORMAL EDUCATION OPPORTUNITIES

The Role of the Critical Care Course

Formal critical care orientation programs have two components: didactic content and clinical content. Formal, didactic critical care orientation programs have been demonstrated to effectively change knowledge (Wynd, 2002) but must be coupled with a strong clinical preceptor program to translate the knowledge into clinical practice.

There is no set curriculum to use when designing a critical care course. However, many institutions have used the AACN Acute and Critical Care Orientation Program (Carlson, 2001) as their template and then made modifications based on the patient populations that the staff cares for. This program consists of instructor materials; student handouts; AV materials in the form of slides and overheads; two final examinations, one for rhythm interpretation and one for the other didactic content; and a competency-based orientation tracking system for the clinical portion of orientation.

Recently, AACN (2005) introduced its Internet-based ECCO program. This program is designed to provide novice nurses the theoretical knowledge required to care for patients in the critical care arena. It consists of nine modules that are organized by body system. It includes testing mechanisms that can be used as both pretests and posttests. A suggested skills checklist is included to assist in guiding the learners' clinical activities.

There are several reports in the literature of metropolitan areas that have formed critical care education consortiums (Jacobsen, Malan, Perkins, & Slatten, 1990; Earp, Capka, Davis, McLain, Ney, & Moorhead, 1992; Sammut, 1994). Working together with other hospitals or perhaps even within the CNS's own health systems allows for sharing of services and provision of content by content experts. In addition to the formal critical care course, the CNS is also involved in planning in-services and all-day programs or seminars.

A strong preceptor program is necessary to build the link between the critical care course work and the practice realities with hands-on application. Suggestions for content in preparing preceptors may include socialization of new staff, skill-building techniques, critical thinking, assignment management, giving feedback, and adult learning principles (Baltimore, 2004). Alspach (2000) has published a number of resources for preceptor programs for both health care professionals and ancillary employees.

Another option for formal educational intervention is the development of self-study materials. These can be created with a variety of components such as journal articles on a topic or audio or videotapes (perhaps obtained at a national conference such as AACN's National Teaching Institute), accompanied by self-assessment questions.

One creative educator uses audiotapes 30- to 60-minutes long to help meet the needs of her off shift staff. The tape is created by CNS/experienced staff on a regular basis and is entitled "Journal tidbits." It consists of an overview of important information gleaned from a variety of nursing journals. It may include items such as medications, treatments, and drug alerts. An inspirational/motivational topic is often included. The focus of the update is on clinical practice and research and highlights a featured article. The article is read out loud. The tape is packaged with a coversheet, including a table of contents and a written summary of feature articles (can be used as a handout for notes).

The usual preparation time is between 2 and 3 hours. Staff can check it out for use at home or in their cars or on breaks. It is approved for continuing education credits, an additional incentive for use (Cooper & Morton, 1990).

EVALUATION

If the CNS has developed the educational plan with the end in mind, the evaluation tools will already be in place and will be focused on the attainment of the expected outcomes. Evaluation of learning includes three stages. First the learning event is evaluated. This many be an in-service evaluation. It might include such questions as: Did the faculty meet the objectives? Was the presentation clear? Second, the outcome for the learning is evaluated. How has learning been incorporated into practice? Finally the impact of the learning is evaluated. Has the change in practice made any difference in patient care outcomes (Dickerson, 2003)?

Evaluation should be systematic; be ongoing; use a multiplicity of resources; and establish, monitor, and evaluate the effectiveness of educational intervention on patient care. If there are appropriate quality indicators, they should be incorporated into the evaluation.

The CNS's ability to identify the impact of educational activities on patient outcomes is vital in this cost-conscious, evidence-based practice environment. As an example, suppose the CNS recognizes the large number of patients in his or her unit who develop renal failure and determines that there is a learning need in the area of renal failure. In assessing the unit, the CNS finds that nearly all patients admitted who might be at risk (as documented in the literature) for the development of renal failure do go on to develop renal failure. The CNS intervenes with a variety of learning opportunities in this area, knowing that the best way to treat renal failure is to prevent it. Follow-up evaluation within a month of intervention shows that only 40% of patients at risk are actually going on to develop renal failure. What a powerful example of how the CNS and his or her interventions are moving patient populations toward better outcomes (and at a reduced cost!).

INTEGRATION OF THE STANDARDS OF PROFESSIONAL PRACTICE

In the late 1990s the AACN board of directors identified the need to develop Standards of Practice and Professional Performance for the Acute and Critical Care Clinical Nurse Specialist (AACN, 1998) and used the Synergy Model for Patient Care to give the standards their framework (Curley, 1998).

Quality of Care

As part of the focus on promoting quality care, the CNS develops criteria to evaluate quality and effectiveness of nursing practice. Looking for relationships between quality indicators and learning needs and using quality indicators as outcome measures are useful in ensuring quality care. Differences in practice and outcomes can trigger need for intervention that begins with designating desired outcomes, identifying practices that do not lead to those outcomes, and designing learning interventions to refocus practice in the direction of best practice. If educational plans are developed using this format, CNSs should be able to show the link between educational intervention and change in practice, a bonus for preserving the CNS role. Yeh, Hsiao, Ho, Chiang, Lin, Hse, & Lin (2004) show the positive link between educational intervention and quality care. Their educational intervention surrounding the use of restraints in the intensive care unit resulted in a change in attitude and practice. This also has implications for reporting CNS activities.

Individual Practice Evaluation

CNSs are responsible for evaluating their own practice in relation to professional practice standards and for taking action to improve their own practice. Feedback should be sought from staff, peers, colleagues, and customers. As CNSs

progress in their roles, it is common for them to believe that more emphasis on education is necessary for success in the role. CNSs have the responsibility to stay current and maintain their own clinical practice. Reading journals and using chat rooms, together with participation in seminars, course work, and other practicums on all of the CNS roles (educator, practitioner, researcher), help the CNS to know the issues.

Just as it is important for the new critical care nurse to have a role model, novice CNSs need a role model to gain feedback on their development. It is essential for an experienced CNS to be that role model and help others develop. One study that looked at development needs of the CNS found peer mentoring extremely valuable. One newer CNS commented, "What would have helped me would have been having regular contact with people already doing this sort of thing" (Bamford & Gibson, 2000).

Collegiality/Collaboration

CNSs work with many members of the interdisciplinary team in assessing, planning, implementing, and evaluating learning needs and intervention for their staff. Few patient care outcomes are solely dependent on nursing. In addition, CNSs are involved in the professional development of others, of their practice, and of their ability to facilitate learning for others.

Ethics

CNSs need to ensure that decisions/actions made on behalf of the patient are done in an ethical manner. As part of this, CNSs should be sure that they establish an ethical educational environment. For example, case studies should not include patient names or any identifying information. The same would be true of ancillary teaching materials such as electrocardiograms or x-ray films.

Research and Research Utilization

In their own practice and as they seek to make possible change in practice through facilitating learning, CNSs are responsible for evaluating nursing practice based on current research. Decisions about interventions to be used should be substantiated by research whenever possible. Creation of an educational plan, as described earlier in this chapter, with the desired patient outcome in mind from the beginning, helps provide for quantitative evaluation of any change in practice.

Often the literature review done before attempting to meet a learning need sparks clinical questions. Evidence-based practice is encouraged by incorporating research findings from published literature into clinical practice. The CNS can do this as she or he works in their learning facilitation role.

SUMMARY

The education facilitation role of the clinical nurse specialist in acute and critical care is extremely important. As acute and critical care nursing practice continues to evolve, become increasingly sophisticated, and move outside of the traditional walls of the hospital, this role will also grow in complexity. Accurate assessment, thorough planning, expert implementation, and consistent evaluation, all with improved patient outcomes in mind, will be essential to the CNS's success.

DISCUSSION QUESTIONS

1. Given the need to provide education on the newly released ACLS guidelines, how could adult learning principles be used?
2. Using a "begin with the end in mind" approach, use the five steps of planning to develop an educational plan for a need identified in your area of influence.
3. Keep track of your consultations for the past week. Identify each one as process, resource, or expert. Evaluate your consultations for any trends.
4. You are a new CNS and are tasked with developing a quality assurance plan for the upcoming year. Your institution is being surveyed by governing bodies with a focus of the survey being placed on your staff's implementation of written standards. Using the questions listed in Table 7-4, prepare an evaluation of your unit's standards.
5. An incident occurred on the intermediate care unit in which a patient received an incorrect dose of a vasoactive medication. The nurse manger asks you to do an in-service on vasoactive medications. Using the APES approach, determine if this is a problem that is appropriate to be addressed best through education.
6. You just completed a class on hemodynamic monitoring for the postanesthesia recovery unit. Develop a plan to determine if your intervention was successful in addressing your pre-identified outcomes.
7. You have determined that your staff need education on evaluating a patient's fluid balance. What would your considerations be when choosing the best venue(s)?

References

Alspach, J.G. (1982). *The educational process in critical care.* St. Louis: Mosby.

Alspach, J.G. (1984). Designing a competency-based orientation for critical care nurses. *Heart & Lung, 13*(6) 655-662.

Alspach, G.A. (2000). *Preceptor Instructor's Manual—For Professional Healthcare Staff.* Aliso Viejo, CA: AACN.

Alspach, G.A. (2000). *Preceptor Handbook—For Professional Healthcare Staff.* Aliso Viejo, CA: AACN.

Alspach, G.A. (2000). *Preceptor Handbook—From Staff Nurse to Preceptor.* Aliso Viejo, CA: AACN.

Alspach, G.A. (2000). *Preceptor Instructor's Manual—Staff Nurse to Preceptor* (6th ed.). Aliso Viejo, CA: AACN.

American Association of Critical-Care Nurses. *Essentials of critical care orientation: An Introduction to critical care.* www.aacn.org, accessed 09/15/2005.

American Association of Critical-Care Nurses. (1998). *Standards of practice and professional performance for the acute and critical care clinical nurse specialist.* Aliso Viejo, CA: Author.

Armstrong, E., & Parsa-Parsi, R. (2005). How can physicians' learning styles drive educational planning? *Academic Medicine, 80*(8), 680-684.

Bachman, J.A., Kitchens, E.K., Halley, S.S., & Ellison, K.J. (1992). Assessment of learning needs of nurse educators: continuing education implications. *Journal of Continuing Education in Nursing, 23*(1), 29-33.

Baker, C.M. (2000). Problem-based learning for nursing: integrating lessons from other disciplines with nursing experiences. *Journal of Professional Nursing, 16*(5), 258-266.

Baltimore, J.J. (2004). The hospital clinical preceptor: Essential preparation for success. *Journal of Continuing Education in Nursing, 35*(3), 133-140.

Bamford, O., & Gibson, F. (2000). The clinical nurse specialist: Perceptions of practicing CNSs of their role and development needs. *Journal of Clinical Nursing, 9,* 282-292.

Bellamy, N., Goldstein, L.D., & Tekanoff, R.A. (2000). Continuing medical education-driven skills acquisition and impact of improved patient outcomes in family practice setting. *Journal of Continuing Education in Health Professions, 20*(1), 52-61.

Benner, P. (1982). Issues in competency-based testing. *Nursing Outlook, 30*(5), 303-309.

Benner, P. (1984). *From novice to expert: Excellence and power in clinical nursing practice.* Menlo Park, CA: Addison-Wesley.

Benner, P., Stannard, D., & Hooper, P.L. (1996). A "thinking-in-action" approach to teaching clinical judgment: classroom innovation for acute care advanced practice nurses. *Advanced Practice Nursing Quarterly, 1*(4), 70-77.

Boulet, J.R., Murray, D., Kras, J., Woodhouse, J., McAllister, J., & Ziv, A. (2003). Reliability and validity of a simulation-based acute care skills assessment for medical students and residents. *Anesthesiology, 99*(6), 1270-1280.

Carlson, K.K. (Ed.). (2001). *AACN's acute and critical care orientation manual* (3rd ed.). Aliso Viejo, CA: American Association of Critical-Care Nurses.

Cavanagh, S.J., Hogan, K., & Ramgopal, T. (1995). The assessment of student nurses' learning styles using the Kolb learning styles inventory. *Nursing Education Today, 15*(3), 177-183.

Chase, C.R. (2001). Learning style theories: Matching preceptors, learners and teaching strategies in the perioperative setting. *Seminars in Perioperative Nursing, 10*(4), 184-187.

Cohen, S.S., Crego, N., Cuming, R.G., & Smyth, M. (2002). The Synergy Model and the role of clinical nurse specialists in a multisystem hospital. *American Journal of Critical Care, 11*(5), 436-446.

Cooper, S.S., & Morton, P.G. (1990). Providing CE to evening and night shift. *Journal of Continuing Education of Nurses, 21*(3), 230.

Covey, S.R. (1989). *The seven habits of highly effective people: Powerful lessons in personal change.* New York: Simon and Schuster.

Cox, C.W., & Galante, C.M. (2003). An MSN Curriculum in preparation of CCNSs: A model for consideration. *Critical Care Nursing, 23*(6), 74-80.

Curley, M.A. (1998). Patient-nurse synergy: optimizing patients' outcomes. *American Journal of Critical Care, 7*(1), 64-72.

DeBourgh, G.A. (2001). Champions for evidence-based practice: A critical role for advanced practice nurses. *AACN Clinical Issues, 12*(4), 491-508.

DeCoux, V.M. (1990). Kolb's learning style inventory: A review of its applications in nursing research. *Journal of Nursing Education, 29*(5), 202-207.

Dickerson, P. (2003). 10 Tips to help learning. *Journal of Nursing Staff Development, 19*(5), 240-246.

DiMauro, K., & Mack, L.B. (1989). A competency based orientation program for clinical nurse specialists. *Journal of Continuing Education in Nursing 20*(2), 74-78.

Earp, J.K., Capka, M.B., Davis, A.E., McLain, R.M., Ney, C.A., & Moorhead, J. (1992). Enhancing quality critical care education: Establishing a consortium. *Continuing Education in Nursing 23*(1),15-19.

Elliott, M. (2004). Reflective thinking: Turning a critical incident into a topic for research. *Professional Nursing, 19*(5), 281-283.

Good, V.S., & Schulman, C.S. (2000). Employee competency pathways. *Critical Care Nurse, 20,* 75-85.

Halm, M.A., Gagner, S., Goering, M., Sabo, J., Smith, M., & Zaccagnini, M. (2003). Interdisciplinary rounds: impact of patients, families, and staff. *Clinical Nurse Specialist, 17*(3), 133-142.

Hanneman, S.K. (1996). Advancing nursing practice with a unit-based clinical expert. *Image Journal of Nursing Scholarship, 28*(4), 331-337.

Jackson, T. (1993) *Activities that teach.* Cedar City, UT: Red Rock Publishing.

Jacobsen, C., Malan, S., Perkins, T., & Slatten, R. (1990). A regional approach to entry-level critical care education. *Focus on Critical Care, 17*(5), 385-386, 388-390, 392-393.

Janing, J. (2001). Linking teaching approaches and learning styles: How can it help students? *Emergency Medical Services, 30*(9), 77-80.

Jannings, W., & Artitage, S. (2001). Informal education: A hidden element of clinical nurse consultant practice. *Journal of Continuing Education of Nurses 32*(2), 54-59.

Jeffries, P.R., Woolf, S., & Linde, B. (2003). Technology-based vs. traditional instruction. A comparison of two methods for teaching the skill of performing a 12-lead ECG. *Nursing Education Perspectives*, 24(2), 70-74.

Kolb, D.A. (1984). *Experiential learning: Experience as the source of learning and development.* Englewood Cliffs, NJ: Prentice Hall.

Long, R.E. (2005). Using simulation to teach resuscitation: An important patient safety tool. *Critical Care Nursing Clinics of North America*, 17(1), 1-8, ix.

McKane, C.L. (2004). Clinical objectives: A method to evaluate clinical performance in critical care orientation. *Journal of Nursing Staff Development*, 20(3), 134-139.

Morton, P.G. (1997). Using a critical care simulation laboratory to teach students. *Critical Care Nursing*, 17(6), 66-69.

Morton, P.G. (2005). An annual employee education calendar as the capstone of educational assessment, planning and delivery. *Journal of Continuing Education*, 36(3), 124-132.

Oermann, M.H., & Jamison, M.T. (1989). Nursing education component in master's programs. *Journal of Nursing Education*, 28(6), 252-255.

Paparella, S.F., Mariani, B.A., Layton, K., & Carpenter, A.M. (2004). Patient safety simulation: Learning about safety never seemed more fun. *Journal of Nursing Staff Development*, 20(6), 247-252.

Sammut, N.A. (1994). Critical care education: A consortium approach. *Journal of Nursing Staff Development*, 10(4), 219-222.

Scherer, L.A., Chang, M.C., Meredith, J.W., & Battistella, F.D. (2003). Videotape review leads to rapid and sustained learning. *American Journal of Surgery*, 185, 516-520.

Scott, R.A. (1999). A description of the roles, activities, and skills of a clinical nurse specialist in the United States. *Clinical Nurse Specialist*, 13(4), 183-190.

Tennant, S. & Field, R. (2004). Continuing professional development: Does it make a difference? *Nurses in Critical Care*, 9(4), 167-172.

Thompson, C. & Crutchlow, E. (1993). Learning style research: A critical review of the literature and implications for nursing education. *Journal of Professional Nursing*, 9(1), 34-40.

Tomey, A.M. (2003). Learning with cases. *Journal of Continuing Education in Nursing*, 34(1), 34-8.

Toth, J.C. (2003). Comparing basic knowledge in critical care nursing between nurses from the United States and nurses from other countries. *American Journal of Critical Care*, 12(1), 41-46.

Vezina, M., Chiang, J., Laufer, K., Garabedian, C., Padre, H., & Sanders, N. (1996). Competency-based orientation for clinical nurse educators. *Journal of Nursing Staff Development*, 12(6), 311-313.

Wheeler, E.C. (1999). The effect of the clinical nurse specialist on patient outcomes. *Critical Care Nursing Clinics of North America*, 11(2), 269-275.

Wiecha, J, & Barrie, N. (2002). Collaborative online learning: a new approach to distance CME. *Academic Medicine*, 77, 928-929.

Wynd, C. (2002). Evidence-based education and the evaluation of a critical care course. *Journal of Continuing Education in Nursing*, 33(3), 119-125, 142-143 (quiz).

Yeh, S.H., Hsiao, C.Y., Ho, T.H., Chiang, M.C., Lin, L.W., Hsu, C.Y., & Lin, S.Y. (2004). The effects of continuing education in restraint reduction on novice nurses in intensive care units. *Journal of Nursing Research*, 12(3), 246-256.

Young, P., & Diekelmann, N. (2002). Learning to lecture: Exploring the skills, strategies, and practices of new teachers in nursing education. *Journal of Nursing Education*, 41(9), 405-412.

Collaboration

Jan Foster

INTRODUCTION

Research has shown that more patients die when nurses and physicians don't communicate and that lower mortality rates are associated with clinical nurse specialist (CNS) responsibility for staff development in a comprehensive, multidisciplinary education support system (Knaus, Draper, Wagner, & Zimmerman, 1986). Collaboration is critical for safe patient care and pivotal to the success of the CNS role. Collaboration is a key tactic to operationalizing other components of the Synergy Model in effecting quality patient care. In the AACN Synergy Model for Patient Care, collaboration is defined as "working with others to promote and encourage each person's contribution toward achieving optimal patient goals" (retrieved June, 2004 from http://www.aacn.org/certcorp.nsf/vwdoc/SynModel/), working with both intradisciplinary and interdisciplinary colleagues. Positive patient outcomes achieved through caring practices, clinical judgment, clinical inquiry, facilitation of learning, responding to diversity, and serving as a moral agent using systems thinking are best realized when the CNS uses expert knowledge and skill in collaboration with other professionals.

In the *Scope of Practice and Standards of Professional Performance for the Acute and Critical Care Clinical Nurse Specialist*, four measurement criteria are described to guide the CNS in collaboration with patients, families, and health care professionals to "create a healing and caring environment" (Bell, 2002). The criteria are: (1) consultation and referral, (2) interdisciplinary collaboration and coordination of patient care, (3) mentoring to nursing students and collaborating with nursing schools for CNS preparation, and (4) collaborating with multiple disciplines in teaching, management, and research activities for quality patient outcomes and a healthy environment (Bell, 2002).

Clinical and social skills, communication, negotiation, and coordination are essential to collaborative practice (Flaherty, 1998). Because CNSs influence change through expertise and role modeling versus administrative authority, they must have articulate communication skills to succeed in the multifaceted role of educator, researcher, consultant, and clinical leader. Integrating the dimensions of the CNS role (i.e., expert clinician, consultant, educator, and researcher) (Sparacino, 2000), the CNS uses collaboration in the three spheres of influence (i.e., patient/family, nursing personnel, and organization) to provide quality care that is the benchmark of every organization. This chapter describes collaboration for advanced practice in acute and critical care and provides examples of structures, processes, and outcomes for which collaboration is instrumental.

COLLABORATION IN EXPERT PRACTICE

Collaboration between health care providers is essential for effective patient care now more than ever before. In the current flurry of safety and quality concerns in health care, collaborative relationships are crucial. Medical errors are responsible for injury in as many as 1 out of every 25 hospital patients, and an estimated 48,000 to 98,000 patients die from medical errors annually (Institute of Medicine, 2002). Most errors are systems-related, not the result of individual negligence or misconduct. The key to reducing medical errors is to focus on improving systems of care delivery. Communication and collaboration among nurses, physicians, pharmacists, and other interdisciplinary team members form the most elemental core of the health care system, critical to error avoidance and safe patient care. A 5% reduction in mortality in magnet hospitals with collaborative relationships between nurses and physicians has been documented through research (Aiken, Smith, & Lake, 1994).

Acute and critical care nurses care for increasingly sick patients with multiple system problems, sometimes with competing management strategies, necessitating consultation from numerous specialists and disciplines. Patients often present with unique and complex situations, requiring the expert knowledge and skill of the CNS. The underlying premise of the Synergy Model is that the competencies and expertise of the nurse should increase as patients' needs intensify in effectively achieving quality patient outcomes (Curley, 1998). Using concepts from Benner (1984), collaboration can be viewed on a hierarchy of novice to expert. The nurse practicing at a novice and advanced beginner level functions largely in a follower and participative role in the collaborative process; the competent and proficient practitioner assumes some leadership responsibility and initiates opportunities for collaboration in specific circumstances in their view of "the whole" with awareness of a broader trajectory; and the CNS at the expert level actively pursues collaborative opportunities involving diverse resources across the system (Table 8-1).

Four approaches to collaboration have been described by Hanson, Spross, & Carr (2000). The first is coordination, in which providers communicate to avoid duplication and maximize efficiency of resources and use of services. Second is consultation, the process of seeking assistance or advice regarding patient care but retaining primary responsibility. Co-management, a third type of collaboration, frequently arises from consultation; each professional maintains responsibility for a specific aspect of care and together the professionals manage the patient. This has been a traditional model for critically ill patients with multiple physician and advanced practice nurse (APN) consultations (e.g., the pulmonologist writes orders for ventilator management, the nephrologist manages the dialysis, and the CNS oversees wound care). Finally, referral is the process of transferring care to another professional when the needs exceed the expertise of the provider.

TABLE 8-1	
Collaboration Across Novice-to-Expert Practice	
Novice advanced beginner	Willing to be taught, coached and/or mentored; participates in team discussions regarding patient care, open to team contributions
Competent proficient	Seeks opportunities to be taught, coached, and/or mentored; initiates and participates in discussions of patient care
Expert	Seeks opportunities to teach, coach, and mentor; facilitates active involvement and contributions of multiple disciplines regarding practice issues to optimize patient outcomes individually and globally

From Benner, P. (1984). *From novice to expert: excellence and power in clinical nursing practice.* Menlo Park, CA: Addison-Wesley.

IMPLEMENTING COLLABORATIVE PRACTICE

The standards of practice for the acute and critical care CNS are derived from the standards of practice for all nurses and include assessment, diagnosis, outcome identification, planning, implementation, and evaluation of care relevant to three spheres of influence to include patients and families, nursing personnel, and organizational systems (Bell, 2002). The CNS uses interdisciplinary and intradisciplinary collaboration at various points throughout this process. Implementation of collaboration in practice is illustrated by a case example describing a research study spearheaded by a pharmacist with a doctorate's degree (PharmD), a CNS with a doctorate's degree (PhD), and a systems analyst. This example illustrates the importance of CNS collaboration to affect positive patient outcomes with regard to medication safety in the acute and critical care setting.

CASE STUDY

The Cerner Millennium Clinical Adverse Drug Event (ADE) Alert Module (Cerner Corporation, Kansas City, MO) consists of 33 ADE alerts based on algorithms that advise the clinician when the rules of the algorithms are met. The ADE Alert Module interacts with the laboratory module in the Cerner Care4 system (Cerner Corporation, Kansas City, MO), allowing for triggers when relevant laboratory values pose potentially unsafe medication administration. In addition, alerts can be constructed around patient characteristics such as age and other prescribed medications that potentiate adverse drug responses. For a system to benefit the nurse or pharmacist, the alerts must be designed liberally enough to include potential medication safety threats to multiple patient populations with co-morbidity and a comprehensive medication database and yet conservatively enough to represent clinical significance. Excessive alerts with ill-defined clinical significance lead to desensitization by the clinician, resulting in ignored clinical alerts and potential threats to patient safety.

The system provides choices in communicating the drug alerts to either the pharmacist or the nurse via pager, text message to the Care4 inbox, or hard copy to a printer. Some alerts are best suited for the pharmacist, who should then collaborate with the physician for decisions such as choice and dosage of drugs. Other alerts related to factors such as patient age and behavior are more appropriate for the nurse to be used in medication administration decision making. Pharmacy, information systems, and nursing collaborate on this project to create the rules for triggering potential adverse drug alerts, determine best communication methods, and identify the most appropriate clinician (pharmacist or nurse) to ensure correct action in response to the alerts.

Assessment

According to the standards of practice for acute and critical care nurses, the acute and critical care CNS collects data that reflect the dynamic nature of patients and systems; identifies factors that either facilitate or act as barriers to proposed changes; and uses and designs methodology to identify gaps in knowledge, skills, and competencies for nurses (Bell, 2002). For this project it was first necessary to assess the current state of affairs with respect to medication safety to determine the potential value of this technology in averting medication errors. The CNS collaborated with risk managers and quality improvement personnel to evaluate data from root cause analyses, variance reporting, and other relevant sources concerning medication safety. Through a systematic approach to data analysis, the collaborators were able to pinpoint problem areas, including identification of drugs commonly associated with errors, type of errors, and patient outcomes.

Diagnosis

The acute and critical care CNS analyzes assessment data to determine the needs of the organization to identify factors that enhance or hamper achievement of desired outcomes for the organization (Bell, 2002). Through a systematic review of medication use, the research team identified the most problematic issues. The highest incidence of medication errors was underdosing, followed by excessive dosing. Providing subtherapeutic medication doses may unnecessarily prolong acute illnesses and invites complications from under treating both acute and chronic illnesses. Excessive doses increase the risk of dangerous side effects and both direct and indirect drug costs. Through collaboration with a PharmD, risk manager, and systems analyst, the CNS "diagnosed" a potential threat to patient safety and quality care associated with inappropriate medication administration that could possibly be resolved with adverse drug alert technology.

Outcome Identification

Expectations of the acute and critical care CNS in outcome identification are identification of risks, benefits, and costs of changes in the system, along with modifications based on needs of the organization (Bell, 2002). In the 1990s a dramatic reduction in CNSs occurred across the nation. Nurse practitioner (NP) programs grew to fill a house-staff physician shortage, and academic institutions were given grant money incentives to educate NPs, replacing CNS curricula. Confusion over the role, inconsistent use of CNSs, and failure to document the impact of the CNS on patient care and within the organization contributed to this mass exit of CNSs from the workplace setting. A renaissance of CNS practice is surging. Driven by a savvy, demanding public for quality, tight health care budgets that demand evidence-based, cost-effective practices in a system with increasingly sick patients among complex technology, organizations have a renewed interest in CNSs. However, despite this demand, CNSs must demonstrate the impact of their practice on patient care outcomes. Only through rigorous, on-going data collection and analysis of outcomes will CNSs maintain their status within the health care system.

An outcome is the end result of an intervention, treatment, or process (Houston & Miller, 1997). Morbidity and mortality have been the hallmark of outcome assessment and reporting for many years. More recently, however, especially important to APNs, additional outcome measures have been identified. Length of stay, nosocomial infection rates, functional status, and patient and nurse satisfaction, to name a few, are often directly impacted by CNS practice. Outcomes selection for measurement should be established with clear rationale, based on variables such as patient population served, known quality problems, and cost outliers. Kleinpell (2003) describes a six-step process for outcome measurement. See Table 8-2 for a summary.

Sources of outcome measures can come from internal or external triggers. Examples of internal triggers include performance improvement data, patient satisfaction scores, and variance reports. External sources include items such as published clinical guidelines, position statements, and regulatory agency mandates (Titler & Everett, 2001).

Once the outcomes for measurement have been identified, the CNS must determine how to measure. Multiple psychometric instruments are available to measure outcomes such as anxiety, pain, sedation, delirium, and satisfaction. However, the most efficient approach and perhaps the most effective is integration of the measurement process into the daily routine (Wojner, 2001). For example, in a study to

---

TABLE 8-2

Steps to Outcome Measurement

Determine indicators or measures of interest
Gather appropriate data
Aggregate and analyze data
Interpret results
Implement practice changes
Regather, analyze, and interpret data

From Kleinpell, R.M. (2003). Measuring advanced practice nursing outcomes: Strategies and resources. *Critical Care Nurse;* Feb Suppl: 6-10.

evaluate the impact of early enteral nutrition in patients following thoracic aneurysm repair, the clinical dietitian records data during routine clinical rounds. Much of the same information is necessary for both the clinical care and research study, and recording the data adds only a few minutes to completing rounds. This is not only wise use of time, but it reframes the way clinicians think, providing ongoing analysis and real-time assessment of clinical outcomes. Personal data assistant (PDA) devices are beneficial for this purpose.

Once outcome data are analyzed, the CNS must then evaluate and implement practice changes accordingly. The reevaluation process propels the entire quality improvement cycle. Identification and measurement of outcomes allows the CNS to examine processes and structures that can be improved on and, in turn, contribute to better outcomes.

In this case example, an organizational outcome was the target: improved medication safety through better processes enhanced by technology, ultimately leading to improved outcomes for patients. The overriding aim of the study was to evaluate the effectiveness of established rules for activating adverse drug alerts and to describe use of the alerts. Specific objectives were to (1) determine the usefulness of the selected alerts to pharmacy and nursing in alerting potentially unsafe medication dispensation or administration, (2) evaluate use of the communication method for the alerts, (3) identify action taken in response to the alerts, (4) determine the response rate for ADE alerts, and (5) capture the number of potentially unsafe medication events averted through use of the system.

In addition to identification of outcomes, this project required close examination of structures and processes related to medication safety. Structural components of the process included the computer system and capabilities, hard-copy physician orders and medication administration records, and the health care professionals participating in and supporting medication administration. Processes identified included order entry, medication dispensation, and administration.

An up-front evaluation of structures and processes helped not only to determine feasibility of the study but also to evaluate the potential for improved medication safety with implementation of the technology.

Planning

Movement toward positive outcomes for acutely and critically ill patients always requires careful planning. The acute and critical care CNS is charged with collaborative planning that contributes to achievement of desired outcomes (Bell, 2002). The sphere of influence for which the CNS engages in planning determines the nature of collaboration. In this case example, all three spheres were affected by the change and required consideration during the planning process. There must be collaboration among pharmacy, nursing, and information technology to determine the most useful adverse drug alerts, personnel to be alerted, and best method of communication. Nurses are key players and should be included in planning the research protocol and eventually implementing the medication safety technology since he or she is the individual charged with responding appropriately to the alert. The patient is the ultimate beneficiary, with safer care brought on by use of the drug alert technology.

Implementation

Implementation of a practice change is often the most challenging. Integrating large, complex initiatives championed by top organizational leaders through the maze of structure and personnel to the bedside level where the impact is felt is a colossal task for any organization. Likewise, there are barriers and challenges to selling a grassroots–originated idea to top administrators and decision makers. The CNS is in a pivotal position and, with knowledge of the system and clinical expertise, is often sought for leadership in organizational change. In fact, during the implementation phase of any project, the expertise of the CNS is most essential. Many protocols are stuck in committees, where the members are victimized by "analysis paralysis." The CNS is well suited to move it forward.

Critically ill patients are vulnerable and may not tolerate subtle changes in care or excess stimulation brought on by research participation. The acute and critical care CNS can determine the burden and tolerance to research participation and assist with developing methods that critically ill patients can endure. In this case example, the CNS was an experienced researcher with knowledge and skill in protocol development. Burden for nursing and pharmacy personnel was a consideration, along with feasibility issues related to current structures and processes. With clinical and research expertise, along with knowledge of medication administration processes and safety issues, the CNS was instrumental in the success of this project.

Evaluation

Evaluation is the foundation for gauging the impact of the CNS on patient and organizational outcomes. The acute and critical care CNS evaluates the effect of interventions on patient care, organizational and nursing personnel outcomes, and costs using multiple sources of data and interdisciplinary collaboration. The evaluation process is based on an analysis of risks, benefits, and cost-effectiveness (Bell, 2002). Aggregation of data is necessary for this process. Applying this case example, aggregate data were analyzed to answer each research question. Some drug alerts were more helpful than others; the best method of communicating the alerts was determined; action taken in response to the alerts was able to be captured; a response rate to the alerts was calculated; and the number of potentially unsafe medication events averted through use of the system was determined. The number and gravity of adverse drug events alerted through use of this technology was a break-through in medication safety.

Evaluation is not limited to outcomes. The CNS is charged with evaluation of the process,

structural components of the system, and any other factors that provide explanations for patient and organizational outcomes. Anticipated results, along with answers for serendipitous findings, are often found in the analysis of data and evaluation of the processes undertaken to elicit change. It is only through the evaluation of processes, structures, and outcomes that the full impact of the CNS on the system can be captured.

STANDARDS OF PROFESSIONAL PERFORMANCE

Quality Care

Quality care is the foundation of CNS practice. The CNS assumes a leadership role in establishing quality initiatives within the three spheres of influence, uses evidence-based recommendations for quality improvement, and collaborates with multiple disciplines to address barriers to quality, cost-effective care (Bell, 2002). *Quality care* is defined by The Institute of Medicine as "the degree to which health services for individuals and populations increase the likelihood of desired health outcomes and are consistent with current professional knowledge" (Donaldson, 1999). The notion of quality encompasses the concept of performance measure based on some predetermined criteria and requires a framework, which provides a method of benchmarking. One of the earlier frameworks was described by Donabedian in 1966, which consisted of a process-structure-outcome orientation. However, the emphasis of quality assessment historically has been on processes and structural components of the health system such as policies and procedures, practice guidelines, standards of care, staffing ratios, technology availability, and documentation systems, to name a few (Donabedian, 1966). In the 1990s a metamorphosis in health care began, due to the reimbursement climate and the Joint Commission on the Accreditation of Healthcare Organization's Agenda for Change (JCAHO, 2004). The link between processes and structures on patient outcomes has since become a major focus in the quest for quality care.

With increased costs of health care and decreasing employer contributions, Internet access contributing to more educated and demanding health care recipients, dissatisfaction with the system, and increasing litigiousness in our society, an "am I getting my money's worth?" mentality has grown. Likewise, competition in the marketplace, tighter reimbursement, and financial failures have driven hospitals and hospital systems to increase the focus on quality outcomes in acute care. Another framework for performance evaluation of quality care uses four categories: clinical, functional, financial, and perceptual (Hegyvary, 1991). This approach allows for the unique view of the user of the data. For example, the financial category would be of interest to the administrator and ultimately the chief financial officer, whereas the perceptual category would be relevant to the patient and manager in evaluating patient and family satisfaction. The CNS, appreciating the different viewpoints of individuals in the system, may design care strategies and data collection tools to evaluate quality outcomes in all spheres.

The American Nurses' Association (ANA) launched the Safety and Quality Initiative in 1994 to investigate the impact of massive restructuring occurring in health care on nursing practice and on the safety and quality of patient care (ANA, 2004a). Nursing-sensitive quality indicators, which are "indicators that capture care or its outcomes most affected by nursing care" (ANA, 2004a), evolved from this project. A database was established and funded by seven state nursing associations, resulting in 10 Nursing-Sensitive Quality Indicators to date. The National Database for Nursing Quality Indicators (NDNQI) is housed at the Midwest Research Institute (MRI) and jointly managed by the University of Kansas School of Nursing. The indicators for acute care are listed in Table 8-3.

A focus on nursing-sensitive indicators for performance evaluation at first glance appears antithetical to collaboration. However, because nurses in acute and critical care work with many

---

TABLE 8-3
Nursing-Sensitive Quality Indicators for Acute Care

Mix of registered nurses, licensed practical nurses, unlicensed staff caring for patients in acute care settings
Total nursing care hours per patient day
Pressure ulcers
Patient falls
Patient satisfaction with pain management
Patient satisfaction with educational information
Patient satisfaction with overall care
Patient satisfaction with nursing care
Nosocomial infection rate
Nurse staff satisfaction

From ANA. (2004a). Nursing-sensitive quality indicators for acute care settings and ANA's safety and quality initiative. Retrieved April, 2004 from http://www.nursingworld.org/quality.

---

members of the health care team who contribute to patient outcomes, it is critical that the unique contributions by nursing be measured in concert with the contributions of the multidisciplinary team (Duffy, 2002). Measurement of outcomes specific to nursing does not imply that other disciplines do not contribute to the overall well-being of the patient. Due to the multisystem problems typical of acutely and critically ill patients, quality patient outcomes result from incremental contributions from multiple disciplines that otherwise cannot be accomplished. For example, patients with atherosclerotic disease undergoing thoracic aortic aneurysm repair may achieve hemodynamic stability largely as a result of vigilant monitoring and assessment by nurses, coupled with fluid and medication therapy authorized by physicians and guided by PharmDs. However, nursing largely commandeers prevention of pressure ulcers, a very costly and quality-of-life detriment that occurs in unstable patients with compromised integumentary perfusion associated with underlying atherosclerotic disease and vascular repair.

The CNS holds clinical expertise, leadership skills, and knowledge of data collection techniques. The CNS is able to navigate the system with knowledge of resources, both material and human. In collaboration with nursing and other team members, the CNS is in an ideal position for evaluation of quality care using both nursing-sensitive and multidisciplinary indicators as performance measures.

Individual Professional Practice Evaluation

Every CNS begins his or her practice with a vision of influencing clinical outcomes; organizational effectiveness, including financial outcomes; and modeling expert care to nursing and other disciplines. It is important not to lose sight of this vision during the melee of day-to-day practice. However, more than vision is necessary for the success of the CNS. Faced with financial constraints in a dynamic health care system in constant flux and in perceived competition with other roles such as physician's assistants and the threat of emerging roles such as the clinical nurse leader (AACN, 2004), CNSs must validate their practice through individual professional practice evaluation. The CNS is charged with evaluating practice within the three spheres of influence to determine value to the organization, benefit to nursing and other disciplines, and impact on patient outcomes.

Professional practice evaluation requires three components: (1) a framework for performance appraisal, (2) establishment of performance expectations, and (3) instruments and strategies for measurement of performance. Evaluation begins with establishment of a theoretical model for evaluation derived from performance expectations. Performance expectations flow from setting goals that fit with the values and mission of the facility, along with the patient population served and nature of services provided.

Several frameworks are derived from the literature. One of the early models described by Hamric (1989) uses a functional approach in which the role and functions are demanded by societal need. The employing agency establishes

the expectations of the CNS role (Hamric, 1989). A second theoretical model emerges from symbolic interactionist theory, with a focus on the individual (Titler & Stenger, 1999). Using this framework, the CNS negotiates the activities of importance in the role and has the freedom to establish relevant performance indicators. A structure-process-outcome approach (Hamric, 1989) is also commonly used to frame CNS performance evaluation. In this theoretical approach, the structure represents the organization in which the CNS is employed. Process includes the many activities in which the CNS engages in order to fulfill the expectations of educator, consultant, researcher, leader, and clinical expert in response to needs arising in the three spheres of influence. Outcome is the measurable change or impact resulting from intervention (Kleinpell, 2003). CNS performance is measured against predetermined criteria from organizational, nursing, and patient spheres.

Evaluation of professional practice requires tools for measurement of performance. Regardless of the theoretical framework used for performance evaluation, a pretest/posttest approach best serves the CNS's ability to demonstrate effectiveness. It is recommended that the CNS collect baseline data during initial employment; or, if time has passed without establishment of a baseline, data should then be gathered before any initiative (Prevost, 2002). For example, the CNS might collect baseline data on select nursing-sensitive indicators such as pressure ulcers, ventilator-acquired pneumonia and other nosocomial infections, and unplanned extubation. Following implementation of process and structural strategies and interventions such as weekly rounds, educational summits, and implementation of evidence-based practice protocols, systematic data collection should be undertaken to evaluate improvements in patient outcome.

Despite a focus on documentation of outcomes, it is also valuable to capture the effectiveness of CNS processes. This can be achieved through traditional performance appraisal tools that highlight items established by the job description. Other methods of documentation include productivity logs and cumulative reports (Prevost, 2002). Productivity logs can be maintained manually on a weekly or monthly basis and account for time devoted to activities, processes, and programs. Data can also be maintained electronically via personal assistant devices or desktop computer devices. This method allows for easy aggregation of data through various software applications.

Cumulative reports facilitate pooling activities and outcome data across multiple CNSs within the organization (Prevost, 2002). Large databases over time can be generated, which enable CNSs to demonstrate cost savings to the institution. For example, the incidence of ventilator-acquired pneumonia can be captured before and after a CNS-driven practice protocol, and the cost savings calculated for ventilator days and intensive care unit (ICU)–related costs. This approach to performance evaluation transcends multiple perspectives, including clinical, functional, financial, and possibly perceptual categories.

Education

The role of educator for the CNS is traditionally one of the most comfortable because patient education is integral to the role of nursing even at the novice level. Standards for the APN mandate the use of current research and other evidence for knowledge and role performance enhancement (ANA, 2004b). The acute and critical care CNS is accountable for current knowledge and competency in the three spheres of influence. In addition, she or he is responsible for advancing knowledge and skills for nurses and assisting them in providing cost-effective quality care to meet a variety of cultural and ethnic requirements (Bell, 2002). CNSs participate in teaching activities in many settings and engage many individuals in addition to patients, including nurses and other health care professionals, undergraduate and graduate students, and communities. The CNS integrates knowledge derived from a theoretical base with clinical experience in both formal and informal teaching opportunities. It is the expert clinical knowledge that distinguishes the CNS educator from the academic educator without a faculty practice or other mechanism for direct participation in clinical care.

Staff Education

The CNS is uniquely positioned to educate nurses and other health care professionals. Combining theory, research, and clinical experience, there are many opportunities for both formal and informal education. The American Association of Critical-Care Nurses (AACN) position statement concerning the critical care CNS role as an educator describes six behaviors expected of the role and includes "assisting critical care nursing staff in the acquisition of practice skills and knowledge" and "contributes to the educational process and professional development of nursing students" (AACN, 1987). (See Table 8-4).

Educational needs of the staff vary, depending on where they are in the trajectory of clinical

---

TABLE 8-4

The Critical Care Clinical Nurse Specialist: Role Definition Position Statement

The Critical Care CNS As an Educator

- Seeks to improve patient and family outcomes through the application of educational concepts and skills
- Assists critical care nursing staff in the acquisition of practice skills and knowledge
- Acts as a role model of professional critical care nursing practice in the community
- Contributes to the scientific nursing literature by publishing scholarly works
- Contributes to the educational process and professional development of nursing students
- Maintains current critical care knowledge and skills in a specialty area

From AACN. (1987). *The critical care clinical nurse specialist: role definition position statement*. Newport Beach, CA: AACN.

experience and expertise. For the novice and advanced beginner, orientation, internships, and preceptor opportunities that provide prescriptive guidance in the form of protocols, policies and procedures, and practice guidelines are appropriate. The competent and proficient practitioner with 2 to 3 years of experience benefits from continuing education and in-service offerings that address decision making in complex patient scenarios. The expert is best served by shared experience and role-modeling as a means of further development to affect systematic change within the organization (Benner, 1984).

Technology and medical device use in clinical practice is ripe territory for CNS expertise. As many as 50 to 80 devices are approved by the Food and Drug Administration (FDA) on an annual basis (Feigal, Gardner, & McClellan, 2003). However, malfunction and operator error may cause harm to patients. Staying abreast of the proliferation of new devices and technology and maintaining expertise in their use is a challenge. CNSs are responsible for achieving and maintaining their own skills, as well as that of nurses, patients, and families. Manufacturer publications, clinical consultants, and other experts are resources for CNSs in technology and device education (Clark, 2003).

Collaboration between the manager, staff, unit educator, and preceptors are vital to success in implementation of the CNS educator role. Educational program development begins with a needs assessment. This can be achieved through informal mechanisms such as clinical rounds, individual consultation, and classroom discussion. A formal needs assessment can be accomplished through a written instrument, either in paper form or on-line. Listing topics relevant to practice in the unit with a Likert response approach is recommended over an open-ended method, which may invite topics that are irrelevant to the knowledge and skills necessary for quality patient care. For example, a neonatal critical care nurse may request in a write-in response an in-service on care of the adult burn patient. The neonatal CNS would be hesitant to honor this request because it is outside the scope of practice for the neonatal ICU and fulfilling the request would not be good use of resources.

Program development follows aggregation of data from needs assessments and review of other sources of determining educational needs such as job descriptions, clinical ladder criteria, new medications, technology, and changes in practice protocols based on newly published literature and research. Competency-based educational programs are commonly used in hospitals to capitalize on previously learned knowledge and skill and ensure appropriate preparation for safe practice. The CNS works in collaboration with the manager and educator to determine the necessary competencies from performance and educational-need standpoints and contributes to the process with knowledge of research and evidence-based practice changes needing to be incorporated, which provide substance for the educational offerings.

Formal program planning consists of objective and content development, determining methodology such as classroom- or computer-based teaching, establishing a timeline, budgeting and calculating a cost-benefit analysis, and developing evaluation methodology, including participant as well as overall program appraisal. Numerous resources are available in the staff development and academic teaching literature for use in educational program development.

AACN is rich with alternative and innovative educational resources. Essentials of Critical Care Orientation (ECCO) (retrieved April, 2004 from http://www.aacn.org) is an Internet-based, interactive program for teaching basics of critical care. It is designed for the novice and is self-paced and provides periodic self-assessments to monitor progress and mastery of information. Content addresses cardiovascular, pulmonary, neurological, renal, hematological, gastrointestinal, endocrine, and multisystem critical care topics. Completion of ECCO prepares the individual with the requisite knowledge for successful completion of the AACN certified critical care nurse (CCRN) examination.

AACN has an abundant selection of personal digital assistant resources, including both hardware and software for use in daily clinical practice (retrieved April, 2004 from http://www.aacn.org). Software includes practice protocols for use in caring for patients with problems in every body system, drug guides, databases, and coding and billing references, to name a few. Numerous other educational resources are available for advanced practice, clinical practice, research, and ethics for CNS use in educating staff (retrieved April, 2004 from http://www.aacn.org,).

Education for Patients and Families
Our society emphasizes health and illness and places responsibility on the individual for maintaining health and well-being. People need information to actively participate in recovery and rehabilitation from critical illness and injury. Client education can assist individuals with adaptation to changes brought on by acute and critical illness, prevent complications, fulfill prescribed treatment regimens, and promote return to functional status and quality of life (Smeltzer & Bare, 2004).

Both the ANA and AACN standards delineate the role of the CNS in client education (ANA, 2004b; Bell, 2002). The CNS is charged with synthesizing learning, motivational, and behavioral theories with relevant client health information when designing and implementing initiatives for health care education (ANA, 2004b). Expert teaching and coaching are an integral part of the CNS educator role for influence within the sphere of patients and families experiencing acute and critical illness (Sparacino, 2000). The CNS is ideally positioned to provide client education consistent with Benner's conception of expert, and is able to view the episode of critical illness or injury in the gestalt (Benner, 1984). Priorities during the critical period are identified, with an eye to the future for predictable learning needs during recovery, rehabilitation, and home care.

The teaching-learning process for acutely and critically ill patients and families can be affected by multiple factors such as readiness to learn, environmental setting, and teaching strategies used. Level of sedation; cognition; physical limitations of pain, injury, and surgery;

and emotional stress are examples of patient characteristics that may create barriers to learning. In addition, cultural variables, educational preparation, and reading skills are important considerations during the client education process (Smeltzer & Bare, 2004). Distractions in the environment such as monitors and other technology, noise, lighting, and frequent disruptions by multiple health care professionals can interfere with client learning. Finally, methods used for client education impact the effectiveness of the teaching-learning process. Group teaching and classes are sometimes useful for standardized procedures and topics such as central intravenous catheter care, intermittent urinary catheterization, glucose monitoring, postoperative cardiovascular surgery care, anticoagulation therapy, and smoking cessation. Moral support and encouragement among group members can benefit retention of learning. However, follow-up with each individual by the CNS is imperative to ensure that learning has occurred and for any additional clarification (Smeltzer & Bare, 2004). Individual, one-on-one teaching is more suitable for unique needs such as wound care, medication therapy, and specific nutritional plans. Teaching aids such as models, pamphlets, audio and videotapes, compact discs, digital video devices, computer-assisted learning modules, and Internet links can be tailored to the content and learner characteristics.

Formal community client education provides an enormous opportunity for CNSs to showcase their expertise and influence the health and well-being of its members. Programs featuring The American Heart Association's guidelines for prevention of cardiovascular disease and stroke (American Heart Association, 2004), diabetic education and prevention, and motor vehicle safety are examples of community education that focus on preventing acute and critical illness and injury, a major tenet of *Healthy People 2010* (U.S. Public Health Service, 2000).

Students
Academic education provides one of the most collaborative opportunities for CNSs. Early in

nursing's history, students were exclusively taught by clinicians. As nursing education migrated toward the university setting, the focus shifted from clinical proficiency to traditional academic learning. Early on, APNs were largely taught by physicians. The need for integrating clinical expertise with formal graduate education emerged as the APN role grew.

Linking practice and education dates back to the 1950s; at the University of Florida the administrator of both nursing education and nursing service envisioned a blend of service and education, which was operationalized by faculty caring for patients in their role of teaching students (Taylor & Marion, 2000). Several other faculty practice models have been described through the years. Currently two basic models of collaborative practice between academia and service organizations exist. In the first, faculty are employed by the educational institution which contracts with a hospital or hospital system for specific functions and roles. In this example the hospital pays the academic facility for services rendered by the faculty. In a second model, the APN is an employee of a hospital or other service-based organization and provides teaching to students in the academic program, both in the classroom setting and in a preceptor role in the clinical setting (Taylor & Marion, 2000). Several other hybrids have emerged during the most recent shortage of nurses and nursing faculty. For example, "loaned faculty" from service organizations are released from their usual responsibilities 1 day per week and provide clinical teaching and supervision to students. The incentive to the hospital is recruitment of the students following graduation, with fewer recruitment and orientation expenditures.

CNSs participate in teaching numerous health care disciplines to nursing students and at both the undergraduate and graduate levels, including medical, occupational and physical therapy, nutrition, and respiratory therapy. Often orientation for rotating residents through the various critical care services is provided by CNSs. Expert clinical knowledge and experience, coupled with good communication and teaching skills,

make the CNS an ideal candidate for teaching in this capacity.

The CNS participates in both classroom and clinical teaching. Classroom participation may include full-time responsibility or episodic guest lecturing on a topic of keen interest. In the clinical setting the CNS may hold full-time or adjunct faculty responsibility, serving in a preceptor role. Clinically precepting graduate students is a common use of CNSs in academic education. In fact, it is a requirement for graduate nursing programs to use only CNSs with appropriate expertise to teach in the CNS program (American Association of Colleges of Nursing, 1996). Preparation of future CNSs is one of the most challenging and most important opportunities for CNSs. It may provide a foundation for collaboration that extends well beyond the preceptored experience, with a potential for future scholarly activities that positively influence care for critically ill patients.

Collegiality

The ANA describes collegiality as a standard of professional practice for the APN as modeling expert practice within an interdisciplinary team to advance the development of advanced nursing practice and influence health care. This occurs through participation within a team, role modeling expert care, and mentoring others (ANA, 2004b). The nature of the acute and critical care setting provides ideal opportunity for collegiality for CNSs. Collegiality may occur through the consultant role. Consultation is defined as a collaborative, interactive process between a consultant and consultee for the purpose of enhancing outcomes for the consultee (Norwood, 1998). It is a systematic problem-solving process, which entails five phases: (1) gaining entry; (2) problem identification; (3) action planning; (4) evaluation; and (5) disengagement (Norwood, 1998). The consultation may be direct patient care oriented; indirect care oriented by providing assistance to the nurse or other caregiver; program focused, when CNS expertise is needed to guide or develop programs in the unit or institution; or administrative/consultee focused to guide processes within the organization (Walsh, 1999). In all instances the CNS collaborates with others to provide a supportive and healthy work environment that serves the best interests of patients and health care professionals.

Another example of collegiality is in the development and facilitation of clinical pathways and care maps. Clinical pathways are inherently multidisciplinary, providing a framework for coordination and communication for all disciplines participating in the care of a patient with a focus on overall outcomes. Pathways facilitate standardization of care and synergy among various caregivers, allowing all to see the contribution by each discipline; "the right hand knows what the left hand is doing." Furthermore, standardization of care allows for data aggregation and evaluation of patient outcomes. For example, development of a cardiac surgery clinical pathway program spearheaded by a CNS yielded multiple practice changes, including earlier extubation and ambulation, decreased use of sedatives, and increased gastrointestinal prophylaxis. Overall outcomes included decreased pneumonia rates, earlier increases in level of consciousness, and improved levels of nausea (Jacavone, Daniels, & Tyner, 1999). Knowledge of research, leadership skill, clinical expertise, and collaboration with other disciplines were key elements in the success of the pathway.

Ethics

Ethics represents the very essence of nursing. All of nursing energy is directed at doing "the right thing for patients." It follows that the standard of professional performance for nurses demands "ethical provisions in all areas of practice" (ANA, 2004b). Ethics is defined as "reasoned inquiry that studies both the nature of and the justification for general principles governing right conduct" (Furrow, 1991). Biomedical ethics is guided by a deontological theory of justice founded on the belief that a covenant or social contract exists between free, equal,

---

TABLE 8-5
Principles of Biomedical Ethics

Autonomy (individual choices and actions should not be constrained by others)

Nonmaleficence (do no harm)

Beneficence (do what is best)

Confidentiality (information will not be revealed)

Distributive justice (burdens and benefits should be allocated fairly and proportionately)

Truth telling (honesty and integrity; disclosure of all pertinent information)

From Furrow, B., Johnson, S., Jost, T., & Schwartz, R. (1991). The study of bioethics. In: *Bioethics: Health care law and ethics.* St. Paul, MN: West Publishing Co.

---

and rational persons and includes six principles (Furrow, Johnson, Jost, & Schwartz, 1991), listed in Table 8-5.

The ANA Code of Ethics provides guidance for fulfilling nursing responsibilities consistent with the ethical obligations of the profession of nursing (ANA, 2001). Provisions of the Code of Ethics include protection of patient dignity, privacy, and confidentiality; maintenance of professional boundaries in therapeutic relationships; advocating for patients; a commitment to practicing self-care; resolving ethical issues with patients and colleagues; and reporting illegal, incompetent, or impaired practice. In addition, ethical conduct for APNs requires CNSs to take an active role in informing patients of risks and benefits of health care regimens and participation in interdisciplinary teams dealing with ethical issues (ANA, 2001).

The ethical issues surrounding end-of-life care is an opportunity for CNSs to positively influence patients, nurses, and the organization. The CNS may be the one who initiates a referral to the ethics committee for evaluation of futility in a critically ill terminal cancer patient or severely brain-injured individual. The CNS may be a member of the ethics committee and participate in evaluation of such cases. Spearheading the development of a multidisciplinary end-of-life framework clearly exemplifies the expectations of the CNS in critical care. Holtschneider (2004) describes the implementation of a unit effort to promote communication among caregivers; family trust through consistency in practice; and most important, compassionate, dignified death without pain and suffering.

Use of narcotics for pain and anxiety and to quell the sensation of air hunger concerns is another ethical principle commonly faced by critical care nurses (Hawryluck & Harvey, 2000). The primary purpose of morphine is to promote comfort through relief of pain and suffering during the dying process; respiratory depression is a secondary or dual effect and is not a limiting factor in the administration of morphine. Ultimately the patient will stop breathing with or without morphine; but giving it will decrease pain, anxiety, the sensation of air hunger, and promote comfort. This fulfills the ethical principle of beneficence that guides nursing care (Hawryluck & Harvey, 2000).

The issue of patient confidentiality has been at the forefront of health care since the enactment of the Health Information Portability and Accountability Act (HIPAA) (Centers for Medicare and Medicaid Services, 2004). The act was designed for patients to ease the transfer of health information across providers and payers while maintaining confidentiality of personal health information. With it has come many challenges for hospitals and all health care professionals. Despite nursing's ethical underpinnings and commitment to patient confidentiality, the HIPAA has created additional challenges, particularly in the domain of quality improvement and research. Careful review by an institutional review board is advised to ensure that data collection procedures and documentation of patient information comply with the federal mandates of HIPAA (Centers for Medicare and Medicaid Services, 2004). For example, informed consent *for participation* in a descriptive, noninterventional study limited to recording of medical record information may not be necessary. However, consent *for recording the information* for purposes other than clinical management is required by the law.

Ethical issues for critically ill patients will continue to mount, with progress in genetic and stem cell research, advances in technology, an aging population amidst a youth oriented culture, and costs of health care and rationing issues, to name a few. CNSs in acute and critical care are well suited to address these complex issues that require collaboration with patients, families, and multiple disciplines within the organization.

Research

Research is fundamental to the success of the CNS. As change agents charged with impacting nursing practice that positively influence patients and health care systems, research is necessary to be effective in the role. All nurses are charged with using the best available evidence and participating in the research process at some level. In addition, CNSs are obligated to synthesize research findings and/or conduct research and disseminate the findings in order to move the science of nursing forward for the benefit of patients (ANA, 2004b). Patients are increasingly well educated about their health and come to the provider demanding specific treatment options. Payers and accreditation bodies such as the Joint Commission on Accreditation of Healthcare Organizations want evidence to show that care delivery is effective clinically and cost-wise (JCAHO, 2004).

Research skills, including utilization, evaluation, and conduct are identified as a core competency by the National Association of Clinical Nurse Specialists (1998) and the American Association of Colleges of Nursing (1996). The Essentials of Master's Education for Advanced Practice Nursing requires research as part of the core of graduate education (American Association of Colleges of Nursing, 1996). Preparation at the master's level is intended to provide the CNS with the necessary skills to critique and synthesize the literature for use in practice to improve outcomes. Some CNSs have doctoral degrees, enabling them to be producers as well as consumers of research.

Application of research encompasses both research utilization and evidence-based practice. Research utilization maintains a narrower focus than evidence-based practice. It is practical application of empirically derived knowledge or using research study findings in a setting unrelated to the original research. Simply stated, research utilization is translation into practice (Titler & Everett, 2001). In contrast, evidence-based practice is broader in scope and achieved through accumulation of knowledge. It begins with a search for the best method for solving a specific problem and entails a systematic review of the literature. The purest form of evidence is derived from rigorous research. The result is practical application and clinical decision making based on the best possible evidence (Titler & Everett, 2001).

Research-based practice requires the CNS to appraise the scientific merit, clinical significance, application to the designated patient population, and readiness for implementation of the evidence. Competency in statistical interpretation and assessment of design and other methods are necessary. In addition, weighing the evidence for decisions to implement in practice requires a systematic, rigorous approach. What is the best evidence and how does one make that determination? Randomized clinical trials are the gold standard. A true experimental design requires manipulation of a variable (treatment or intervention), randomization to the treatment or intervention group, and a control group for comparison. However, randomized clinical trials are not always achievable in clinical research because of patient variables, ethical issues, and other factors. Other levels of supporting evidence must be relied on for changing practice; as a result, nursing science is slow to move forward.

Several models to evaluate the available evidence are described in the literature. One framework (Table 8-6), developed by the American Association of Critical-Care Nurses, describes the level of scientific information available for the phenomenon of interest to determine the usefulness in practice, based on quantity of published studies (Lynn-McHale & Carlson, 2001).

TABLE 8-6
Levels of Scientific Information

I. Author/manufacturer recommendation only
II. Theory-based, no research data to support, data or recommendations from expert consensus group may exist
III. Laboratory data only, no clinical data to support
IV. Limited clinical studies to support
V. Clinical studies in more than one or two patient populations and/or situations
VI. Clinical studies in a variety of patient populations and situations

Adapted from Lynn-McHale, D.J., & Carlson, K.K. (2001). *American Association of Critical-Care Nurses (AACN) Procedure manual for critical care* (4th ed.). Philadelphia: Saunders, xv-xvi.

The Stetler Model (Stetler, 2001) uses a similar framework with the evidence scored according to design of published research studies (Table 8-7). Using either framework, the CNS conducts a systematic review of the literature, tabulates the evidence, and is required to interject judgment about implementing the change in practice. Following implementation, the CNS is charged with ongoing evaluation of outcomes, along with process and structural improvements to yield the best quality of care. The evidence-based practice movement

TABLE 8-7
Hierarchy of Evidence

I. Metaanalyses of controlled studies
II. Individual experimental studies
III. Quasi-experimental studies
IV. Nonexperimental studies
V. Program evaluations, research utilization studies, quality improvements, case reports
VI. Opinions of respected authorities and expert committees

From Stetler, C.B. (2001). Updating the Stetler Model of research utilization to facilitate evidence-based practice. *Nursing Outlook,* 49(6):272-279.

pressures CNSs to work collaboratively with a multidisciplinary team in the development of practice derived from rigorous research.

Conductors of research are also encouraged to collaborate in the research process. To affect meaningful change and quality improvement, the disciplines who participate in the care of acute and critically ill patients must engage in the research process at all stages. People bring different skill sets and knowledge to the clinical care of the patient; likewise a variety of expertise enriches the research process and leads to generation of knowledge and solutions for clinical problems. Nurse-sensitive outcomes are best recognized by the CNS, as are the most feasible and least burdensome methods. Working with experts in design and statistical analysis, as well as other health care professionals, facilitates quality investigations that contribute to science and provide further evidence that can be used to impact practice.

Technology assessment and product evaluation is another opportunity for CNSs to collaborate in the research process. The FDA approves 8000 products annually (Feigal, Gardner, & McClellan, 2003). However, new devices are less likely than new drugs to have clinical safety established before widespread use; as a result, problems sometimes occur when used for patients. With implementation of a program for medical device reporting of adverse events, manufacturers have an opportunity take corrective actions, including product recall. Over 1000 devices are recalled annually (Feigal, Gardner, & McClellan, 2003). However, rather than a model of "disseminate, report, recall, and correct," a model of "trial, correct, and disseminate" is a better standard.

Knowledge of a systematic approach to evaluation methodology, confidence with technology, collaborative skills, and clinical expertise place the CNS in an ideal position for technology assessment and product evaluation. Criteria to be considered when evaluating products, technology, and medical devices include patient safety, utility, ease of use for the practitioner, effect on patient and organizational processes and outcomes, cost-benefit ratios, and ethical considerations (Clark, 2003). Conducting formal product evaluations before purchase can be instrumental in creating a safer environment for patients and reducing costs to the organization.

Research skill is a competency for CNSs that should continue to develop after graduate school. Using knowledge derived through rigorous scientific inquiry promotes standardization in care and collaboration among multiple disciplines and facilitates capturing of outcomes in individual patients and populations. Evidence-based quality care follows.

In conclusion, collaboration for CNSs facilitates success in the role and harbors numerous benefits for patients and providers. Improvements in patient care and satisfaction, reduction in mortality, numerous examples of patient outcomes, and increased security for patients when their caregivers collaborate have been reported (Sullivan, 1998). Benefits for providers include increased sharing of responsibility and expertise, greater communication and satisfaction with problem solving, increased personal and professional satisfaction, and greater mutual respect and trust. Collaboration also bridges disparity in the cure-care paradigm, avoids redundancy while expanding care, and provides opportunities for providers to influence health policy (Sullivan, 1998). Clearly, acute and critical care CNSs can make their optimal contribution to the recovery of acutely and critically ill and injured patients through collaboration with patients, families, and other health care providers. "No [wo]man is an island" (John Donne).

DISCUSSION QUESTIONS

1. You are charged with implementation of a system wide change in medication administration. Develop a plan for how this collaborative plan can be implemented including the disciplines that will be involved as well as the needed interventions.

2. Describe three collaborative projects in critical care and identify the appropriate outcome measures.

3. How do the nursing sensitive quality indicators contribute to collaboration with other disciplines?

4. Illustrate the five steps of the consultative process within the framework of a clinical issue.

5. Explain the collaborative processes needed for implementation of a clinical pathway project.

References

Aiken, L. H., Smith, H. L., & Lake, E. T. (1994). *Lower Medicare mortality among a set of hospitals known for good nursing care. Medical Care, 32*(8), 771-787.

American Association of Colleges of Nursing. The clinical nurse leader: Developing a new nursing role. Retrieved July 2004 from http://www.aacn.nche.edu/NewNurse/index.htm.

American Association of Colleges of Nursing. (1996). *The essentials of master's education for advanced practice nursing.* Washington, D.C.: Author.

American Association of Critical-Care Nurses. (1987). *The critical care clinical nurse specialist: role definition position statement.* Newport Beach, CA: Author.

American Heart Association. Get with the guidelines. Retrieved July, 2004 from http://www.americanheart.org/presenter.jhtml?identifier=1165.

American Nurses Association. (2001). *Code of ethics with interpretive statements.* Washington, D.C.: Author.

American Nurses Association. (2004a) Nursing-sensitive quality indicators for acute care settings and ANA's safety and quality initiative. Retrieved April, 2004 from http://www.nursingworld.org/quality.

American Nurses Association (2004b). *Scope and Standards of Practice.* Washington, D.C.: Author.

Bell, L. (2002). *Scope of practice and standards of professional performance for the acute and critical care clinical nurse specialist.* Aliso Viejo, CA: American Association of Critical-Care Nurses.

Benner, P. (1984). *From novice to expert excellence and power in clinical nursing practice.* Menlo Park, CA: Addison-Wesley.

Centers for Medicare and Medicaid Services. The Health Insurance Portability and Accountability Act of 1996 (HIPAA). Retrieved July, 2004 from http://www.cms.hhs.gov/hipaa/. Cerner Corporation, Kansas City, MO.

Clark, A.P. (2003). Malfunction prevention and technology expertise, legal and ethical dimensions of CNS practice. *Clinical Nurse Specialist, 17*(3), 126-127.

Curley, M. (1998). Patient synergy: Optimizing patients' outcomes. *American Journal of Critical Care, 7*(1) (electronic version). Retrieved March, 2004 from http//:www.aacn.org/certcorp/certcorp.

Donabedian, A. (1966). Evaluating the quality of medical care. *Milbamnk Memorial Fund Quarterly, 44*(2), 166-206.

Donaldson, M.S. (Ed.). (1999). *The National Roundtable on Health Care Quality, Institute of Medicine. Measuring the quality of health care.* Washington, D.C.: National Academy Press.

Duffy, J.R. The clinical leadership role of the CNS in the identification of nursing-sensitive and multidisciplinary quality indicator sets. *Clinical Nurse Specialist, 16*(2), 70-76.

Feigal, D.W., Gardner, S.N., & McClellan, M. (2003). Ensuring safe and effective medical devices. *New England Journal of Medicine, 348,* 191-192.

Flaherty, M.J. (1998). Collaboration: Clinical nurse specialists can lead the way. *Clinical Nurse Specialist, 12*(4), 160-163.

Furrow, B., Johnson, S., Jost, T., & Schwartz, R. (1991). The study of bioethics. In: *Bioethics: Health care law and ethics.* St. Paul, MN: West Publishing Co.

Hamric, A.B. (1989). A model for CNS evaluation. In Hamric, A.B., Sprouss, J.A. (Eds.). *The clinical nurse specialist in theory and practice.* (2nd ed). Philadelphia: Saunders.

Hanson, C.M., Spross, J.A., & Carr, D.B. (2000). In Hamric, A.B. Spross, J.A., & Hanson, C.M. (2000). *Advanced nursing practice an integrative approach.* Philadelphia: Saunders.

Hawryluck L.A., & Harvey, W.R. (2000). Analgesia, virtue, and the principle of double effect. *Journal of Palliative Care, 16* Suppl, S24-S30.

Hegyvary, S.T. (1991). Issues in outcome research. *Journal of Nursing Quality Assurance, 5*(21), 1-6.

Holtschneider, M. (2004). Guidelines aimed at improving practice around end-of-life care. *AACN News, 21*(4): 4.

Houston, S., & Miller, M. (1997). The quality and outcomes management connection. *Critical Care Nursing Quarterly*, 19, 80-89.

Institute of Medicine (2002). *Care without coverage: Too little, too late*. Washington, D.C.: National Academy Press.

Jacavone, J., Daniels, R., & Tyner, I. (1999). CNS facilitation of a cardiac surgery clinical pathway program. *Clinical Nurse Specialist*, 13(3), 126-132.

Joint Commission on the Accreditation of Healthcare Organization: Agenda for Change. Retrieved April, 2004, from http://www.JCAHO.org/agendaforchange/main/html.

Kleinpell, R.M. (2003). Measuring advanced practice nursing outcomes: Strategies and resources. *Critical Care Nurse*; Feb Suppl: 6010.

Knaus, W.A., Draper, E.A., Wagner, D.P., & Zimmerman, J.E. (1986). An evaluation of outcome from intensive care in major medical centers. *Annals of Internal Medicine*, 104, 410-418.

Lynn-McHale, D.J., & Carlson, K.K. (2001). *American Association of Critical-Care Nurses (AACN) Procedure manual for critical care* (4th ed.). Philadelphia: Saunders, xv-xvi.

National Association of Clinical Nurse Specialists (NACNS). (1998). *Statement on clinical nurse specialists practice and education*. Harrisburg, PA: NACNS, 1-28.

Norwood, S. (1998). *Nurses as consultants*. Menlo Park, CA: Addison-Wesley.

Prevost, S. (2002). Clinical nurse specialist outcomes: vision, voice, and value. *Clinical Nurse Specialist*, 16(3), 119-124.

Smeltzer, S.C., & Bare, B.G. (2004). Health education and health promotion. In *Brunner and Suddarth's textbook of medical-surgical nursing* (10th ed). Philadelphia: Lippincott, Williams, & Wilkins, pp. 45-56.

Sparacino, P. In Hamric, A.B., Spross, J.A., & Hanson, C.M. (2000). *Advanced nursing practice an integrative approach*, pp. 381-405. Philadelphia: Saunders.

Stetler C.B. (2001). Updating the Stetler Model of research utilization to facilitate evidence-based practice. *Nursing Outlook*, 49(6):272-279.

Sullivan, T. J. (1998). *Collaboration: A healthcare imperative*. New York: McGraw-Hill Health Professions Division.

Taylor, D., & Marion, L. (2002). In Hamric, A.B., Spross, J.A., & Hanson, C.M. *Advanced nursing practice an integrative approach*, pp. 381-405. Philadelphia: Saunders.

The AACN Synergy Model for Patient Care. Retrieved March, 2004 from http://www.aacn.org/certcorp.nsf/vwdoc/SynModel/.

Titler, M.G., & Stenger, K.M. (1999). Role evaluation for the critical care clinical nurse specialist. In American Association of Critical Care Nurses (Eds.). Gawlinski, A., & Kern, L.S., *The clinical nurse specialist role in critical care*, Philadelphia: Saunders, pp. 275-292.

Titler M.G., & Everett, L.Q. (2001). Translating research into practice. Considerations for critical care investigators. *Critical Care Nursing Clinics of North America*, 13(4), 587-604.

U.S. Public Health Service (2000). *Healthy people 2010: Understanding and improving health*. Washington D.C., U.S. Government Printing Office.

Walsh, S. (1999). The critical care clinical nurse specialist role in consultation. In American Association of Critical Care Nurses (Eds.). Gawlinski, A., & Kern, L.S. *The clinical nurse specialist role in critical care*, Philadelphia: Saunders, pp. 143-154.

Wojner, A. (2001). *Outcomes management: Application to clinical practice*. St. Louis: Mosby.

Systems Thinking

Mary Fran Tracy
Ruth Lindquist

INTRODUCTION

Today clinical nurse specialists (CNSs) are functioning in highly complex health care environments. Issues facing CNSs in their roles include patients with multiple interacting disease conditions and patients and families with diverse backgrounds and complex dynamics. The context of health care includes nursing shortages and aging nurses. Environments can be characterized as having information overload, increased use of technology, and intricate though not well-articulated relationships among health care organizations along the health care continuum. In light of the complexity and demand, there seem to be fewer and fewer resources to provide quality care and meet specifications of ever-changing regulatory requirements. CNSs are recognized as leaders in health care who can achieve positive outcomes for patients, staff, health care organizations, and the nursing profession. A key to effectiveness and creating positive outcomes in this current health care environment is the CNSs' ability to know their system and use systems thinking to address and resolve patient issues. CNSs translate issues from organizational, nursing, staff, and patient perspectives using systems thinking.

Systems thinking is part of the repertoire of CNSs' unique set of skills derived from experience and advanced educational preparation that enables them to look beyond the immediate situation and circumstance and to use more global thinking to lead to creative and innovative solutions. Use of systems thinking may be viewed as expanding effectiveness and capacity to serve patients and the institution. It is viewed by some as the most rewarding aspect and best part of the role. CNSs often use systems thinking to serve as change agents within an organization.

This chapter defines systems thinking, identifies activities to consider in developing a systems thinking approach, and offers examples of tools and resources to assist CNSs in the process of systems thinking. Things that contribute to the development and use of systems thinking, including systematic use of the nursing process within the context of the AACN Synergy Model for Patient Care, are reviewed. A case study illustrating systems thinking is presented.

DEFINITION

Systems thinking is defined as applying a broad outlook that encompasses information and resources beyond the immediate environment that results in innovative problem resolution or the advancement of practice (Bell, 2002; National Association of Clinical Nurse Specialists, 2004). CNSs who use systems thinking develop and implement a wide variety of strategies in work and anticipate the consequences of change (Bell, 2002). Through this broad anticipatory outlook, CNSs can develop proactive strategies and the ability to critically evaluate what is working well, determine what needs to be improved, and implement an efficient process for improvements to achieve quality, cost-effective outcomes (National Association of Clinical Nurse Specialists, 2004). It has been stated that systems thinkers need to ask the difficult questions and challenge the status quo (Cassidy, 1996).

Advanced practice nurses are well educated in the nursing process and typically apply it in their clinical practice while working directly one-on-one with patients and staff and in the resolution of unit and institutional problems. CNSs use systems thinking to take the nursing process from a micro level (i.e., one-on-one with patients) and translate it into a macro level (i.e., system-wide) as they gain experience. CNSs are valuable providers in health care organizations; thus they may be asked to lead efforts both within and outside of their immediate specialized area of clinical expertise because of their leadership and their ability to use systems thinking expertise. CNSs do not necessarily need to be content experts to facilitate projects but rather can use these facilitation skills to complete broad-based projects that rely on the expertise of others. Over time, novice CNSs learn that they do not need to have all the answers (Bierema, 2003) but instead need to have key abilities to collaborate, know resources, use inquiry, ask the right questions, and communicate effectively.

Experienced CNSs use the whole repertoire of CNS competencies outlined in the Synergy Model in a systems-thinking approach when addressing problems or developing policies, including clinical judgment, patient advocacy, clinical inquiry, facilitator of learning, and a caring collaborative approach (Bell, 2002). Systems thinking requires analytic skills, pattern recognition, attention to organizational ethics, and sensitivity and awareness of organizational culture.

Systems thinking is used to resolve problems and to gather and apply information. It must be timely and encompass essential detail and depth to be effective. Carefully calculated risk taking is part of the CNS role and the process of problem solving. Decisions are made using the best information available to the CNS at the time. An understanding of system and health care trends may lead to greater understanding and generation of more relevant and successful solutions. Although information is seldom complete, the CNS who uses systems thinking will have anticipated potential pitfalls, have backup plans in place, and be confident that she or he has used the best judgment along with available information to make the best possible decision. Ideally this results in more effective, meaningful, and stable solutions.

The wide array of requirements by regulatory agencies (e.g., Joint Commission on Accreditation of Healthcare Organizations [JCAHO] and the Centers for Medicare and Medicaid Services) necessitate systems thinking by CNSs when looking to resolve issues related to patient care. Resolution of patient care issues frequently involves multiple disciplines, solutions that work across patient populations, and standardization of care whenever possible. It also makes fiscal sense to try to thoroughly investigate and resolve problems through systems thinking. Proper systems thinking ensures that the needs of the system and interests of the patient are in balance and requires an understanding of competing priorities.

CNSs are involved in many projects as they evolve from novice to expert. These types of projects include product evaluation, problem resolution, quality improvement projects, change processes, error reduction initiatives, and the creation and modification of care delivery models. Their success in resolving problems relies not only on their problem-solving abilities but also on their level of expertise as it evolves over time.

CNS LEVEL OF EXPERTISE

CNSs learn and grow with experience. The CNS role evolves and develops with the person, role, and institution. Benner's theory of nurses' development from novice to expert is applicable to the nurse in the CNS role as well (Benner, 1984). Novice CNSs need time to learn about the three spheres of influence—patient, nursing personnel, and organization—in which they will be practicing. Depending on experience, typically the CNS focuses on learning about the patient population he or she is working with in the specific environment and establishing a respectful, trusting relationship with the nursing staff. At this point systems thinking is usually low level and limited to projects focused in the isolated environment of the unit with the CNS as the primary resource. Strategies used fit within the system. They are limited, and attention is intermediate, focused on people and components in the immediate environment rather than on the broad and holistic view and (Bell, 2002). The novice nurse may not have the complete picture of the whole and may not understand the broad relationships of the immediate circumstances to other less obvious factors that are salient to the problem and its solution.

CNSs who are new to the role may take some time in learning how things work in their environment, the kind of impact they can make, and how to advance nursing and systems processes. As CNSs progress in experience, they begin to make connections between the component parts of issues in the local environmental context within the broader system; they are able to anticipate likely outcomes over space and time. As experience increases, there is a broadening of the array of potential strategies to address the issue, including seeing potential for negotiation despite lack of negotiating skill. CNSs start to look to other resources beyond themselves and envision the patient/family as transitioning beyond the immediate environment. CNSs who are mature in the role have earned the respect of their colleagues and are seasoned and appreciate the system (Bell, 2002).

The experienced CNS generally uses a fully developed systems thinking approach to problems and strategic planning. Strategies are developed and implemented by integrating an holistic perspective encompassing a broadly inclusive outlook. The expert CNS can think "outside the box" in negotiating with or on behalf of patients and families (Bell, 2002). Experienced CNSs can recognize opportunities to acquire unique resources and can anticipate future needs

and challenges of both individual patients and populations. They can see commonalities and opportunities for collaboration between what are apparently diverse populations (e.g., how standards can be consistent for nursing practices in obstetrics and bone marrow transplant or between pediatrics and adults). They also recognize when an issue is so vastly different between populations that a population-specific or even a patient-specific approach is in the best interest of patients.

Care-related insights grow as the CNS develops in the role. A novice CNS may assume that technological advances are always better and improve practice and patient care. However, an experienced CNS knows that, although technology can at times improve practice, it can also resolve one issue while perhaps introducing even more deleterious issues not anticipated if not fully evaluated before implementation.

As CNSs progress from novice to expert, much growth occurs that contributes to further evolve capacity for systems thinking. Expert CNSs are open to and readily seek diverse opinions and views as they recognize that this results in stronger solutions. Expert CNSs also assess the culture of the organization within which they are functioning, recognizing that the organization's mission, vision, values, and strategic priorities will all impact their practice.

With experience, the CNS becomes more sensitive and responsive to information collected during a change of adoption of a new procedure. The CNS can then use judgment as to whether to proceed with the change as planned, alter the implementation plan, or determine that the change should be deferred because of timing or shifting prioritization of the problem or issues.

The CNS who adeptly uses systems thinking can accurately evaluate the system environment to judge when to assertively advocate for an outcome and when to adjust the plan because timing or priorities are not right. Systems thinking is implemented most effectively in practice in an ongoing way as advanced practice nurses carry out the nursing process from assessment to evaluation at the macro level.

IMPLEMENTATION WITHIN THE DIMENSION OF PRACTICE

Assessment

A key step in the initiation of any project or problem-solving effort is the comprehensive assessment of the issue or area of concern. The identification of key stakeholders, including those who will be impacted, is an important step to take to decide who should be involved in the project or problem-solving process. Accurate proactive identification may reduce the risk of potentially excluding key stakeholders who could derail the process at a later time if they do not understand the plan or who have contrary viewpoints and action. It is also important to get a wide range of perspectives since, without these perspectives, the project would not be fully informed. Different viewpoints should not be ignored or dismissed. Further, it may be strategic to engage "naysayers" in the problem solving.

It is important to assess the scope of the project to enable estimates of time and costs to provide for appropriate allocation of resources and to develop reasonable timelines. Identifying ground rules of any project or program is a key step to take before beginning. For example, knowing whether the solution needs to be budget neutral or not is essential to be able to successfully formulate a plan or propose a solution. It is helpful for CNSs to proactively identify the level of authority they or their group has in working on the solution to determine whether it is expected that they will gather data only, make recommendations to a higher authority, or have full authority to decide on a plan and act to implement it for problem resolution (Manthey and Miller, 1994). Assessment is a critical step to take before project initiation to understand and know the organizational culture. With this knowledge, CNSs can determine whether the project aligns with organizational strategic priorities, as well as unit, staff, or patient priorities. Not only does the CNS use the system and its resources, but the CNS's actions may add to or build his or her understanding of the structure of the organization. Alignment with priorities of stakeholders makes it more likely to have resources allocated to the effort and the attention needed to successfully implement the work to achieve the desired outcomes. A successful comprehensive assessment is followed by a fully informed diagnosis that is "on target" and centered on the problem to be addressed in context of the system as a whole.

Diagnosis

The second step in problem solving with a systems approach is the full and accurate identification of the most essential issue in formulating a diagnosis. This step ensures that the diagnosis is built on the full and solid assessment of the system and relevant circumstances. A good diagnosis is necessary for future steps that focus on the development of innovative solutions to address the problem or project. There is nothing as discouraging as implementing a costly or time-insensitive solution that doesn't solve the "real" practice problem faced because the diagnosis missed the central issue or problem. Selected tools to help in the identification of the central or true problem are described later in this chapter.

Having all key stakeholders at the table as the information is processed and the problem is diagnosed may sharpen the diagnosis. Inclusion and consideration of diverse viewpoints at this point are valuable in making the diagnosis, identifying what the issues are, and identifying desired outcomes. In complex organizations such as health care environments, there is often not one cause or one diagnosis that can be made. It is important to take the time to fully assess the problem and then study the data acquired to understand the situation and its context. Ultimately the CNS and the project team must proceed with their best judgment as to the proper diagnosis, which in effect targets the problem as it defined. The diagnosis must flow directly from the assessment and not from pet ideas for solutions.

Outcome Identification

The more clearly that desired outcomes are identified early in the process (before planning and implementation), the easier it is to identify approaches to implement actions that are likely to succeed in achieving the outcomes desired. CNSs who use systems thinking are able to consider a range of possible scenarios of potential consequences that may result from their contemplated actions. During the process of implementation, if anticipated outcomes are not materializing as intended, the plan may be modified. Likewise, if the anticipated outcomes are shaping up as planned, implementation efforts may be sustained or increased.

Once the outcomes are identified, systems thinking CNSs will also be cognizant of other alternative outcome opportunities as interim analyses are conducted at predetermined phases throughout the process. This is especially true in the planning phase, in which actions are selected and standardized or individualized to the patient, the unit, or the hospital.

Planning

The planning phase includes evaluation and gathering of support and resources. Budgets are created, and communication of the planned work is structured and systematic. Throughout this phase the team continues to think through the work to the plausible outcomes and anticipates adverse consequences that may be easier or less costly to address in the planning phase (preventive planning) than to remedy during full implementation. It is important to plan for interim reevaluation(s) to be sure that the work is achieving intended effects and so that adjustments can be made along the way to ensure intended results. The timing of these depends on the project, the judgment of the team, and the phases of the project. Good planning includes the evaluation of the strengths and weaknesses of alternative strategies and the selection of the option judged to be the most likely to bring about the desired outcomes. A good plan serves as a useful, sufficiently detailed blueprint for the actions of implementation.

Implementation

The smooth implementation of the planned effort may be impeded by a number of factors—foreseeable and unforeseeable. In cases in which the problem addressed is significant and the solution broad ranging or the effects evident only after some time, one may need to wait a significant amount of time for the results of the effort to be evidenced. In such cases it is wise to give the effort enough time to work to be open to the likelihood that the effort will work in the end. However, during this process it is necessary to consider the potential need to refine strategies and to address barriers that arise. These must be anticipated when possible and identified as soon as there is evidence of their presence. Barriers to implementation include such things as:

- Resistance of staff to change and engagement in new behaviors or practices
- Changes in approval or regulations
- Cost increases or overruns
- Loss of interest and support

Likewise, some facilitators support effective implementation that ought to be considered. These include the following:

- Inclusiveness of individuals involved and affected as much as possible
- Careful judgment in the timing of implementation
- Clear and respectful communication to stakeholders affected
- Appropriate and adequate education
- Gathering of resources needed
- Nimbleness in changing course or modifying the plan as reality warrants
- Openness to change and refinement and a continuing evaluation of the effects of the refinement

The CNS must be open to hearing about negative impact of the change and may decide to tolerate it because it may be related to change in and of itself versus making a change in course or abandoning the plan altogether. This latter is difficult to do but may ultimately be the best course of action in some circumstances. Throughout the project good communication with constituencies may foster support and enable the project to come to successful completion. However, to accurately determine the effects of the project, an evaluation plan must be conducted.

Evaluation

During the evaluation phase a complete review of the outcomes of the effort is accomplished, and conclusions from the work are derived. If a good plan was developed before initiation of the work, the process of evaluation is facilitated. Development of an evaluation plan before implementation facilitates the evaluation at the conclusion of the project. Some adjustments may need to be made to accommodate the modifications in the implementation activity. An essential step is to evaluate whether the outcome goals have been achieved by assessment to determine whether criteria that have been set were achieved and, if so, to what degree. If outcomes have been achieved, the project is complete. If outcomes have not been achieved or have only partially been achieved, the process of assessment and planning begins again either to further revise the plan that has been implemented or to select another plan for implementation. In some cases the end point may need to be revised. Often a judgment is needed about when the work is considered complete. It is important to make sure that the necessary objectives have been accomplished.

Once the evaluation is completed, it is important to disseminate the findings of the work. If the project was significant, perhaps the findings of the work and the process could be disseminated beyond the unit (e.g., throughout the institution via a poster display or institutional newsletter). If the project uses a novel approach or reflects "best practices," dissemination beyond the institution may be indicated. Other institutions

in the area may be interested in the findings; or the process and outcomes of the work may be of interest to professional audiences, and an abstract could be submitted at a professional nursing meeting or an interdisciplinary meeting. Perhaps publication of the process and outcomes and the experience of implementation may be of interest to readers of professional clinical journals or educational journals.

One step often overlooked is that of celebration. It is important that the team and the CNS be rewarded for work well done. It is also important to present a summary of the work and effort to supervisors so that proper credit may be given for work done.

Examples of key systems thinking questions that CNSs can use when initiating a project are listed in Box 9-1. To illustrate steps in the process, a case study of a performance improvement project headed by a CNS is presented in Table 9-1.

Standards of professional performance are never static and need specific goals and direction for full integration. Many interesting and unexpected challenges surface when working at a systems thinking level. Systems thinking opens new dimensions in professional practice. New layers and levels of complexity within the system are encountered. The rewards garnered through systems thinking are substantially different from those of focused daily unit practice. There is a need for translation of goals and objectives with other disciplines. Collaborative relationships develop; it is necessary to understand alternate perspectives and ways of addressing problems. The priorities of the other disciplines may be different and foreign to the CNS. However, the integration of systems thinking into ones' professional practice and practice standards is likely to contribute to improved quality of care through usual processes.

INTEGRATION OF STANDARDS OF PROFESSIONAL PERFORMANCE

Quality Care

Quality care is the main goal of practice. Systems thinking broadens the identification

BOX 9-1

Examples of Key Questions in Project Planning

Assessment
- Who should be involved or consulted? Who are key stakeholders? Who will be impacted?
- What is the scope of the project?
- What level of authority will you or the project team have?
- What are the ground rules or requirements (e.g., budget implications)?
- How does this project align with organization, department, or unit priorities?

Diagnosis
- What is the real issue to be addressed?
- What are the formal and informal power bases?

Outcomes
- What are the impacts of the potential solutions?
- What are the potential consequences of the solutions and potential resulting issues?

- What are the consequences of individualization versus standardization?

Planning
- At what points will interim evaluations be done?
- What are the strengths and weaknesses of alternatives?

Implementation
- What are the barriers and facilitators to implementation?
- Who needs to be educated and informed?
- Who needs communication about the solutions or as progress is made?

Evaluation
- How will the solution be evaluated?
- What criteria will be used to judge success?
- How will you disseminate the results?

TABLE 9-1

Case Study of a CNS-Led Oral Care Protocol Implementation

Process Stage	Systems Thinking Context
Assessment	
Expectation that nursing has unit-based continuous quality improvement projects	Alignment with organizational priorities
CNS-led brainstorming of Nursing Practice Council members to identify potential projects	Engagement of stakeholders
Oral care and its role in development of ventilator-acquired pneumonia (VAP) identified as high priority	Engagement of stakeholders Alignment with organization and regulatory priorities (JCAHO)
CNS-taught staff to do literature search and critique of research	Engagement of stakeholders Advance nursing practice beyond daily clinical skills
Initial contact with Infection Control, Cardiopulmonary Services, Organizational Learning, Performance Improvement, Nurse Managers, Corporate Materials	Key stakeholders Alignment with organizational priorities
Diagnosis	
Identification of all potential issues related to oral care, including staff knowledge deficit, lack of standards, oral care product availability and ease of use, extent of problem, documentation that supports standard of care	Full exploration and delineation of problem
Developed and conducted survey of current staff practices with large variation noted	Exploration and delineation of problem

Continued

TABLE 9-1	
Case Study of a CNS-Led Oral Care Protocol Implementation—cont'd	
Process Stage	**Systems Thinking Context**
Outcomes	
Protocol development	Standardization of care
Cost-benefit analysis (increased cost of product; decreased cost of VAP)	Engage materials financial consultant
Baseline VAP rates data	Engage Infection Control Data tracking
Commitment of all adult intensive care units (ICUs) to use same protocol	Standardization vs. individualization
Planning	
Product evaluation	Right tools Address barriers
Buy-in from all adult ICUs in health system's five hospitals	Standardization of product
Changing documentation in computerized charting	Address barriers
Education in-service planning	Engage stakeholders Education
Staff buy-in, including ancillary staff and aides	Engage stakeholders
Develop audit tool	Data tracking Evaluation tool
Develop timeline for implementation of all components (product, protocol, charting, education)	Preparation and prioritization Ensuring all steps have been considered
Negotiate accountability for product distribution	Engage involvement of unit materials supply personnel
Implementation	
Oral care protocol compliance annual staff performance goal by Nurse Managers	Engage stakeholders Alignment priorities
Listen for feedback	Interim evaluations
Evaluation	
Audit protocol compliance through charting	Evaluation of criteria achievement
Post implementation VAP rates	Evaluation of criteria achievement
Consider application for evidence-based practice (EBP) award	Dissemination of findings Celebrating success
Submission of abstract presentation at EBP conference	Dissemination of findings Celebrating success

and scope of what can be accomplished to achieve quality practice and patient care. Continuous quality improvement (CQI) is a good example. Using systems thinking in CQI embraces a fuller set of criteria from which judgments of effect may be made. Further, results of the CQI process using systems thinking tends to be more robust. With a systems approach, benchmarking is broadened from the unit or department perspective to a standard within a hospital, across hospitals, or within consortiums. The depth and scope of the impact are expected to be enlarged and enduring, and the result likely to impact more than one practice discipline. Identification of "best practices" is another way to improve quality of care. Best practice data may be shared and expanded to other systems where the adoption can result in improved patient outcomes.

The systems thinker recognizes that controlling the organization or its parts is impossible; rather the goal should be the ability to predict based on longitudinal patterns and behaviors (Bierema, 2003). Many techniques and tools can be used in the quality process that advance systems thinking. These include things such as root cause analysis, flowcharting, and Fishbone diagrams (Pande, Neuman, and Cavanagh, 2002). Specific tools can be useful for specific problems or phases of a process (Table 9-2). They support a systematic way to explore the full extent of an issue.

TABLE 9-2
Selected Examples of Quality Improvement Tools

Type of Tool	Use	Application
Pareto charts	Compares frequency and/or impact of types or causes of a problem Allows focus on prioritization of issues	Setting priorities Defining problems Determining root causes
Run charts	To measure and track key input, process or output over time	Identify trends and patterns Determining potential root causes Follow-up and verification of results
Histograms	To show the range, amount, and patterns of variation in a group of data	To see range and distribution of continuous factors To see how many defects occur in a group of items To see how key characteristics in a group are distributed
Fishbone or Ishikawa diagram	To identify the cause of a problem by applying the experience and expertise of a group in structured brainstorming	Determining major causes Determining potential root causes Determining solution options Planning a process change or solution
Relations diagram	To help a team identify the drivers (root causes) of a complex problem	To understand complex relationships To reach consensus within a team on key causes or drivers to investigate further
Scatter plots	To measure and identify possible relationships between variables	Provide data to confirm a hypothesis that two variables are related Evaluate strength of a potential relationship Follow up to cause-and-effect analysis
Stratified charts	To look for patterns in data that link to root causes	Used primarily to see if theories about causes or patterns are supported by data
Flowcharts	To visually represent the steps/tasks, sequences, and relationships within a process or system	Identify problems Define a process Analyze potential areas for improvement and simplification

A systems thinking perspective on cause-and-effect relationships is different from the traditional perspective in that cause and effect are viewed as interdependent and circular rather than as a linear relationship (Pickett and Kennedy, 2003). The identification of common denominators that underlie adverse occurrences can be useful in efforts to improve quality of care. Insights may be gained as to the causality of problems and prospects for their resolution through examining practices and outcomes both upstream and downstream from the adverse events.

Although these practices are commonly used by CNSs, how does the CNS determine how successful and effective he or she is in using systems thinking? Self-assessments and evaluation by supervisors or peers may be useful.

Individual Practice Evaluation

Novice CNSs can use mentoring relationships as a means to gain expertise and evaluate their skills as systems thinkers. Mentors can assist in professional growth and offer perspectives that are key in developing systems thinking skills.

When systems thinking is used effectively, networks of professional colleagues are established within and outside of nursing as the CNS seeks to gain insight through the inclusion of multiple perspectives and ideas. Information, help, and support flow in and out of the CNSs' domain. Such a network comprises key people who may be practice authorities. Affiliation with these individuals enriches CNSs' careers and the potential to make contributions to practice. Their professional effectiveness and resourcefulness are augmented through the experts that they have cultivated and have at hand.

As CNSs grow in systems thinking, it is imperative that they use critical self-reflection to evaluate how their behaviors and assumptions impact the problem-solving process (Bierema, 2003). Introspection and self-evaluation of their performance can be difficult but are needed to continue to develop as a leader in systems thinking.

Education

The systems thinker makes the most of education by considering its effectiveness in broader terms. Education is not planned in a silo, but efforts are made to use education to its fullest possibilities. When developing education, CNSs are constantly aware of others who may benefit from the education—nurses in other units, professionals in other departments, patients in other but similar populations, and nurses or patients at other hospitals. The systems thinking CNS also looks at the ever-increasing education needed by nurses beyond their immediate, population-focused clinical knowledge and skills. With the increasingly complex health care environment, the systems thinking CNS is proactive and visionary in providing education for nurses to develop the skills needed for the future. Such CNSs find creative ways to develop nurses and oneself professionally through a combination of education and experience. They realize that relying on clinical experience alone can be limiting in the increasingly complex health care environment (Bierema, 2003). The systems thinking CNS can incorporate principles useful in areas outside of health care to health care issues and education as appropriate.

Collegiality

Collegiality is a characteristic of the systems thinking nurse. Collegiality is reflected in the tone with which nurses relate to others within the same discipline, as well as across disciplines. Collegiality is reflected in the development of resources. It is reflected in engagement and mature interest in shared success, whether it be ones' own or that of ones' colleague. Collegiality thrives when individuals respect the skills and talents of others and value and foster the leadership skills and potential of one another. There is mutual interest and investment in practice of one another. One example was a city in which a strong collegial network of CNSs had been established to form a mutually beneficial and helpful resource for professional practice in the geographic area. When the CNS has been collegial and built networks, the richness of the network can be brought to bear on problems and issues such that many minds are focused on its resolution and the intellectual pool on which to draw is enlarged. Networking with CNS colleagues can be done in person, over the phone, and through the use of listservs or email.

It is essential that a CNS build a network in her or his own institution to help others appreciate CNS skills in achieving positive outcomes. This is done through interactions that promote others to seek her or his opinion and involvement. Having CNSs included early in change processes that impact nursing practice and patient care is imperative to the achievement of positive results. It can be frustrating when a CNS is consistently brought into a project in its late stages only to have to point out gaps in the plan that can have deleterious consequences if not addressed. If this happens frequently, the CNS can start to appear to function as a barrier when he or she could have been a viewed as a facilitator if consulted earlier. To prevent this from occurring, CNSs need to help educate others about their roles and expertise. One tool that highlights how to encourage others about how and when to involve CNSs is presented in Fig. 9-1.

Collegiality is a tone set in interactions. There is a willingness to engage and consider respectfully with the other to move toward a mutually desired outcome. Collegiality can be expressed by the novice or the expert. It is based on respect and appreciation of what each individual has to offer. Collegiality means that one is open to the perspective of others, a crucial component of systems thinking. To achieve this, CNSs must help others understand their role and their unique skills, including the ability to make decisions and actions of ethical nursing practice and patient advocacy.

Ethics

Ethics is always at issue in work using resources and completed in the context of competing priorities. Commonly competing demands exist in settings and among contingencies comprising the human environment of institutions. For example, there may be competition between patients' needs versus nurses' needs versus the needs of the institution. The best interests of the patient, nurse, and system are considered in light of available resources and specified goals. Ethical considerations are eminent when an expert opinion is not popular or acceptable to some stakeholder or contingent within the institution.

Patient advocacy is almost by definition a systems thinking phenomenon. It connotes the promotion of the rights and interests of the patient within the system of care when a patients' rights or well-being are at risk within that system.

Nurses and CNSs are challenged continuously to reduce costs and to manage resources responsibly. It is incumbent on CNSs to show the results of their labor and of their expenditure of these resources. They are challenged to maintain and improve the quality of care. In this process there is an exchange of resources and competition for resources to address needs within and across units. Decisions are hard to make because goals are not always aligned. It is clear that there must be an evidence base to support the use of resources. One might challenge the use of untested interventions that use human or financial resources so that efficient and effective practice is the norm. Systems thinking requires that evidenced-based practice be the norm and that a broad analysis of risks and benefits will promote ethical practice.

Collaboration

Systems thinking does not support an individualistic approach. Collaboration is a process of working together in a particular activity. A partnership is formed that is most successful if it benefits both or all parties that are involved. Successful collaborations can be forged when all parties are in agreement as to the goals of the project within the system. Collaborations are beneficial when the work and minds of many are brought together to address a common problem. It is helpful to have common goals and

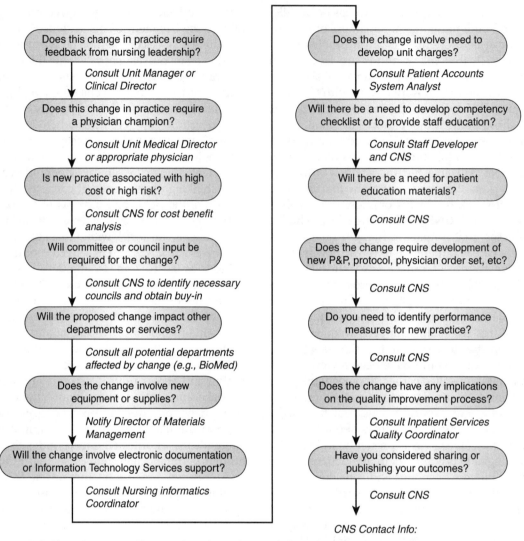

FIG 9-1 JPS Clinical Practice Change Algorithm. This is a resource tool and is not meant to take the place of critical judgment. (Hanson, D. [personal communication, March 4, 2004]; Hanson, D., & Harrington, L. (2003). Clinical practice change algorithm, John Peter Smith Health System, Unpublished figure.)

perspectives established at the outset to unite the parties in the systems approach. Successful teams tend to have high levels of trust, share a vision, use ground rules, learn from errors, be able to challenge each other openly, and feel empowered to take risks (Cassidy, 1996).

Collaborations wrought by systems thinking are fueled by progress toward goals that are mutually set and values that are shared. Often

mutual agreement can be extended to other areas of concern and interest. Systems thinking is useful for many project areas in which CNSs are involved. For example, when adopting new equipment in a unit, a CNS with systems thinking recognizes that this equipment is used throughout the institution. Thus it may be efficient to plan implementation of educational programs together with other units. Or such collaborations may be set by institutional planning, enabling CNSs and professionals from a variety of areas to work together to do systems planning. This activity can foster systems thinking for future strategic activities.

Research

Research is an important role function of the CNS. Systems thinking highlights the importance of evidence-based practice (EBP) as it fosters an awareness of practice outside ones' immediate environment. Numerous tools are available to promote EBP. EBP and clinical resources are easily accessible on the Internet and listed in Table 9-3.

As data are consistently gathered for EBP, it can be a challenge to manage the references and

information acquired. Electronic tools are available to help track these references and organize the evidence found.

The analytical skills of CNSs are vital in systems thinking processes. As more data and information are gathered, the CNS can be overwhelmed with the amount of information, some of it conflicting. In addition, systems thinking fosters the development of more comprehensive efforts in problem solving and analytical processing and helps to prioritize and evaluate the meaning of the data (McDaniel, 2003a).

CNSs may also use systems thinking in their conduct of research. One important practice is to conduct replication studies to determine the relevance of findings in the literature to specific clinical populations, or evaluation studies may be used to determine whether EBPs that are

TABLE 9-3

Selected Resources for Evidence-Based Practice

Resource	Purpose of Site	Web Address
Joanna Briggs Institute	Some systematic reviews as well as links to evidence-based practice (EBP) resources and hints on how to evaluate Internet information	www.joannabriggs.edu.au
Academic Center for Evidence-Based Nursing	Links to EBP resources and education about EBP	www.acestar.uthscsa.edu
Agency for Healthcare Research and Quality	Sponsors and conducts research that promotes evidence-based information on outcomes, quality, cost, use, and access to health care	www.ahcpr.gov
National Guideline Clearinghouse	Database of EBP guidelines developed by associations, health care organizations, institutes, and governmental agencies	www.guideline.gov
Cochrane Database	Provides access to systematic reviews of interventions and promotes evidence in the form of clinical trials	www.cochrane.org
National Library of Medicine	Provides free online access to Medline	www.ncbi.nlm.nih.gov/PubMed
Healthcare Cost and Utilization Project	Collection of health care databases and software tools that include longitudinal hospital care data, medical practice patterns, and outcomes of treatments	www.ahcpr.gov/data/hcup

adopted, for example, are from the literature or successful experience of others.

Resource Utilization

CNSs have accountability for responsible use of resources, including those of the patient, the population, nursing staff, and the institution. This is true when considering competing priorities in the context of limited budgetary resources. It is in a CNS's best interest to become familiar with the financial tools and software used in his or her institution. Although it is unlikely that the CNS will become an expert in those tools, partnering with a financial expert will facilitate full evaluation of the resources used and required by the particular population and unit. CNSs need to be able to understand the financial data well enough to interpret whether it is accurately reflecting what he or she is seeing in clinical practice and to address discrepancies or misinterpretations when they occur. In addition, the CNS can readily track her or his own population and project data with hardware and software, including Excel spreadsheets, statistical packages (SPSS or SAS), and databases. These databases can have shared access by one or two users or more broad access across the institution. A well constructed database permits the sorting of fields to present reports to assist in and to inform decision making that can have a large impact.

In addition to tracking fiscal outcomes, other useful outcomes may relate to efficacy and satisfaction. An example of this could be decreasing unnecessary waste by using research related to changing invasive tubing. Resource costs of intravenous tubing replacement can be optimized through knowledge of the length of time that the tubing can remain in place before colonization and infection occur. Further, cost-benefit evaluations can be tracked and monitored; it may be systematically determined that a product that has the lowest cost may not perform as well as a more costly product and vice-versa. The margins in these cases may be revealed with good data.

Data must be selected with forethought and relevant to the needs of the unit and the context of the larger system. Managing relevant data is critical for the CNS who is trying to evaluate a problem (McDaniel, 2003b). Technology solutions are increasingly valuable and necessary because of the increasing amount of data generated and available. Wise use of technology may be timesaving and increase efficiency of work. For example, the use of handheld personal data assistants may be used to track data as it is generated. The planned selection and purchase of such technology requires good systems thinking and coordination among the end users so that the range of needs is served.

CONCLUSION

CNSs have the greatest capacity to function and perform at optimal levels when decisions are informed by systems thinking and a broader perspective on problems faced. Systems thinking can result in solutions woven together by professionals from a number of disciplines working together. Systems thinking can improve and expand on needs of a broader constituency and render the solution more durable and useful to institutions. Best practices may result in synergistic effects that increase the quality of care and the health of the institution. Solutions that are the result of a systems approach may create an articulation of service components that result in greater efficiencies and transformation of practice and policies within an institution. With the systems based "big picture," CNSs' efforts are more likely to have an impact on a patient population, multiple units, or an institution as a whole rather than single individuals or single units.

Systems thinking opens up new perspectives and integration in an organizational structure of an institution. It may give greater meaning to the work of the CNS and may result in broad impact institutionally. Conversely, the broad solutions of a larger context may have impact on individuals and be brought back to the bedside to directly improve patient care.

Keeping abreast of current trends beyond ones' own clinical area enriches perspectives and expands which resources are brought to the point of care. Systems thinking is a process in which the CNS may gather information to enhance and broaden understanding. It may result in an enlarged influence within an organization; efficacy of organizations may be enhanced; and the role of the CNS as an effective change agent is enhanced.

DISCUSSION QUESTIONS

1. Describe the skill progression of a CNS from novice to expert through the development of systems thinking.
2. Discuss the leadership role of the CNS in systems thinking.
3. List key points to consider in each phase of a project when using systems thinking.
4. Discuss the potential consequences of not using systems thinking when implementing practice changes.

References

Bell, L. (Ed.). (2002). *Scope of practice and standards of professional performance for the acute and critical care clinical nurse specialist.* Aliso Viejo, CA: American Association of Critical-Care Nurses.

Benner, P. (1984). *From novice to expert: Excellence and power in clinical nursing practice.* Menlo Park, CA: Addison-Wesley.

Bierema, L.L. (2003). Systems thinking: A new lens for old problems. *Journal of Continuing Education of the Health Professions,* 23(Supp 1), S27-S33.

Cassidy, J. (1996). Systems thinking helps leaders handle change. *Health Progress,* 77(1), 44-45.

Manthey, M., and Miller, D. (1994). Empowerment through levels of authority. *Journal of Nursing Administration,* 24(7/8), 23.

McDaniel, A.M. (2003a). Using technology to advance the knowledge work of clinical nurse specialists: Part II: Transforming data into information and knowledge. *Clinical Nurse Specialist,* 17(3), 123-125.

McDaniel, A.M. (2003b). Using technology to advance the knowledge work of clinical nurse specialists: Part I: Organizing data. *Clinical Nurse Specialist,* 17(2), 78-80.

National Association of Clinical Nurse Specialists. (2004). Statement on clinical nurse specialist practice and education. (2nd ed.). Harrisburg, PA: Author.

Pande, P.S., Neuman, R.P., & Cavanagh, R.R. (2002). *The six sigma way team fieldbook.* New York: McGraw-Hill.

Pickett, R.B. & Kennedy, M.M. (2003). Systems thinking and managing complexity, Part one. *Clinical Leadership Management Review,* 17(1), 34-38.

Advocacy and Moral Agency: Quintessential Nursing

Linda J. Bell
Ramón Lavandero

Remove advocacy and one emasculates nursing. Deploring the unsanitary conditions of 19th-century hospitals and identifying four essential elements in the health of hospitals, Florence Nightingale implanted advocacy in the essence of modern nursing. Not only did Nightingale promote the health of patients and their care environments, she championed the cause of evidence-based health care, contributing a large sum to endow the first professorship in applied statistics at Oxford University. It was never established "because the subject wasn't covered in university examinations, a major criterion for deciding which subjects to teach" (Dossey, 2000).

In contemporary nursing Virginia Henderson's widely espoused definition of nursing, a foundational source of the American Association of Critical-Care Nurses (AACN) Synergy Model for Patient Care, moved advocacy and moral agency front and center as cardinal components of the role of a clinical nurse specialist (CNS):

> The unique function of the nurses [she writes] is to assist the individual, sick or well, in the performance of those activities contributing to health or its recovery (or to peaceful death) that he [sic] would perform unaided if he had the necessary strength, will, or knowledge.

And to do this in such a way as to help him gain independence as rapidly as possible (Henderson, 1966).

Expanding on the principle that helping patients to communicate with others is an element of basic nursing care, Henderson points to this interpreter-communicator role as essential because *separation from family and friends and the fear of altered relationships are responsible for much of the suffering attendant on sickness* (Henderson, 1997).

DEFINING ADVOCACY AND MORAL AGENCY: WHY IT IS IMPORTANT

Leah Curtin proposes that nursing distinguishes itself not by its functions but by a philosophy of care (Curtin, 1979). Since they seek the welfare of others, Curtin suggests, nurses ultimately pursue a moral end, making nursing a moral art in which the goal is that of seeking what is good. This goal is reached by nurses' relationship with others by carrying out the fundamental role of advocate. The role of advocacy is not one more function added to a steadily growing list, she suggests. Rather, advocacy embraces all of nursing's functions because it lays the foundation by which nurse and patient "freely determine the form [their] relationship is to have" (Curtin, 1979). Curtin's framework allows for several definitions of advocacy to co-exist. Advocacy has been defined as "active support; the act of pleading or arguing in favor of something, such as a cause, idea or policy" (American Heritage, 2004). The word derives from the Latin *advocare* meaning "to call to one's aid" (Random House, 2006). The AACN defines advocacy as "working on another's behalf and representing the concerns of the patient, family, and community" (Bell, 2002).

Advocacy and moral agency have been codified in several ways. Nurse Practice Acts in many American states consider advocacy to be one of nurses' roles. The third statement of the American Nurses Association (ANA) Code of Ethics for Nurses states that "the nurse promotes, advocates for and strives to protect the health, safety and rights of the patient" (ANA, 2004).

Considered as a person's "ability to act upon or influence a situation," moral agency can be shown when a CNS engages, responds, and transforms a situation on behalf of a patient, family, colleague, or system (Hardin & Kaplow, 2005). Patricia Benner describes "skillful moral comportment" as expertise that nurses develop through experience. Benner defines ethical comportment as "the embodied, skilled know-how of relating to others in ways that are respectful and support their concerns" (Benner, 1991). Along with thoughts and feelings such as words, intentions, beliefs, and values, comportment includes physical actions such as stance, touch, and orientation.

A qualitative study by Lindahl and Sandman examined the role of advocacy in critical care nursing. They suggest that advocacy assumes meaning from the moral and existential response between two human beings. It occurs as "an outspoken demand of another human being whose autonomy is threatened" (Lindahl & Sandman, 1998). Further validating Curtin's premise that the nurse and patient decide the nature of their relationship, the researchers

identified seven themes representing a range of advocacy roles: building a caring relationship, carrying out a commitment, empowering, making room for and interconnecting, being a risk taker, being a moral agent, and creating a trusting atmosphere conducive to recovery (Lindahl & Sandman, 1998).

Skilled listening is critical when assessing the need for advocacy and moral agency. And listening implies risk because listening means getting involved, especially if one disagrees with what is being said (Burghardt, 2000). The Canadian philosopher Bernard Lonergan proposed a practical approach listening, calling it transcendental because it is not limited to a specific field. Simply put, Lonergan's approach has four principles: be attentive, be intelligent, be reasonable, be responsible (Lonergan, 1971). *Being attentive* means giving full rein to one's experience, gathering the data and facts. *Being intelligent* necessitates moving beyond raw data to understand what is going on and why. *Being reasonable* represents judging the situation with wisdom, which may require soliciting consultation from others with greater experience or objectivity. Finally, *being responsible* means acting with discernment and sincerity. Burghardt cautions that fear can limit what someone hears (i.e., fear of not knowing what actions one can and should take) (Burghardt, 2000).

A CASE FOR ADVOCACY: SETTING THE STAGE

The following case vividly illustrates how advocacy and moral agency permeate every level of health care, from the microsystem at a patient's bedside to the macrosystem of an entire health system. This case does not include the interventions of the CNS but provides an optimal scenario to demonstrate the application of the CNS role in the health care environment.

An intensive care unit (ICU) nurse receives morning report from the night shift nurse. Five days earlier this 76-year-old man had abdominal surgery and had been extubated for 2 days. He had been up in the chair and talking with his family the day before. During the night his blood pressure slowly dropped, even after several fluid boluses, and he became increasingly obtunded. After report, the nurse assesses the patient as responsive only to noxious stimuli. The surgeons replace a positional arterial line and establish central venous access for fluid management. Vasopressors are started. During these procedures it also is determined that the patient requires intubation. The physician notifies one daughter by telephone that her father's condition is deteriorating. There is no advance directive in the patient's record.

The arterial line replacement is in progress, and the anesthesiologist has arrived to perform the intubation when two daughters and a son-in-law come into the room. "What are you doing? He has an advance directive and wouldn't have wanted any of this!" the daughter states. The physicians ask the charge nurse to have the family step out while they complete the procedures, and then there will be time to talk. The advance directive cannot be found, nor does the patient's record have a physician's note about advance directives. After the patient has been intubated, one physician speaks alone with the family. They agree that no further resuscitative efforts will be made but also that no therapies will be withdrawn until the patient can be evaluated more extensively.

While one physician is talking with the family, a second physician completes suturing the arterial line, and the nurse reassesses the patient. The patient is mechanically ventilated and not triggering the ventilator. Despite large-volume fluid infusions and vasopressors, the blood pressure remains low.

The family has not yet been allowed to see the patient. However, the second physician proceeds to talk with them about amending the plan of care to allow aggressive treatment since it appears to this physician that the patient is responding to verbal commands. The family visits the patient and find that he does not respond to their voices or touch. They return to the waiting room, agonizing between the possibility of their father's survival with aggressive

treatment and disregard for his wishes. Their brother died of leukemia at a young age and their mother of end-stage lung disease 5 years earlier. This familiarity with complex care is also helping them to ask medically appropriate questions.

The charge nurse invites the family back into the patient's room, even though visiting times and number of visitors are usually restricted. They talk with the bedside nurse about their father and what he would want, asking for more information about the continued therapy. One daughter asks what the nurse would do if this was her father. "I don't know your dad," the nurse says. "This is my first day caring for him. But I can tell you that we will probably get him through today and maybe tomorrow. Yet, even if he survives, he will not be the same man you brought in when he leaves the hospital." The family thanks the nurse for her honesty and decides that aggressive treatment would not be in their father's best interest since full recovery is unlikely.

When the family tells the physician of their decision, he returns to advocate for continued aggressive therapy. The family insists that no further therapy be instituted and preferably that current therapy be withdrawn. The unhappy physician finally agrees and writes orders to titrate sedation and decrease both blood pressure and ventilatory support. The bedside nurse intervenes so the charge nurse will extend visiting time from the unit policy of two visitors for 15 minutes up to four times per day. This allows the family to ask questions, tell stories, and say goodbye to their father. The daughters choose to leave, preferring not to be with their father when he dies. The son-in-law and grandsons elect to stay, fondly talking about the patient's life and his presence in their lives as a "man's man." They stay until he dies, shed some tears, and leave, saying that, in the end, they have persevered to honor his needs.

INTEGRATION OF STANDARDS OF PRACTICE

The standards of practice for the acute and critical care CNS role parallel the familiar elements of the nursing process: assessment, diagnosis, outcome identification, planning, implementation, and evaluation. As set forth by the AACN, they have been applied to the unique exigencies of advanced nursing practice and span three spheres of influence: patient and family members, nurses, and organizational systems (Bell, 2002).

When assessing the need for advocacy and moral agency, the CNS should be guided by an ethic of open-mindedness. Defined by ethicist David Thomas in his practical guide titled *The Ethics of Choice*, this ethic states that "it is ethical to be open to the possibility that your view is incomplete and therefore capable of expansion and improvement. It is unethical to ignore information that could allow you and/or your organization to grow" (Thomas, 2003).

ANALYSIS OF A CASE FOR ADVOCACY: CNS PERSPECTIVE

Analysis of *A Case for Advocacy* offers the opportunity of examining against the standards of practice the impact that a CNS could have in each sphere of influence. A note of caution: when committed to writing, a case study will appear to be linear and sequential. In reality, a CNS moves back and forth among each standard and each sphere of influence, responding to the demands of the situation. For clarity, the appropriate standard and sphere(s) of influence are identified as the analysis progresses.

In this scenario the CNS would first step back to identify and evaluate the various perspectives present at this patient's bedside (assessment—patient/family/nurse). There is no advance directive available for immediate review; thus the patient's family would be considered the patient's proxy. His wife is deceased; two daughters are the closest living immediate family. Both daughters are present and agree about what the patient would/would not want, so there is no need to mediate family differences. It would be appropriate for the CNS to clarify the bedside nurse's understanding of issues surrounding patient proxy.

This can be done at the moment or by debriefing with the nurse later on (assessment—nurse).

Additional factors confound the situation. The physician first acts based on the only available information (i.e., that, in the absence of advance directives and before the family arrived, this patient would have been a candidate for complete resuscitation). The physician made decisions about clinical interventions based on that assumption. Confronted with disagreement from family, his inclination was to proceed with the clinical interventions, leaving the bedside nurse to solve the dilemma of determining a course of action. The physician is clearly uncomfortable having the family present since they disagree with the interventions. The CNS could help the bedside nurse to understand the appropriateness of continuing emergent therapy until further discussion with the family can take place (AACN, 2004; Meyers, Eichhorn, Guzzetta, et al., 2000). The bedside nurse would need to understand that future dialogue with the physician will be necessary for family members to be present during procedures and resuscitation efforts. Through these actions the CNS provides a safe environment for continuing dialogue with the family, physician(s), and the nurse. Ultimately the CNS could facilitate interdisciplinary philosophical dialogue directed at reaching a unit norm and processes to facilitate family presence and open visiting since this cannot be arbitrarily instituted during an emergent situation (Hamric & Reigle, 2005). The CNS can use the current case situation as a springboard for this future dialogue (outcome identification—nurse/nursing personnel/organizational system).

Once the immediate situation has been defused, the CNS can spend time discussing the patient's wishes with the family. This dialogue can help to identify how communication has broken down and the family's immediate expectations and concerns. Family dialogue can uncover additional information that can be conveyed to the physician before his next interaction with them (diagnosis—patient/family).

Dialogue will also allow family members to ask questions about precipitating events and possible outcomes. This information can be shared with the physician and bedside nurse, enabling them to clarify any questions the family may ask at the bedside. This opportunity for dialogue continues to support a safe environment for all of the participants (implementation—patient/family, nurse, and organizational system).

The goal of these ongoing interactions with family members, bedside nurse, and physician is to bring everyone into consensus about the best course of action for the patient (outcome identification—patient/family, nurse/nursing personnel). Effective communication and true collaboration with everyone involved will be required to discern progress. As the CNS moves through these interactions, she or he can role model and coach behaviors for the bedside nurse, the patient's family, and the physician. This requires the CNS to skillfully integrate education and past experiences while separating his or her perceptions or biases and the participants' emotions and agendas in each interaction. The CNS has the best opportunity to advocate for the patient (i.e., to take on the patient's perspective given his inability to do so) while gaining an understanding of the additional perspectives represented at the bedside and all those represented in patient's care (assessment, outcome identification—patient/family, nurse/nursing personnel).

Once urgent patient care needs have been met, the bedside nurse and the CNS can continue to discuss what is known about the patient and family. Clearly family relationships have been strong since family members have been visiting and calling for condition updates. The daughters could speak about "how he was yesterday" because they had been with the patient. Understanding these relationships provides useful insight so the CNS can determine how best to approach the family. It also helps the CNS to provide the physician with information that will facilitate decision making for optimal patient and family outcomes (planning—patient/family).

It is essential for the CNS to facilitate dialogue between the physician and the patient's family. Although the physician may need to attend other patients, his personal communication will help to provide connection and context for the family members. Initial dialogue with the patient's family and physician should take place in a private space away from the bedside so everyone can focus on the discussion at hand. The CNS can best facilitate the dialogue in the role of patient advocate; calling to mind that it is the patient's interests that must be served while clarifying potential misunderstandings among the participants (Hamric & Reigle, 2005) (implementation—patient/family).

If at all possible, the bedside nurse should be present during the family dialogue, providing another opportunity for the CNS to role model and coach advocacy behaviors. However, unit staffing and patient acuity may not allow the bedside nurse to participate, in which case the CNS should provide the nurse with information about the discussion and its outcomes, allowing time for the nurse to seek clarification and ask questions (implementation—nurse/nursing personnel). Optimally the CNS would also validate shared understanding with the physician after every family conference to ensure common goals and strategies for continuing care.

The CNS can prepare the bedside nurse for the family's presence and be available to help answer any questions. As facilitator and advocate, she or he is in the best position to clarify family understanding of exactly what has been done, what it is possible to do, and the potential outcomes of those actions (intervention—patient/family, nurse/nursing personnel). The CNS is also present to witness dialogue between family members and with the patient, providing additional understanding of any underlying issues that may need to be addressed (assessment—patient/family).

In this case it became clear that the physician's immediate goal of care for the patient differed from the daughters' long-term goal for their father. The women talked about previous experiences with the health care system (i.e., witnessing the death of their mother and their younger brother, both of whom had long-term chronic diseases). The challenge for the CNS and the bedside nurse is to verify for the physician that the family truly does understand the potential outcomes he discussed with them (implementation—patient/family, nurse/nursing personnel).

The CNS must also advocate for effective end-of-life care once the decision to discontinue aggressive therapy is reached (implementation—nurse/nursing personnel, organizational system). End-of-life care includes care for both the patient and the family. The family's willingness and/or desire to be present during the patient's final hours must be assessed and supported (outcome identification, implementation—patient/family). The CNS and bedside nurse may be called on to give family members permission either to be absent or present, providing equal support to both choices. Validation that either option is acceptable will allow family members to participate in end-of-life care in the way that best meets individual needs.

Advocacy for the patient's end-of-life care includes assessment of sedation and pain management along with other comfort needs. The CNS can help the bedside nurse to evaluate current medical orders to identify any additional requirements while the physician is still readily available (assessment—patient; implementation—nurse/nursing personnel).

The circumstances leading to the decision for end-of-life care in an ICU can create moral distress and place a tremendous emotional burden on a bedside nurse. The CNS must pay attention to issues that arise for the nurse and the unit personnel. These issues can arise from physician-nurse interactions; hospital and unit policies about family presence; experience level of the nurse/comfort in managing this type of patient care, and ability to adjust patient care based on the acuity of the patient and experience of the nurse. Each issue needs to be identified and addressed so the nurse and unit personnel can be debriefed appropriately.

The CNS has the ability and accountability to ensure both the identification and the interventions best suited to everyone involved (evaluation—nurse/nursing personnel, organizational system). An outcome of this evaluation may lead to the development and implementation of a structured protocol for end-of-life care, ensuring that each patient and family will be evaluated and provided for appropriately. In addition, the CNS has the opportunity to follow up on satisfaction data for end-of-life care, which provides the patient and family perspective (assessment, outcomes—patient/family, organizational system).

INTEGRATION OF THE STANDARDS OF PROFESSIONAL PERFORMANCE

A CNS has the opportunity of role modeling and further influencing advocacy in the patient/family, nurse/nursing, and organizational or system level spheres (NACNS, 2004). The uniqueness of the CNS role allows movement among and between spheres of influence, making those advocacy activities deeply felt. It is the CNS's ability to role model behavior in all three spheres that will pave the way for the next generation of strong advocates for patients and families, health care organizations, and the nursing profession. For acute and critical care the AACN standards of professional performance for CNSs are used as guideposts in implementing and evaluating the role (Bell, 2002).

Quality Care

The acute and critical care CNS systematically develops criteria for, and evaluates the quality and effectiveness of, nursing practice and organizational systems (Bell, 2002).

A CNS is accountable for ensuring that his or her practice meets the standards of professional performance. In the preceding patient scenario, the CNS can monitor and evaluate both the quality of nursing care provided and the interdisciplinary actions/interactions that occur.

This includes an evaluation of his or her own practice to ensure that both the CNS scope of practice as an advanced practice nurse and the bedside nurse's scope of practice are acknowledged and maintained. Neither of the nurses should seek to exceed or abdicate his or her responsibilities to the patient, the family, the physician, or each other.

Individual Practice Evaluation

The acute and critical care CNS evaluates his or her practice in relation to professional practice standards and relevant regulations (Bell, 2002).

When debriefing about the patient scenario just described, a CNS must assess his or her own individual actions. As part of this accountability for individual practice evaluation; the CNS will use nursing's Code of Ethics with Interpretive Statements (ANA, 2004) to ensure that practice meets the standards expected of the professional nurse. To provide the broadest scope of evaluation, the CNS may request additional clarification and feedback from the bedside nurse, physician, and perhaps the family to identify areas for improvement. The feedback ethic defined by David Thomas is a useful yardstick: "It is ethical to request, encourage and deliver feedback on all facets of individual and organizational performance. It is unethical to ignore, discourage or fail to give feedback" (Thomas, 2003).

Education

The acute and critical care CNS acquires and maintains current knowledge and competency in the three spheres of influence in acute and critical care nursing (Bell, 2002).

Topics for further education of a practicing CNS often involve clinical practice issues. For example, to effectively advocate in the case described previously, a knowledgeable CNS would need to be familiar with current recommendations for effective decision making in end-of-life care in acute and critical care. Mastering strategies for creating a work environment that supports nurses' advocacy efforts would be a

second topic. But where does a CNS or, for that matter, any nurse learn about advocacy and moral agency? Two experiential studies, one with a robust study sample of 62 nurses, sought to answer this question and identify recurring themes about what advocacy involves. The researchers found that the learning is situationally dependent and rather haphazard, not systematically included in nursing education programs (Foley, Minick, & Kee, 2002). They identified safeguarding as an overarching pattern with four related themes: protecting, attending the whole person, being the patient's voice, and preserving personhood (Foley, Minick, & Kee, 2000).

Accordingly, CNSs, especially those new in the role, need to focus attention on honing their competency in advocacy and moral agency while acquiring supportive collateral skills (e.g., skill in professional visibility that uses what Bernice Buresh and Suzanne Gordon term the *voice of agency,* someone who "is instrumental, through whom power is exerted" [Buresh & Gordon, 2006]). The voice of agency will become invaluable as the CNS learns how to be influential, overcoming barriers and teaching others to do the same (Sullivan, 2004). Equally important will be skill in holding successful crucial conversations when stakes are high (Patterson, Grenny, McMillan, & Switzler, 2002) and navigating crucial confrontations when faced with bad behavior, broken promises, and expectations gone bad (Patterson, Grenny, McMillan, & Switzler, 2005).

Collegiality

The acute and critical care CNS contributes to the professional development of peers, colleagues, and others (Bell, 2002).

Lucille Joel advances the intriguing notion that advocacy is a duty of citizenship in the nursing profession. Joel cites the 18th century French writer Alexis de Tocqueville who distinguished between inhabitants and citizens. "Inhabitants become complacent towards the future," she quotes from de Tocqueville. Applied to nursing, "we find ourselves in a profession where most members are content to be inhabitants," she expands. Nurses "find it difficult to identify with newcomers to the profession, seeing it as a bother to precept their practice or develop their qualities of professional citizenship" (Joel, 1998). As role models, teachers, coaches, and mentors, CNSs fulfill a critical role of guiding new nurses into full citizenship within their profession.

CNSs are obligated to be role models of collegiality, not only with nursing peers but among all the professional disciplines participating in patient care. This means that interactions with the physician will be respectful even in disagreement. Interactions with nursing peers ought to be sensitive to unit traditions and structure, enlisting managers and other unit leaders in areas of policy and professional change (Monicken & Zwygart-Stauffacher, 2006). Modeling skills in mediation and advocacy for patient populations increases the likelihood of engaging physician support. Involving professionals such as respiratory care, social work, and pastoral care in developing patient-specific and unit-based plans acknowledges their expertise in specific care management interventions. A CNS can also bring great value and expertise to organizations such as the Center for Patient Partnerships, an interdisciplinary center of the Schools of Law, Medicine and Public Health, and Nursing at the University of Wisconsin-Madison, that trains professional and graduate-level students from a diversity of disciplines in the art and science of patient advocacy and patient-centered care (Center for Patient Partnerships, 2007).

Ethics

The acute and critical care CNS's decisions and actions are made on behalf of patients, family members, nursing personnel, and organizational systems and are determined in an ethical manner (Bell, 2002). The nurse promotes, advocates for, and strives to protect the health, safety, and rights of the patient (ANA, 2004).

CNSs anticipate ethical conflicts that may arise in the health care environment and plan

for resolution (NACNS, 2004). When carried out in clinical practice, nurse competencies, such as advocacy and moral agency, derive from patients' needs and range in expertise from competent (Level 1) to expert (Level 5) as shown in Box 10-1. Notable in this continuum is

---

BOX 10-1

Levels of Nurse Expertise in Advocacy/Moral Agency

Level 1: Competent

Works on behalf of patient

Assesses personal values

Aware of ethical conflicts or issues that may surface in clinical setting

Makes ethical and moral decisions based on rules

Represents patient when patient cannot represent self

Aware of patient's rights

Level 3

Works on behalf of patient and family

Considers patient values and incorporates them into care even when they differ from personal values

Supports colleagues in ethical and clinical issues

Moral decision making can deviate from rules

Demonstrates give and take with patient's family, allowing them to speak for/represent themselves when possible

Aware of patient's and family's rights

Level 5: Expert

Works on behalf of patient, family, and community

Advocates from patient's and family's perspectives, whether similar to or different from personal values

Advocates ethical conflict and issues from patient's and family's perspective

Suspends rules to allow patient and family to drive moral decision making

Empowers the patient and family to speak for/represent themselves

Achieves mutuality within patient and professional relationships

Bell, L. (Ed.). (2002). *Scope of practice and standards of professional performance for the acute and critical care clinical nurse specialist.* Aliso Viejo, CA: American Association of Critical-Care Nurses.

how a competent nurse makes ethical/moral decisions based on rules, whereas an expert nurse suspends rules so patients and families can drive the decision making.

Advocacy and moral agency represent the quintessence of nursing. However, each time a CNS fulfills those roles she or he is challenged to reaffirm a commitment to the profession. Advocacy and moral agency are risky activities (Mallik, 1997). The risk-taker often lacks the safety net afforded by adequate support systems, especially when the situation challenges personal values. In short, acts of advocacy often demand moral choices from the individual nurse (Mallik, 1997). The risk taken when engaging in advocacy and moral agency is consistent with the proposition stated earlier that advocacy lays the foundation for the relationship between patient and nurse. This points to the link between advocacy and justice when justice is defined as "fidelity to the demands of a relationship" (Burghardt, 2000).

Personal and professional ethics require a CNS to identify ethical issues. The advanced practice role also requires a CNS to advocate for ethical issues to be resolved (Hamric, 2005). A CNS can only be a bystander when the participants are functioning within a healthy work environment and excelling in ethical decision making. Even then a CNS will have assessed both the nursing personnel and the organizational system supporting them. After debriefing all involved in this case, a CNS would proceed as an authentic leader, aware of the value she or he brings to the situation, to dialogue with nurses, physicians, and other organizational leaders to implement policy changes that support family presence in all of the hospital's critical care units (Stannard & Hardin, 2005).

Collaboration

The acute and critical care CNS collaborates with patients and their family members and health care personnel in creating a healing and caring environment (Bell, 2002).

Collaboration in meeting the patient's and family's needs in this or any other situation requires a CNS to truly listen and clarify perceptions of what is happening at the time. Lonergan's approach described earlier can be an especially useful framework. In the case presented previously, the CNS guides the physician, bedside nurse, and family members to reach consensus while sustaining respect for every person's opinion. Collaborating with the family to find resources that meet their psychosocial needs may include accessing the social worker and/or pastoral support. Even with the best intentions, interdisciplinary collaboration often receives lip service. CNSs are well positioned to model true collaboration. As described in the *AACN Standards for Establishing and Sustaining Healthy Work Environments*, this means collaboration in which each professional's unique knowledge and abilities is respected with safety and quality as the agreed-on outcomes (AACN, 2005).

Research

The acute and critical care CNS uses, participates in, and disseminates research to enhance practice (Bell, 2002).

Seeking best practice and using available research to implement evidence-based practice is a strong component of CNS practice. For example, culling evidence to develop a collaborative unit policy that supports family presence offers a CNS a valuable opportunity of translating research into practice and supporting planned change. Published reports about nurse advocacy present mostly theoretical analyses, opinion pieces, and case studies (Segesten, 1993). Empirical studies are scarce. CNSs can help to identify applied topics that will benefit from further inquiry (e.g., advocacy/moral agency in hospitals using the Synergy Model as a conceptual framework; differences in advocacy/moral agency between teaching and nonteaching hospitals; analysis of nurses' advocacy activities and their effect; and how nurses learn advocacy [Kerfoot, Lavandero, Cox,

Triola, Pacini, & Hanson, 2006; Reinhard, Grossman, & Piren, 2004; Snowball, 1996]). CNSs also can participate when studies are conducted and translate the results for use in clinical practice.

Resource Utilization

The acute and critical care CNS influences resource utilization to promote safety, effectiveness, and fiscal responsibility in the planning and delivery of patient care (Bell, 2002).

Efforts to support practical resource utilization can be fraught with challenge in advocacy issues. Patients and their families may perceive that resources that could help them are being withheld when there is disagreement over patient outcomes. For example, the decision to not resuscitate may be interpreted as resulting in reduced care. Among nurses, advocating for a match between nurse competencies and patient needs may be seen as playing favorites when assigning patients. A CNS has the opportunity to role model and coach communication and negotiation skills to best meet patients' and families' actual and perceived needs (Tschudin, 1994). A CNS also can model appropriate use of internal resources such as ethics committees or risk management and legal consultants and external resources such as professional organizations, government officials, and community agencies to facilitate resolution of issues of advocacy or moral agency (Becker, Kaplow, Muenzen, & Hartigan, 2006).

Advocacy and moral agency represent a distinctive nursing contribution to the care equation. They draw equally from a CNS's professional knowledge and skill as from his or her personhood. Successful advocacy and moral agency can be exhilarating. Failure can be devastating. Whichever the case, the CNS is always challenged to remain faithful to the demands of the nurse-patient relationship.

Therefore advocacy happens at the interface between the strictly correct and the personally possible (Tschudin, 1994).

DISCUSSION QUESTIONS

1. How would the CNS modify or change any of the identified actions if there was a patient in the next bed?
2. What actions could have been taken to provide advocacy for the other patient?

References

American Association of Critical-Care Nurses. (2005). *AACN standards for establishing and sustaining healthy work environments: A journey to excellence.* Aliso Viejo CA: Author.

American Association of Critical-Care Nurses. (2004). *Practice alert: Family presence during CPR and invasive procedures.* Retrieved February 4, 2007, from http://www.aacn.org/AACN/practice Alert. nsf/Files/FP/$file/Family%20Presence%20During%20CPR%2011-2004.pdf.

The American Heritage Dictionary of the English Language (ed 4). (2004). Boston, MA: Houghton Mifflin Company. Retrieved February 4, 2007, from http://dictionary.reference.com/browse/advocacy.

American Nurses Association. (2004). *Code of ethics for nurses with interpretive statements.* Washington DC: American Nurses Publishing.

Becker, D., Kaplow, R., Muenzen, P.M., & Hartigan, C. (2006). Activities performed by acute and critical care advance practice nurses: American Association of Critical-Care Nurses study of practice. *Am J Crit Care, 15,* 130-147.

Bell, L. (Ed.). (2002). *Scope of practice and standards of professional performance for the acute and critical care clinical nurse specialist.* Aliso Viejo, CA: American Association of Critical-Care Nurses.

Benner, P. (1991). The role of experience, narrative, and community in skilled ethical comportment. *Adv in Nurs Sci, 14*(2), 1-21.

Buresh, B., & Gordon, S. (2006). *From silence to voice: What nurses know and must communicate to the public* (ed 2). Ithaca NY: ILR Press.

Burghardt, W.J. (2000). *Hear the just word and live it.* New York NY: Paulist Press.

Center for Patient Partnerships. Retrieved February 4, 2007, from http://law.wisc.edu/patientadvocacy/index.html.

Curtin, L.L. (1979). The nurse as advocate: A philosophical foundation for nursing. *Adv in Nurs Sci, 3*(1), 1-10.

Dossey, B.M. (2000). *Florence Nightingale: Mystic, visionary, healer.* Springhouse PA: Springhouse Corporation.

Foley, B.J., Minick, P., & Kee, C.C. (2000). Nursing advocacy during a military operation. *Western J Nurs Research, 22,* 492-507.

Foley, B.J., Minick, P., & Kee, C.C. (2002). How nurses learn advocacy. *J Nurs Scholarship, 34*(2), 181-186.

Hamric, A. B. & Reigle, J. (2005). Ethical decision making. In Hamric, A.B., Spross, J.S., & Hanson, C.M. (Eds.) *Advanced practice nursing: An integrative approach.* (ed 3). St. Louis: Elsevier Saunders.

Hardin, S.R., & Kaplow, R. (2005). *Synergy for clinical excellence: The AACN Synergy Model for Patient Care.* Sudbury MA: Jones and Bartlett.

Henderson, V. (1997). *Basic principles of nursing care.* Geneva, Switzerland: International Council of Nurses.

Henderson, V. (1966). *The nature of nursing: A definition and its implications for practice, research and education.* New York: Macmillan Publishing Co.

Joel, L.A. (1998). On citizenship in a great profession. *Am J Nurs, 98:*4, 7.

Kerfoot, K., Lavandero, R., Cox, M., Triola, N., Pacini, C., & Hanson, M.D. (2006). Conceptual models and the nursing organization: Implementing the AACN Synergy Model for Patient Care. *Nurse Leader,* August, 23-29.

Lindahl, B., & Sandman, P.O. (1998). The role of advocacy in critical care nursing: a caring response to one another. *Intens Crit Care Nurse, 14:*179-186.

Lonergan, B. (1971). *Method in theology.* Toronto, ON: University of Toronto Press.

Mallik, M. (1997). Advocacy in nursing—a review of the literature. *J Adv Nurs, 25:* 130-138.

Meyers, T.A., Eichhorn, D.J., Guzzetta, C.E., et al. (2000). Family presence during invasive procedures and resuscitation: The experiences of family members, nurses, and physicians. *Am J Nurs, 100:*2, 32-42.

Monicken, DR, & Zwygart-Stauffacher, M. (2006). Multifaceted Roles of the APN. In Mirr Jansen. M. P.

& Zwygart-Stauffacher (Eds.). *Advanced Practice Nursing: Core concepts for professional role development.* (ed 3) New York: Springer Publishing.

National Association of Clinical Nurse Specialists. (2004). *Statement on clinical nurse specialist practice and education.* Harrisburg PA: Author.

Patterson, K., Grenny, J., McMillan, R., & Switzler, A. (2002). *Crucial conversations: Tools for talking when stakes are high.* New York, NY: McGraw-Hill.

Patterson, K., Grenny, J., McMillan, R., & Switzler, A. (2005). *Crucial confrontations: Tools for resolving broken promises, violated expectations and bad behavior.* New York, NY: McGraw-Hill.

Random House Unabridged Dictionary. (2006). New York, NY: Random House, Inc. Retrieved February 4, 2007, from http://dictionary.reference.com/browse/advocate.

Reinhard, S.C., Grossman, J., & Piren, K. (2004). Advocacy and the advanced practice nurse. In Joel, L.A. (Ed.). (2004). *Advanced practice nursing: Essentials for role development.* Philadelphia PA: FA Davis Company.

Segesten, K. (1993). Patient advocacy: An important part of the daily work of the expert nurse. *Scholarly Inquiry for Nursing Practice, 7,* 129-135.

Snowball, J. (1996). Asking nurses about advocating for patients: Reactive and proactive accounts. *J Adv Nurs, 24,* 67-75.

Stannard, D., & Hardin, S.R.. (2005). Advocacy/moral agency. In Hardin, S.R., & Kaplow, R. (Eds.). *Synergy for clinical excellence: The AACN Synergy Model for Patient Care.* Sudbury MA: Jones and Bartlett.

Sullivan, E.J. (2004). *Becoming influential: A guide for nurses.* Upper Saddle River NJ: Pearson Prentice Hall.

Thomas, D. (2003). *The ethics of choice: The handbook.* Omaha NE: David Thomas.

Tschudin, V. (1994). *Deciding ethically: A practical approach to nursing challenges.* London: Baillière Tindall.

Caring Practices

Elizabeth M. Nolan

INTRODUCTION

Definition

The AACN Synergy Model for Patient Care defines caring practices as a "constellation of nursing activities that respond to the uniqueness of patients, families, colleagues. Caring practices create a compassionate and therapeutic environment aimed at promoting comfort and preventing suffering" (www.certcorp.org). Caring can be integral to everything the nurse does as has been suggested in studies to identify caring behaviors (Larsen, 1986; Mayer, 1987). Although the topic of caring practices can encompass all dimensions of practice, it is helpful to focus on common issues associated with caring that arise in acute and critical care nursing practice. In describing the levels of practice (Box 11-1), the Synergy Model addresses specifics—a safe physical environment, death as an outcome of illness, compassion, and individualized care throughout the health care continuum. Other issues identified in caring practices include body image, loss, healing, and powerlessness (Maloney-Harmon, 1999).

The primary research journal for critical care nurses, the *American Journal of Critical Care*, has an ongoing column by Patricia Benner, "Current Controversies in Critical Care," that often focuses on this dimension, which is further evidence of the importance of caring practices in patient care. In addressing issues such as death, human dignity, respect, and equity in care, Benner (2003) provides a context for caring, citing a more extensive definition of caring:

'Caring' is a word for being connected and having things matter works well because it fuses thought, feeling and action, knowing and being. And the term caring is used appropriately to describe a wide range of involvements from romantic love, to parental love, to friendship, from caring for one's garden to caring about one's work, to caring for and about one's patients.

Caring is primary because it sets up what matters to the person or what counts as stressful and what options are available to the person for coping. In this way, caring (having things matter to one), puts the person in a place of risk and vulnerability. Relationships, things, events, and projects do not show up as stressful unless they matter. If the person does not care, an event cannot be stressful. But the notion of caring is such that it also sets up what coping options are available and acceptable to the person.

Caring sets up the condition that something or someone outside the person matters and creates personal concerns. It sets up a world and makes meaningful distinctions, and it is these concerns that provide motivation and direction for persons. Meaninglessness (a place of not caring) and

BOX 11-1

Levels of Caring Practices

Constellation of nursing activities respond to the uniqueness of patients, families, colleagues. Caring practices create a compassionate and therapeutic environment aimed at promoting comfort and preventing suffering.

Level 1

Focuses on the usual and customary needs of the patient; no anticipation of future needs; bases care on standards and protocols; maintains a safe physical environment; acknowledges death as a potential outcome.

Level 3

Responds to subtle patient and family changes; engages with the patient as a unique patient in a compassionate manner; recognizes and tailors caring practices to the individuality of patient and family; domesticates the patient's and family's environment; recognizes that death may be an acceptable outcome.

Level 5

Has astute awareness and anticipates patient and family changes and needs; fully engaged with and sensing how to stand alongside the patient, family, and community; caring practices follow the patient and family lead; anticipates hazards and avoids them and promotes safety throughout patient's and family's transitions along the health care continuum; orchestrates the process that ensures that patient's/family's comfort and concerns surrounding issues of death and dying are met.

From www.certcorp.org.

anomie (the loss of a feeling of belonging) are the positions most bereft of coping options, because nothing stands out as more or less important or inviting. Nothing really matters. In the modern sense, the person is free from care and attachments. But this is a negative freedom that makes all options look equally plausible and provides no direction for choosing one project over another.

In our modern era, in which care and caring are devalued, it can look as if "caring" is a problem or *the* problem. From a place of care, the person cannot claim complete autonomy or be the absolute center of giving. This runs counter to the dominant quest in the culture of extreme individualism (i.e., the quest to be the master of one's own destiny, controlling all options, including feelings and response to events). This version of untrammeled or negative freedom in which the person finally loses all bonds and is free from every care would not create the positive freedom to choose and to act, even if people were ever really able to be so disconnected.

Caring allows the person to focus on the event or the one cared for rather than on personal threat. For example, family members may be quite heroic in their caregiving for a loved one with a serious illness. To someone not in the situation, this kind of caregiving often appears courageous; but the one caring is simply doing the only thing he or she can do. There seems to be no other option compatible with being who this person is (i.e., a person who cares for this family member). When people are praised for their courage, devotion, and so on, in caring for a seriously ill loved one, they typically respond, "I just did what I had to do." Walking away or not caring is not an option.

This enabling condition of connection and concern is also why caring is primary. Caring (about someone or something) places the person in the situation in such a way that he or she can prioritize. This is what enables people to discern problems, to recognize possible solutions, and to implement those solutions.

Finally, caring is primary because it sets up the conditions of possibility of giving and receiving help.

The same act done in a caring and noncaring way may have quite different consequences. A caring relationship sets the conditions of trust that enable the ones cared for to appropriate the help offered and feel cared for (Benner, 2003a).

The last sentence summarizes why caring practices do much more than meet psychosocial needs. This has been evident in studies that have sought patients' perspectives on nurses' caring behaviors. Patients rated "knows how to give shots, IVs" highest, whereas nurses ranked "listens to the patient" highest (Mayer, 1987). In exploring this topic with patients, they expressed the view that injections hurt, and, if nurses care about patients, they would learn to give injections as painlessly as possible. This makes sense since the nurse-patient relationship is a partnership. Just as patients need to trust that the nurse will safely meet their needs (i.e., safely infuse vasopressors and check hemodynamic pressures), nurses need to trust that patients will participate by reporting symptoms and cooperating with treatments (i.e., report chest pain or resist self-extubation).

CNS Level of Expertise

The preparation and role focus of the clinical nurse specialist (CNS) facilitate innovations in practice. Since the advent of critical care units, advanced practice nurses have conducted research examining facets of caring practices such as easing transfer out of the intensive care unit (ICU) (Schwartz & Brenner, 1979) and assessing family needs (Molter, 1979). The topics so often associated with caring practices have continued to be a focus: visitation practices (Simpson, 1991; 1996); family presence (Meyers et al., 2004); family-centered care (Slota, 2003); death and dying (Campbell & Thill, 1996); and innovations to help patients coping with pain, fear, anxiety, or loss (Puntillo et al., 2002). Although the studies to better understand exactly what it is that nurses do that make patients feel cared for began with cancer patients (Larson, 1986; Mayer, 1987), this work has expanded, examining patients of different cultures, ages, and medical conditions

(Gardner et al., 2001; Widmark-Petersson, von Essen, & Sjoden, 1998). The quest to better understand the dimension of caring continues, and CNSs endeavor to integrate what is known in all three spheres of practice.

IMPLEMENTATION WITHIN THE DIMENSION OF PRACTICE

Assessment

The CNS's sphere of influence regarding patient assessment has a micro and macro aspect: micro refers to a CNS conducting assessments as part of direct patient care, and macro refers to CNSs working at a unit or organizational level to influence all nursing assessments. CNSs may influence an institution's or a unit's choice of an assessment framework (e.g., body systems with categories such as respiratory and neurological or Gordon's Functional Health Patterns with categories such as cognition and perception and activity and exercise (Gordon, 1982). Table 11-1 illustrates the eleven functional health patterns identified by Gordon and suggests assessment data related to caring practices that might emerge from any one of the patterns. Selection of a particular assessment approach stems from the belief that the chosen framework will provide a more comprehensive and meaningful patient assessment. Regardless of the framework used, all assessments have biopsychosocial dimensions, with psychosocial data providing a baseline for caring practices.

Given that care is a multidisciplinary enterprise, relevant data may come from a variety of sources, including but not limited to the nursing assessment. For example, notes of physicians, social workers, or dietitians and conversations with pastoral care, family, and friends may offer additional perspectives about the patient and family. Data elements to consider in the assessment of caring needs are:

- The source of admission: where the patient came from—home, another health care facility, or even the street.

TABLE 11-1	
Gordon's Functional Health Patterns	
Gordon's Functional Health Patterns	**Caring-related Assessment**
Health perception and management	Perception of health? Reason patient sought medical care? What has patient being doing for this? Has it worked? What are goals for this hospital stay?
Activity and exercise	Ability to participate in care, dependency needs.
Nutrition and metabolism	Preferred foods. Culture, ethnicity, religion or spiritual aspects? Withholding food or fluid—is it ever permitted?
Elimination	Rituals or routines? Desired level of privacy?
Sleep and rest	Usual patterns? What facilitates rest/sleep?
Cognition and perception	Pain and comfort? Past history—efficacy of treatments? Visual or hearing impairments? Cognitive functioning—ability to handle complex information (e.g., condition, medical equipment) to participate in care.
Self-perception and self-concept	Illness impact on patient's self view? On others' view of patient—are there threats? Loss of job, friends, family?
Roles and relationships	Significant others in patient's life—role of patient? Proxy decision makers? Abuse-neglect issues?
Coping and stress management	Usual patterns? Self-awareness? Substance abuse? How patient shows stress, fear, anxiety. Social support—whom does patient identify? Are they available?
Sexuality and reproduction	Need for intimacy—gender issues, sexuality(heterosexual, homosexual, or bisexual). Concerns rereproduction—impact of treatment on fertility, risks of treatment on fetus.

Gordon, M. (1982). Nursing diagnosis: Process and application. In Carpenito, L.J. (1993). *Nursing diagnosis: Application to clinical practice* (Ed 5). Philadelphia: J.B. Lippincott.

- Advance directives: data about the patient's choice of proxy decision maker and preferences for care.
- Goals for the admission: what caused the patient to come to the hospital? Did the patient come willingly or unwillingly?
- Emergency contact: did the patient come alone? If the patient has someone to contact, has the person been contacted? Will the person be readily available?
- Values and beliefs: cultural, religious, spiritual beliefs about life and death.
- Learning: interest and ability to learn, past health behaviors.

- Dependents: does anyone rely on patient for care or assistance? If so, how is care managed without patient's presence?

Exploring an array of data sources can enable the nurse to have a more encompassing picture of the patient and make the assessment process more efficient and effective.

Excellent resources for nurses seeking information about how religious beliefs and culture may influence care are available in pocket guides (see the following list). One guide (Minarik, Lipson, and Dibble, 1996) addresses death rituals, birth rituals, illness beliefs, health practices, family relationships, food practices, communication, symptom management, spiritual/religious orientation, and cultural/ethnic identity.

Box 11-2 illustrates the use of a culture reference for Chinese-Americans (Chin, 1996). Rather than create or perpetuate stereotypes, this information can enhance nurses' understanding about beliefs by providing a starting point from which they can seek further information to see if the generalization actually fits the patient and family. This exploration can be incorporated into assessment.

The following sources are also useful:

- Rundle, A., Carvalho, M., & Robinson, M. (Eds.). (2002) *Cultural competence in health care: A practical guide.* San Francisco, Josses-Bass.
- D'Avanzo C.E., & Geissler E.M. (2002). *Pocket guide to cultural assessment* (ed. 3). St. Louis: Mosby.
- Minarik, P.A., Lipson, J.G., &. Dibble, S.L. (1996). *Culture and nursing care: A pocket guide.* San Francisco, CA: UCSF Nursing Press.

BOX 11-2

Cultural Profiles: Chinese Americans

Cultural/Ethnic Identity
- Preferred term: Chinese, Chinese American
- History of immigration
- 1840–1882: Chinese laborers came to United States for jobs; many employed to work on railroads
- 1882 Chinese Exclusion Act: suspended immigration of Chinese to America
- 1924 National Origins Quota Act: annual quota = 105 Chinese
- 1965 National Origins Quota Act abolished

By 1970 U.S. Chinese population increased by 84%. Chinese health practices vary according to length of time in United States. Three major groups and health practices are:

1. Early immigrants: immigrated 40 to 60 years ago; strongest believers in Chinese folk medicine
2. Newer immigrants: immigrated in the past 20 years; combine both Chinese folk and Western medicine practices
3. First and second generation Chinese Americans: mostly oriented to Western medicine

Communication
- *Major language(s) and dialects.* Cantonese and Mandarin are the most common.
- *Literacy assessment.* Ability to speak or read varies with individuals. Elderly Chinese (especially women) may be unable to read or write. Ask questions to ascertain understanding but not questions that require only yes or no answer.
- *Nonverbal communication.* Eye contact and touching are more common among family members and close friends; eye contact is avoided with authority figures as a sign of respect. Keeping respectful distance is recommended. Asking questions is seen as disrespectful; silence may be a sign of respect.
- *Use of interpreters.* Family members are usually available for interpreting needs, but professional interpreters are recommended for translation about complicated medical procedures. Avoid male interpreters for older female patients because of modesty issues.
- *Greetings.* Chinese people are often shy, especially in unfamiliar environment; socializing and friendly greetings are helpful. Address older patients by Mr./Mrs. and last name. Use of first name could be viewed as disrespectful among older individuals.
- *Tone of voice.* Chinese language is very expressive and often appears loud to non-Chinese people. Often this "loudness" is carried through to the English language and may appear unintentionally abrupt.
- *Orientation toward time.* Being on time is not valued by traditional Chinese societies. Reinforce the importance of being on time for medical appointments.
- *Consents.* Involve the oldest male of the family with consent explanations, especially with young females. Out of respect, Chinese patients may not ask questions but may nod politely at everything

Continued

BOX 11-2

Cultural Profiles: Chinese Americans—cont'd

being said. Assess understanding by asking clear questions.

- *Privacy*. Privacy is very important; Chinese people are usually extremely modest. To "save face," Chinese people may not want to disclose personal information to health providers. Involve close family members when necessary.
- *Serious or terminal illness*. Some families may prefer to be present when addressing information concerning serious or terminal illness. Ensure involvement of head of household (usually eldest male member of the family).

Activities of Daily Living

- *Modesty*. Chinese people are extremely modest, especially women. Avoid assigning male nurses to female patients.
- *Skin care*. Good hygiene is important; there are no special needs. Allow family to assist with bathing.
- *Hair care*. Patients may not want to wash hair while sick.
- *Nail care*. There are no special needs.
- *Toileting*. Privacy is important; using toilet is preferred to use of bedpan or urinal.
- *Special clothing or amulets*. Good luck articles (e.g., jade, rope around waist) may be worn to ensure good health and good luck. Avoid removing articles; if removal is required, encourage family members to take articles/jewelry home for safety.
- *Self-care*. Most Chinese patients prefer to perform their own activities of daily living, but some older men may expect to be cared for by family members or staff.

Food Practices

- *Usual meal pattern*. Chinese usually eat three meals a day, the largest at dinner. *Special utensils*. Provide chopsticks, if available.
- *Food beliefs and rituals*. Food is viewed as important in maintaining balance of Yin (cold) and Yang (hot) in the body. Imbalance of Yin and Yang is believed to cause illness. Food is also used to treat illness and disease. Patients may refuse certain foods because of beliefs about illness and which foods should be used to treat it. Obtain dietary consultation when appropriate to determine food preferences and diet restrictions.

Encourage families to bring in food from home if possible.

- *Usual diet*. Rice and noodles are important staples in the Chinese diet. Meat usually is not eaten in large quantities, and patients may prefer beef cooked until well done. Vegetables are frequently eaten mixed with meat to maintain the balance of Yin and Yang. Chinese prefer vegetables cooked, not raw.
- *Fluids*. Chinese people drink plenty of hot liquids, especially tea, when sick. Hot beverages are preferred because of belief that cold water shocks the system.
- *Food prohibitions*. Food is considered Yin (cold) or Yang (hot) depending on the Yin or Yang energy it is thought to yield when metabolized. Yin foods include fruits, vegetables, cold liquids, and beer. Yang foods include meats, eggs, hot soup and liquids, and oily and fried foods. Illness caused by Yang excesses are treated with Yin foods, and Yang foods are avoided, and vice versa.
- *Food prescriptions*. Based on information above, family members may bring in special foods to help treat illnesses. Consult with Dietary to ensure compliance with diet. Some Chinese also use herbal preparations and special soups to treat illnesses. Sometimes it is difficult to determine the content of these special preparations.

Symptom Management

- *Pain*. Patient may not complain of pain; be aware of nonverbal cues to assess pain. Offer pain medications instead of waiting for patient to ask for them. Some patients may use acupressure or acupuncture to treat pain or illness.
- *Dyspnea*. Caused by too much Yin. Some patients treat with hot soups/broths and wear warm clothes.
- *Nausea/vomiting*. Caused by too much Yin. Patients treat with hot soups/broths.
- *Constipation/diarrhea*. Caused by too much Yang. Some patients treat with fruits, vegetables, and other Yin foods.
- *Fatigue*. Caused by too much Yin. Treat with hot soups/broths. Ginseng is a common remedy.
- *Depression*. Mental health problems and depression are viewed as shameful and not readily discussed.

BOX 11-2

Cultural Profiles: Chinese Americans—cont'd

- *Self–care for symptom management.* Most Chinese treat minor symptoms with food remedies as discussed earlier. However, many major illnesses (e.g., cancer, heart disease) are ignored until advanced; some patients will seek Western medicine for treatment.

Birth Rituals/Care of the New Mother/Baby

- *Pregnancy care.* Believe that certain activities affect baby during pregnancy (e.g., going to the zoo during pregnancy will cause baby to look like one of animals). Pregnancy is considered a "cold" condition, and Yin foods should be avoided (e.g., eating watermelon during pregnancy will cause the baby to have asthma).
- *Labor practices.* No special practices.
- *Role of the laboring woman during birth process.* Although Chinese are stoic in nature, it is acceptable for Chinese women to exhibit pain by moaning, etc., during childbirth.
- *Role of the father and other family members during birth process.* Usually female family members are present during birth process. Father and other male members do not normally play an active role.
- *Vaginal vs. cesarean section.* Vaginal delivery is preferred.
- *Breast-feeding.* Breast-feeding is usually preferred over bottle feeding unless the mother works. While breast-feeding, the mother is expected to ingest Yang ("hot") foods to strengthen the health of the baby.
- *Birth recuperation.* During the first 30 days' postpartum, the mother's pores are believed to remain open, and cold air can enter the body. Based on this belief, a new Chinese mother may be forbidden to go outdoors or take a shower or bath. Diets high in Yang foods (e.g., meat, eggs, liver), and Yin foods may be avoided. Many mothers ingest specially prepared soups and broths containing pigs' feet and chicken.
- *Problems with baby.* New baby is center of focus and attention in the Chinese family. Problems with the baby should be addressed with the head of household and treated with utmost importance.
- *Male and female circumcision.* Although female circumcision is not performed, male circumcision is quite common.

Death Rituals

- *Preparation.* Chinese patients may be fatalistic when faced with terminal illness and death and may not want to talk about it. Family may prefer that the patient not be told about terminal illness or may prefer to tell the patient themselves.
- *Home versus hospital.* Many believe that people go to hospitals to die because dying at home brings bad luck. Others believe that the spirit might get lost if death occurs in the hospital.
- *Special needs.* Special amulets and cloths may be brought from home to be placed on the body.
- *Care of the body.* Some families prefer to bathe their family member after death.
- *Attitudes toward organ donation.* The Chinese believe that the body should be kept intact. Organ donation is not common.
- *Attitudes toward autopsy.* The body should be kept intact; thus autopsies may not be allowed.

Family Relationships

- *Composition/structure.* Extended families are common. Two or three generations often live in the same household. The wife is expected to become part of husband's family. Gay and lesbian relationships are not acknowledged and are considered shameful for the family.
- *Decision making.* Patriarchal society. Oldest male makes decisions.
- *Spokesperson.* Usually oldest male in household.
- *Gender issues.* Males are usually more highly respected and valued than females.
- *Caring role.* Caring role usually the responsibility of a female in household (mother, wife, daughter, daughter-in-law).
- *Expectations of and for children.* Children are highly valued in Chinese families and expected to respect their elders. Education is highly valued. Children who do not do well in school bring shame to the family.
- *Expectations of and for elders.* Elders are very respected and honored. In extended care families, grandparents are often responsible for care of grandchildren.
- *Expectations of adults in caring for children and elders.* Families are expected to care for children and elders rather than leave them in day

Continued

BOX 11-2

Cultural Profiles: Chinese Americans—cont'd

care or institutions. Mothers often are expected to stay at home to raise their children if another family member is not available to baby-sit.
- *Expectation of visitors*. It is common for great numbers of family members/friends to visit Chinese patient. It is considered polite for visitors to bring food or gifts.

Spiritual/Religious Orientation
- *Primary religious/spiritual affiliation*. Many Chinese are Buddhists. Catholic and Protestant religions also are common.
- *Usual religious/spiritual practices*. It is common for Chinese families to honor their ancestors, especially during major holidays such as Chinese New Year. Incense burning and eating special foods usually occurs during special occasions. Good luck symbols may be displayed in homes.
- *Use of spiritual healing/healers*. Some Chinese use herbalists and acupuncturists in conjunction with Western medicine or before seeking medical help. Rarely a healer is sought to rid psychiatric patients of evil spirits.

Illness Beliefs
- *Causes of physical illness*. Most physical illnesses are caused by imbalance of Yin and Yang in the body.
- *Causes of mental illness*. Mental illness is thought to be caused by a lack of harmony of emotions. In some cases, it is thought to be caused by evil spirits. Mental wellness occurs when psychological and physiological functions are integrated.
- *Causes of genetic defects*. Genetic defects are usually blamed on the mother, generally something she did or ate.
- *Sick role*. Sick role is common in the Chinese patient. Family is expected to take care of patient, and patient takes passive role in his or her illness.

- *Home and folk remedies*. Ginseng root is a commonly used home remedy for a number of ailments, including anemia, colic, depression, indigestion, impotence, and rheumatism. Other Chinese remedies include deer antlers for strengthening bones and treating impotence, turtle shells to stimulate weak kidneys and to remove gallstones, and snake flesh for healthy eyes and clear vision.
- *Acceptance of procedures*. Some Chinese are fearful of having blood drawn, believing that it will weaken the body. Many Chinese avoid surgery because of the belief that the body needs to be kept intact so the soul will have a place to live when making future visits to earth.
- *Care seeking*. Many Chinese use home remedies for minor ailments such as colds and skin diseases. Most Chinese seek Western doctors for more serious ailments such as cancer. In making a decision for seeking care, advice of relatives and friends is sought. Professional Chinese practitioners prescribe herbs and acupuncture based on diagnosis involving Yin/Yang and energy balance.

Health Practices
- *Concept of health*. Health is maintaining balance between Yin and Yang influences, not only in the body but in the environment. Harmony with body, mind, and spirit is important to maintain.
- *Health promotion and prevention*. Preventing illness and promoting good health means that one should eat a diet balanced with Yin and Yang foods. It is also important to maintain harmony with family and friends.
- *Screening*. When screening Chinese patients, be aware of Chinese beliefs and health practices. Allow family involvement and participation and respect privacy issues. For communication barriers, interpreters are recommended.

From Chin, P. In J.G. Lipson, S.L. Dibble, & P.A. Minarik. (1996). *Culture and nursing care: A pocket guide*, San Francisco, CA: UCSF Nursing Press.

Given the nature of illnesses that bring patients to acute and critical care settings, physiological data may be more readily available than psychosocial data. This can make the assessment of patients' unique needs more challenging.

However, in the absence of other data, nurses can be guided by evidence-based data on patient and family needs during critical illness.

The Critical Care Family Needs Inventory (CCFNI) (Box 11-3) identified five common

---

BOX 11-3

Critical Care Family Needs Inventory

Support

1. To be told about someone to help with family problems
2. To talk about negative feelings such as guilt and anger
3. To be encouraged to cry
4. To be told about other people who could help with problems
5. To be told about chaplain services
6. To have someone help with financial problems
7. To be alone at any time
8. To have another person with the relative when visiting the critical care unit
9. To have the pastor visit
10. To have a place to be alone while in the hospital
11. To have directions as to what to do at the bedside
12. To talk about the possibility of the patient's death
13. To have friends nearby for support
14. To have someone be concerned with the relative's health
15. To have explanations of the environment before going into the critical care unit for the first time

Comfort

16. To have the bathroom near the waiting room
17. To have comfortable furniture near the waiting room
18. To have a telephone near the waiting room
19. To have good food available in the hospital
20. To be assured it is all right to leave the hospital for awhile
21. To feel accepted by the hospital staff

Information

22. To know why things were done for the patient
23. To know how the patient is being treated medically
24. To know exactly what is being done for the patient

25. To know about the types of staff members taking care of the patient
26. To know which staff members could give what type of information
27. To help with the patient's physical care
28. To talk to the doctor every day
29. To have a specific person to call at the hospital when unable to visit

Proximity

30. To visit at any time
31. To see the patient frequently
32. To receive information about the patient once a day
33. To have visiting hours changed for special conditions
34. To be called at home about changes in the patient's condition
35. To be told about transfer plans while they are being made
36. To have the waiting room near the patient
37. To have visiting hours start on time
38. To talk to the same nurse every day

Assurance

39. To have questions answered honestly
40. To have explanations given that are understandable
41. To be assured that the best possible care is being given to the patient
42. To know specific facts concerning the patient's progress
43. To feel that hospital personnel care about the patient
44. To know the prognosis
45. To feel there is hope

Importance—rated on a scale of 1-5 (most important to not applicable)

Needs — rated on a scale of 1-4 (never – always)

Reprinted with permission, Nancy C. Molter & Jane Stover Leske, 1983.

needs of families: support, comfort, information, proximity, and assurance (Molter, 1979; Molter & Leske, 1986). Initially developed with adults, the CCFNI has been modified for assessing the needs of parents of critically ill neonates (Ward, 2001) and more recently to assess families' needs while in the emergency department (Redley & Beanland, 2004). The CCFNI has been translated into the Dutch language as well as Chinese and French, providing a reliable and valid tool to measure family needs (Bijttebier et al., 2000; Leung, Chien, & Mackenzie, 2000; Azoulay et al., 2001). Because the CCFNI has 45 items, it is not generally used as part of an admission assessment. However, asking a family to complete the CCFNI might provide greater insights and understanding regarding their needs for caring practices, which is valuable information for nurses as well as everyone else on the team.

Clinicians are using the CCFNI to identify families' needs, and they are using the scale to determine how well these needs are met (Mendonca & Warren, 1998; Kosco & Warren, 2000). After families specify their needs via the CCFNI, they rate how well these needs have been met. It seems likely that many families could provide these data since the reading level of the CCFNI is lower than fourth grade level. Completing the CCFNI could be offered to families as an option rather than a requirement. Another strategy to integrate the CCFNI in practice is to use it to benchmark performance and set goals when improvement is needed. For example, the CCFNI could be used to provide baseline data, and items rated high in importance could be selected for a shorter tool. These items could become part of a unit comment card asking families to rate how well these needs are being met.

Patient satisfaction has been cited as a nurse-sensitive outcome (Urden, 2001). Widely used in health care, patient satisfaction tools generally contain elements of caring practices, asking about nurses' friendliness, their attitude toward patients and family, their attention to spiritual and emotional needs, their effectiveness in keeping patients and families informed, and pain management. Subscales from patient satisfaction tools can be developed, using the items most related to caring practices influenced by the nurse. The subscales can then be used to provide baseline and future monitoring data as improvement strategies are identified and implemented to better meet patients' and families' needs. An advantage of using patient satisfaction measures to assess performance is that the data are collected and analyzed centrally and nurses can focus their attention on implementing caring practices to enhance patients' and families' satisfaction with care.

Chart audits are another source of data when assessing patient populations, although regrettably the patient record is often lacking data regarding the assessment, interventions, and evaluation of caring practices provided to acute and critically ill patients. Thank-you cards to staff and patient satisfaction surveys are more likely sources of data on what that staff does that make patients feel that the staff cares for them. Developing effective strategies to facilitate documentation of caring practices is an opportunity for the CNS.

Although many standard assessment tools (e.g., the Glasgow Coma Scale [neurological status], the Braden Scale [skin], and the Richmond Scale [sedation]) are routinely used as part of nurses' assessment, easy-to-use, standard assessment tools to assess dimensions of caring practices are not yet available or part of admission assessment forms. Although pain scales are widely used, scales to measure rest, comfort, and coping are not routine. It seems likely that, as easy-to-use scales focusing on caring practices become available, they will be commonplace in nursing assessment.

Diagnosis

Once assessment is complete, identifying the diagnoses, desired outcomes, and interventions follows. Initiatives to develop standard nursing language have produced standardized diagnoses (North American Nursing Diagnosis

Association [NANDA]) (NANCA, 2003), outcomes (Nursing Outcomes Classification [NOC]) (Johnson, Maas, & Moorhead, 2000), and interventions (Nursing Interventions Classification [NIC]) (McCloskey & Bulechek, 2000).

Just as CNSs can influence the choice of an assessment framework, they can also influence the adoption of standard nursing language within their organization. The use of standard nursing language is a way to connect all three spheres of practice.

In analyzing assessment data, nurses can draw on approved nursing diagnoses, confirming the appropriateness of the diagnosis by checking the defining characteristics and the related factors. Nursing diagnoses rather than medical diagnoses are particularly well suited to address issues salient to caring practices. Of the NANDA-approved diagnoses, fourteen might be considered in addressing caring practices (Box 11-4).

For the selected diagnosis to be valid, the defining characteristics and the related factors for that diagnosis must be supported by the assessment data. The exercise of selecting a diagnosis and confirming its appropriateness

---

BOX 11-4

Nursing Diagnoses

- Altered Family Processes
- Anticipatory Grieving
- Anxiety
- Chronic Pain
- Defensive Coping
- Fatigue
- Fear
- Hopelessness
- Knowledge Deficit
- Pain
- Powerlessness
- Sleep Deprivation
- Social Isolation
- Spiritual Distress

NANDA Nursing diagnoses 2003-2004: Definitions and classification, NANDA Staff, Philadelphia, North American Nursing Diagnosis Association, 2003.

---

supports an evidence-based approach to practice. Table 11-2 illustrates how one might attempt to use the defining characteristics and related factors to validate the choice of a nursing diagnosis.

TABLE 11-2

NANDA Diagnosis

Assessment Data	NANDA Diagnosis	Defining Characteristics	Related Factors
Patient John Q: Spouse died 2 days before admission. Tearful. Quiet. Has no appetite. States "when she died, a part of me died too." And "my kids don't want me to go back home. They think the house is too much for me."	Grieving	Verbal expression of distress at loss; anger; sadness; crying; difficulty in expressing loss; alterations in eating habits, sleep or dream patterns, activity levels or libido; reliving of past experiences; interference with life function; alterations in concentration or pursuit of tasks	Actual or perceived loss, which may include loss of people, possessions, job, status, home, ideals, or parts and processes of the body

NANDA Nursing diagnoses 2003-2004: Definitions and classification, NANDA Staff, North American Nursing Diagnosis Association, 2003.

If the defining characteristics and related factors are consistent with the data in the assessment, the nurse can be assured that the selection of "Grieving" as a diagnosis is appropriate.

Outcome Identification

Identifying outcomes follows diagnosis and precedes interventions. In selecting outcomes for the patient/family, nurses can draw on the outcomes listed in the NOC system. For caring practices, 18 could be considered (Box 11-5). Following up on the John Q case described in Table 11-2, with the diagnosis of Grieving, several outcomes might be used such as Grief Resolution or Anticipatory Grieving (Table 11-3).

For each outcome (NOC), several indicators are listed, but not all are required. Nurses' clinical judgment determines which indicators will best reflect the desired outcome for a particular patient. Although any or all of the indicators for Grief Resolution could be selected, not all must be selected. In the case of the John Q example, the outcome of Grief Resolution could list two indicators.

The patient will (before discharge):

- Express feelings about the loss of his wife.
- Express positive expectations about the future.

Each indicator is rated on a scale of 1 to 5 (1: never demonstrated; 5: consistently demonstrated). The nurse may not expect that John Q will consistently express positive expectations about the future but perhaps will begin to express positive expectations. The ability to rate the outcome on a scale of 1 to 5 enables nurses to document progress toward a goal, a realistic approach given average length of stay in acute and critical care units.

Planning, Implementation, and Evaluation

Once outcomes are identified for the patient, interventions to consider are listed in the NIC. Each intervention includes a list of activities that can be done as part of that intervention. The nurse selects from the list of activities those that are appropriate; not all activities listed are required. The NIC interventions appropriate to caring practices are listed in Table 11-3. Box 11-6 illustrates some NIC interventions and activities that could be used in practice.

Standard nursing language is relatively new and may seem awkward to nurses who have used other frameworks for documentation. Organizations can facilitate use through the development of tools to facilitate the adoption of NIC/NOC/NANDA in practice. Fig. 11-1 illustrates a care plan developed by a thoracic surgery ICU team who identified anxiety as a nursing diagnosis common to their patient population. Rather than list every defining characteristic for anxiety, every possible outcome and indicator, or every possible intervention and activity, these clinicians individualized the nursing language for the thoracic surgery patient population. This strategy influences all three spheres

---

BOX 11-5

Outcomes

- Anxiety Self-Control 1402
- Cognitive Orientation 0901
- Comfort Level 2100
- Communication 0902
- Compliance Behavior 1601
- Coping 1302
- Fear Self-Control 1404
- Grief Resolution 1304
- Hope 1201
- Knowledge: Treatments and Procedures 1814
- Pain—Psychological Response 1306
- Pain Control 1605
- Quality of Life 2000
- Rest 0003
- Role Performance 1501
- Self-Direction of Care 1613
- Spiritual Health 2001
- Will to Live 1206

Johnson, M., Maas, M., & Moorhead, S. (Eds.). (2000). *Nursing outcomes classification (NOC)* (ed.2). St. Louis: Mosby.

TABLE 11-3

Assessment with Diagnosis and Possible Outcomes and Interventions

Assessment	Diagnosis (NANDA)	Outcome (NOC)	Intervention (Activities)
Patient John Q's spouse died 2 days before admission. Tearful. Has no appetite. States "when she died, a part of me died too." And "my kids don't want me to go back home. They think the house is too much for me."	Grieving	**Grief Resolution** with plan for a positive future as evidenced by the following indicators (select only those apply): • Express feelings about loss • Verbalize acceptance of loss • Describe meaning of loss or death • Reports decreased preoccupation with loss • Expresses positive expectations about the future Each indicator is rated on a scale of 1-5 (1: never demonstrated; 5: consistently demonstrated)	**Active Listening** (attending closely to and attaching significance to a patient's verbal and nonverbal messages) • Encourage expression of feelings • Display an awareness of and sensitivity to emotions • Determine the meaning of the message by reflecting on attitudes, past experiences, and the current situation **Support System Enhancement** (facilitation of support to patient by family, friends, and community) • Determine adequacy of existing social networks • Monitor current family situation • Explain to family how they can help

BOX 11-6

Interventions (Planning)

- Active Listening
- Calming Technique
- Guided Imagery
- Medication Administration
- Music Therapy
- Pain Management
- Patient Rights Protection
- Post-Mortem Care
- Presence
- Reality Orientation
- Referral
- Religious Ritual Enhancement
- Resiliency Promotion
- Security Enhancement
- Sedation Management
- Self-Awareness Enhancement
- Sibling Support
- Simple Massage
- Sleep Enhancement
- Socialization Enhancement
- Spiritual Support
- Support System Enhancement
- Telephone Follow-up
- Touch
- Truth Telling
- Visitation Facilitation
- Values Clarification

McCloskey J.C., & Bulechek G.M. (Eds.). (2000). *Nursing interventions classification (NIC)* (ed. 3). St. Louis: Mosby.

Anxiety [1]		**Today's Date:**

Instructions: **(1)** Stamp with patient name. **(2)** Select Defining Characteristics, Etiology, Interventions, Activities, Patient Outcomes to monitor. **(3)** Score patient outcomes a minimum of Q 12 hours (AM/PM). **(4)** Date/Time/Initial and SOAP note as appropriate.

Defining Characteristics	**Interventions**	**Activities**
☐ Threat or change in role status	☐ Anxiety reduction	☐ Explain all procedures, including sensations likely to be experienced during a procedure
☐ Threat to or change in health status		☐ Administer medications to reduce anxiety, as appropriate
☐ Awareness of physiological symptoms		☐ Provide factual information concerning diagnosis, treatment, and prognosis
☐		☐ Instruct pt. on the use of relaxation techniques
☐		☐ Encourage pt. and family* to verbalize feelings, perceptions, and fears
☐		☐ Control stimuli, as appropriate, for patient's needs
☐	☐ Coping Enhancement	☐ Assess pt.'s understanding of disease process
☐		☐ Help pt. to identify information that interests them most.
Etiology		☐ Provide pt. with realistic choices about certain aspects of care.
		☐ Encourage relationships with persons who have common interests, goals, and experience.
		☐ Assist pt. to identify and use available support systems.
		☐ Encourage family involvement.

Patient Outcomes

	Update every 12 hours minimum (AM/PM)	AM	PM	AM	PM	AM	PM	AM	PM	AM	PM	AM	PM	AM	PM
☐ Anxiety Control		1 = Never Demonstrated		2 = Rarely Demonstrated		3 = Sometimes Demonstrated		4 = Often Demonstrated		5 = Consistently Demonstrated					
	☐ Uses effective coping strategies														
	☐ Behavioral manifestations of anxiety absent														
	Comments														
☐ Coping	☐ Identifies multi-coping strategies														
	☐ Uses effective coping strategies														
	☐ Reports decrease in stress														
	Comments														
☐ Acceptance: Health Status		1 = None		2 = Limited		3 = Moderate		4 = Substantial		5 = Extensive					
	☐ Expressed feelings re: health status														
	☐ Recognition of reality of health situation														
	Comments														
See Progress Note/24-Hour Flowsheet		☐	☐	☐	☐	☐	☐	☐	☐	☐	☐	☐	☐	☐	☐
2004	Month/Day →														
Time															
Initials															

☐ See Progress Note: Date Problem Resolved: _____   Signed by: _____

BP = blood pressure, BSP = body secretion precautions , C.O. - cardiac output, C.I. = cardiac index, ECG = electrocardiogram, family = family or significant other, Hgb = hemoglobin, IER = in expected range, I & O = Intake and Output, LOC = level of consciousness, PAWP = pulmonary artery wedge pressure, PVR = pulmonary vascular resistance, S/S = signs and symptoms, SVR = systemic vascular resistance, WNL = within normal limits

References: <u>NANDA, Nursing diagnoses: definitions and classification</u>, 1999-2000, Philadelphia, PA. <u>Nursing Interventions Classification, 3ʳᵈ Ed.</u>, 2000, Edited by: McCloskey, J.C., Bulechek, G..Mosby, Inc.: St. Louis, MO. <u>Iowa Outcomes Project: Nursing Outcomes Classification, 2ⁿᵈ Ed.</u>, Edited by: Johnson, M., Maas, M., Moorhead, S.   maf/11:04 AM11/21/06

FIG 11-1   Anxiety care plan using NANDA, NOC, and NIC for thoracic surgery patients.

of practice: the patient for whom the care plan is implemented; nurses caring for thoracic surgery patients; and the organization—facilitating communication not only to nurses but to coders, quality abstractors, and future researchers.

Use of standard nursing language (SNL) builds the evaluation component into care as outcomes are rated on a regular basis. Lack of progress in achieving outcomes makes it obvious that something is wrong—either interventions/activities are not being implemented, or, if so, they are ineffective. Use of SNL may expedite awareness that progress is not being made since the nurse must regularly rate progress on achieving the outcome; ideally this would trigger initiatives that may prove more effective. For example, in the case of John Q, interventions involve his family. If staff is unable to reach his family; or if John Q becomes even more tearful, anorexic, and loses weight; a reappraisal of the plan is warranted.

Referring to the care plan for anxiety (see Figure 11-1), one of the activities for coping enhancement is "encourage family involvement." In a study of visitation, Slota (2003) noted the importance of consistency in establishing flexible visitation yet cited the variability among nurses, even when the unit had agreed on a unit policy. If, despite the care plan, staff is inconsistent in their encouragement of family involvement, progress in achieving the outcome may be stunted. However, since progress is being measured using SNL, not only may the issue not be ignored, but it may surface more readily and be effectively addressed.

Many NIC interventions have been the subject of study in critical care. One example is the NIC *presence*, defined as being with another, both physically and psychologically, during times of need (McCloskey & Bulechek, 2000). Studies that have centered on visitation from the perspective of patients and families seek to better understand and promote presence. Yet best practices related to this intervention seem slow to be implemented in practice. Although work began in 1980s to address family presence during cardiopulmonary resuscitation (CPR), many years have elapsed since the issue has caught on (Hanson & Strawser, 1992). Family presence is not the norm.

In a study examining current practices regarding family presence during invasive procedures and cardiopulmonary resuscitation, there was evidence that clinicians' attitudes are becoming more open (MacLean et al., 2003). Although written policies were rare ($\approx 5\%$), about half of the respondents reported that family presence was permitted. The nurses in

this study were evenly split regarding their preferences for written policies. They reported that about a third of families asked to be present during cardiopulmonary resuscitation, and about two thirds during invasive procedures. The comments offered by nurses in the study reflected the perspective that family presence is an essential element to caring practices for the patient and family:

- Provides emotional support for patients and patients' families
- Provides a positive experience for patients' families, patients, and staff
- Provides guidance and increases family understanding of the patient's situation
- Helps patients' families make decisions about resuscitation
- Helps patients' families know that everything was done to save their loved one
- Facilitates closure and healing (MacLean et al., 2003).

Given the association of caring practices to issues of loss and healing, the intervention of presence would seem to be effective. In addition to examining nurses' perspectives on family presence, the perspectives of family members and physicians have been studied (Meyers et al., 2004). Opinions of families and staff were sought following their presence (either visual or physical) during CPR or an invasive procedure. All family members thought the experience was helpful and would do it again. Nurses were more likely than faculty or residents to favor family presence during CPR. Some staff feared disruption as a possible result of family presence, although there was no evidence of that during the study. By involving the multidisciplinary team members, this work is illustrative of expanding the sphere of influence in promoting caring practices. Within weeks of its publication, the Advisory Board (www.advisory.com) reviewed the article in its weekly Nursing Executive Watch, expanding the readership far beyond journal subscribers, a factor that should enhance awareness and perhaps expedite acceptance.

Bereavement Programs demonstrate caring for the patient through care of grieving family and friends. Interventions often begin in the hospital and continue for a period of time after the patient's death. Table 11-4 illustrates programs offered in the ICUs and acute care units at one medical center. Programs facilitate staff in following up with families and expressing their own sense of loss. Programs generally provide survivors' relatives with information that is practical (e.g., how to get a death certificate, information about autopsy, whom to notify of the death), as well as information on grief and loss (e.g., how to talk to children about death, handling the holidays, finding support groups) (i.e., information known to be important to bereaved relatives) (Warren, 2002). The Advisory Board identified the Bereavement Program in Table 11-4 as a best practice (www.advisory.com).

TABLE 11-4			
Bereavement Programs, University of Michigan Hospitals & Health Centers, Ann Arbor, Michigan			
	Pediatric Acute Care Units	**Cardiac ICU/ Adult Acute Care Units**	**Oncology Units and Cancer Center**
Name of program (if it has one)	Bereavement Program Upon the Death of Your Child	Bereavement Program Upon the Death of Your Loved One (adapted from program developed in pediatrics)	UM Comprehensive Cancer Center— Coping Through Transitions (CTT)
Description	The aim of the program is to consistently educate, inform, and support family members of patients who die in acute/critical care	Same as pediatric program; begun in 1994	Begun in 1993; offers assistance and information for those experiencing loss related to cancer
	Desired outcomes: Families are aware of practical information (e.g., funeral arrangements, death certificate), at time of death		
	Families learn about grieving process		
	Families feel support and empathy from UH staff		
	Begun in 1980s		
When does intervention begin?	At/near the time of death	At/near time of death	Staff support/education: along cancer continuum
			Family: at/near time of death

TABLE 11-4

Bereavement Programs, University of Michigan Hospitals & Health Centers, Ann Arbor, Michigan—cont'd

	Pediatric Acute Care Units	Cardiac ICU/ Adult Acute Care Units	Oncology Units and Cancer Center
What is done at the actual time of death? (include the name of any materials given to the family)	Folder to family (booklet *Upon the death of your child*, bookmark, and individualized materials determined by the unit).	Folder to family (booklet *Upon the death of your loved one,* http://www.med. umich.edu/1libr/aha/ umgrief.pdf, bookmark) Funeral home information available (listed by name and by town, phone/fax no.) Phone card provided (45 min.)	At time of death and/or time of notification of death, follow-up varies. Many deaths take place at home or out of the cancer center and/or patient unit. Once CTT notified, generally cards are sent by individual teams/units. Each card includes a unique water-color flower design.
Describe any contact that occurs after death	Sympathy card sent within 2 weeks of death. Cards with unique message sent at 3, 6, and 12 mos.	Sympathy card sent within 2 weeks of death. Cards with unique message sent at 3, 6, and 12 mos.	Bereavement pack is sent when notification of death occurs, usually between 1 and 6 months after the death. Pack includes CTT booklet, cover letter with contact information, and listing of other available resources. Appropriate materials are mailed with pack as needed (e.g., Support Group Flyers, Support for Coping with the Holidays and special times of the year, Helping Children Cope with Death, Art Therapy, Resources, Journaling Resources) http://www.cancer. med.umich.edu/ clinic/coping.htm
Who leads the initiative?	Nursing staff	Staff nurse/unit host for each unit. Program oversight by CNS.	Advanced Practice (AP) Nurse

Continued

TABLE 11-4		
Bereavement Programs, University of Michigan Hospitals & Health Centers, Ann Arbor, Michigan—cont'd		
	Pediatric Acute Care Units	**Cardiac ICU/ Adult Acute Care Units**	**Oncology Units and Cancer Center**
Who participates in the initiative?		Nursing staff primarily but all disciplines welcome	Individual Teams/Central Grief and Loss Office including clerical staff, nursing staff, physicians, AP nurses, physician assistants, art therapist, social work
Additional events?		No	Annual Candle Lighting for Hope and Remembrance—for cancer survivors/ bereaved family and friends Annual Staff Support Event—"Sheltering Wings" Butterfly release Monthly Staff Grief and Loss Rounds
Contact		Enolan@umich.edu	Susan Wintermeyer-Pingel MS, APRN, BC Coordinator, UM Comprehensive Cancer Center's Grief and Loss Program (734) 615-6952 swpingel@umich.edu

Assessment and diagnosis through implementation and evaluation are all part of the nursing process, something that is not at all new to patient care. What may be new are tools such as SNL, and evidence-based resources for assessment and intervention that have yet to be implemented in practice. The CNS armed with current knowledge of caring practices and expertise in influencing change can be instrumental in influencing the environment—for one patient and family, a patient care unit, a nursing department, or an organization.

INTEGRATION OF THE STANDARDS OF PROFESSIONAL PERFORMANCE

The Standards of Professional Performance for the CNS in acute and critical care delineate the multifaceted role of the CNS, with standards addressing eight dimensions: quality of care, individual practice evaluation, education, collegiality, ethics, collaboration, research, and resource utilization. This expands the vision of the CNS role beyond the traditional clinical practice, research, and education focus that often framed a CNS performance plan and subsequent evaluation.

The CNS may influence the spheres of practice by attending to all eight dimensions of the standards. As noted earlier, caring practices may be concerned with death and bereavement, family visitation and presence, comfort measures such as music therapy, promotion of sleep and rest, or amelioration of fear and anxiety. In making an impact on caring practices, the CNS will likely need to mindful of all eight dimensions.

Quality Care

The quality initiatives that permeate health care address several aspects salient to caring practices. Performance improvement topics of national interest include pain management, patient satisfaction, patient education, advance directives, safety, and palliative care. Regulatory standards speak to this as well. The Joint Commission for the Accreditation of Healthcare Organizations (JCAHO) (www.jcaho.org) has standards for providing care and improving organizational performance. JCAHO describes their standards as goals and their elements of performance (EPs) as steps to achieve the goals. Table 11-5 illustrates some of the 2005 JCAHO Provision of Care standards and EPs that have elements salient to caring practices. In reading the EPs for PC 15.2 (see Table 11-5), one might see the influence of the work of Schwartz and Brenner (1979) that addressed transfer out of the ICU and how best to prepare patients and families.

JCAHO's section on improving organizational performance standards speaks to an organization's responsibility to collect data to monitor performance. Educational preparation prepares the CNS to critique research, acquire knowledge of current literature, design projects, and communicate findings surrounding caring practices. Regulatory standards such as JCAHO offer the CNS an opportunity to apply this knowledge and expertise to the everyday work

TABLE 11-5
2005 JCAHO Provision of Care Standards and Elements of Performance

PC No.	Standard (Goal)	Elements of Performance (EP) (Steps to Achieve the Goal)
2.2	The hospital defines in writing the data and information gathered during assessment and reassessment.	The information defined by the hospital to be gathered during the initial assessment includes the following, as relevant to the care, treatment, and services: • Physical assessment, as appropriate • Psychological assessment, as appropriate • Social assessment, as appropriate • Each patient's nutrition and hydration status, as appropriate • Each patient's functional status, as appropriate • For patients receiving end-of-life care, the social, spiritual, and cultural variables that influence the perceptions and expressions of grief by the patient, family members, or significant others

Continued

TABLE 11-5	
2005 JCAHO Provision of Care Standards and Elements of Performance—cont'd	

PC No.	Standard (Goal)	Elements of Performance (EP) (Steps to Achieve the Goal)

6.10	The patient receives education and training specific to the patient's needs and as appropriate to the care, treatment, and services provided.	1. Education provided is appropriate to the patient's needs.
		2. The assessment of learning needs addresses cultural and religious beliefs, emotional barriers, desire and motivation to learn, physical or cognitive limitations, and barriers to communication as appropriate.
		3. As appropriate to the patient's condition and assessed needs and the hospital's scope of services, the patient is educated about the following:
		  • The plan for care, treatment, and services
		  • Basic health practices and safety
		  • The safe and effective use of medications
		  • Nutrition interventions, modified diets, or oral health
		  • Safe and effective use of medical equipment or supplies when provided by the hospital
		  • Understanding pain, the risk for pain, the importance of effective pain management, the pain assessment process, and methods for pain management
		  • Habilitation or rehabilitation techniques to help them reach maximum independence possible

8.7	Comfort and dignity are optimized during end-of-life care.	1. To the extent possible, as appropriate to the patient's and family's needs and the hospital's services, interventions address patient and family comfort, dignity, and psychosocial, emotional, and spiritual needs, as appropriate, about death and grief. 2. Staff is educated about the unique needs of dying patients and their families and caregivers.
15.2	The transfer or discharge of a patient to another level of care, treatment, and services, different professionals, or different settings is based on the patient's assessed needs and the hospital's capabilities.	1. The patient's needs for continuing care to meet physical and psychosocial needs are identified. 2. Patients are told in a timely manner of the need to plan for discharge or transfer to another organization or level of care. 3. Planning for transfer or discharge involves the patient and all appropriate licensed independent practitioners, staff, and family members involved in the patient's care, treatment, and services.

TABLE 11-5

2005 JCAHO Provision of Care Standards and Elements of Performance—cont'd

PC No.	Standard (Goal)	Elements of Performance (EP) (Steps to Achieve the Goal)
15.2 cont'd		4. When the patient is transferred, information provided to the patient includes the following: • The reason for the transfer • Alternatives to transfer, if any 5. The discharge planning process is initiated early in the care, treatment, and services process. 6. When the patient is discharged, information to patients includes the following: • The reasons for the discharge • The anticipated need for continued care, treatment, and services after discharge 7. When indicated, the patient is educated about how to obtain further care, treatment, and services, to meet his or her Identified needs. 8. When indicated and before discharge, the hospital arranges for or helps the family arrange for services needed to meet the patient's needs after discharge. 9. Written discharge instructions in a form the patient can understand are given to the patient and/or those responsible for providing continuing care (www.jcaho.org).

of the organization. The more closely a CNS's efforts are linked to the goals and interests of the organization, the more likely the CNS can engender support for an initiative. Resources within an organization's quality improvement (QI) office may be available to the CNS. Examples of such resources are statistical consultation, access to existing data sources, and perhaps resources for data collection or presentations. Although a CNS may not have the resources or organizational commitment to complete a research study, since QI projects are mandated in health care, the CNS has opportunities to explore mutual areas of interests. Long interested in the comfort of children, CNSs Merkel and Voepel-Lewis (1997) partnered with colleagues and developed a scale for measuring pain in children. Heightened interest in pain management has placed the issue on the priority list for most organizations and regulatory agencies.

CNS-led initiatives are evident in all spheres of influence. Coalescing interdisciplinary rounds has been noted for its effectiveness in communication among the team and alerting staff to patient problems (Halm et al., 2003). National initiatives to improve the quality of care such as the American Heart Association's Get With the Guidelines (www.americanheart.org) and the American College of Cardiology's Guidelines Applied in Practice (GAP) Initiative (http://www.acc.org/gap/gap.htm) often require a nurse champion on site, commonly a CNS (Mehta et al., 2002).

In 2003 there were 123 abstracts on creative solutions at the National Teaching Institute. Many addressed dimensions of caring practices, and QI principles/frameworks were evident. Dickerson & Lester (2003) addressed the challenge of meeting family needs, given the acuity of their unit. By developing a role for a family liaison who could orient families to the unit/organization and who could facilitate communication between families and staff nurses, physicians, social workers and pastoral care, they were able to improve family and staff satisfaction. Pate & Crider (2003) described collaboration between pediatric ICU staff and child-life therapists in helping friends and family cope with the death of a child. They described activities such as making molds of the child's hand or providing paint and a bed sheet to loved ones who make handprints for a "blanket of love" that is placed over the patient. Petlin, Becker, & Powers (2003) responded to survey data from cardiac surgery patients that revealed some dissatisfaction with care and forgotten discharge instructions. Their intervention (i.e., follow-up telephone calls) was effective in reaching ≈90% of their patients. By reinforcing education, problem solving, and answering questions, they were able to improve satisfaction. Further, by tabulating the topics that most frequently caused confusion or questions, they were able to revise their discharge instruction booklet to more clearly provide this information. What is common to these creative solutions is evaluation to determine their effectiveness.

Since QI is a regulatory requirement and an expectation of the CNS role, organizational QI tools and resources are likely available to the CNS. Standards can be used to strengthen interest and attention to caring practices and in some cases overcome barriers to implementation. Although QI is multidisciplinary, nurses (often CNSs) are designated leaders in QI initiatives, empowering the CNS as an agent of change.

Individual Practice Evaluation

Prevost (2002) proposed a data set template that could be used to demonstrate the outcomes of CNS practice, using categories such as demographic, clinical, fiscal, and satisfaction. Although one might not immediately link caring practices and fiscal outcomes, interventions that promote comfort or facilitate decisions about care may well decrease the cost of care. A recent study reviewing 552,157 deaths noted that 22% of the deaths occurred in the ICU (Angus et al., 2004). Hospitalized patients who died inside the ICU had an average length of stay (aLOS) of 12.9 days, longer than patients who died outside the ICU (8.9 aLOS). Costs were higher for ICU as well: $24,951 for ICU and $8548 for non-ICU. Given the authors' projection that half a million patients die annually in the ICU, there was an almost $8 billion difference in cost. Given the value that families place on communication, one could speculate that dialogue about patients' preferences and needs could result in a patient dying in a low-tech area, ideally the home, with hospice. Facilitating this admittedly difficult dialogue would be within the role and expertise of the CNS. The CNS might evaluate this contribution in terms of care, but assessing the impact of cost would also be of value.

Prevost (2002) also outlined a productivity log that could be used by the CNS to document the number of patients seen, interventions done, learners taught, and goals accomplished. Organizations use a variety of approaches to annual employee evaluation. When flexibility exists, the CNS might propose the use of the American Association of Critical-Care Nurses (AACN) Standards of Professional Practice; or, given the opportunity to provide a self-evaluation, the CNS can use the Standards as a framework within which to enumerate the many contributions done within the evaluation timeframe. In this way, the standards can serve as a benchmark for evaluating the comprehensiveness of practice.

Education

Education, a traditional focus of the CNS role, includes formal and informal opportunities for educating patients, staff, and community. Most activities in patient care have an education component. This standard speaks to the CNS as a both a teacher and a learner. Writing about evidence-based medicine, Sackett et al. (2000) noted "the disparity between our diagnostic skills and clinical judgment, which increase with experience, and our up-to-date knowledge and clinical performance which decline." A challenge for the CNS is ensuring that knowledge and performance of caring practices are current or, if they are not current, being able to access resources effectively. Expertise in hospice, palliative care, pain management, cultural competence, spirituality, mental health, or alternative therapies might all benefit the acute or critical care CNS who can develop strategies to keep current on these topics or network with colleagues who can offer this expertise. Computers can facilitate access to resources whether through listserves, e-mail, journals, or professional organizations. Direct access to data on quality (i.e., www.qualitymeasures.ahrq.gov/; ethics, www.utoronto.ca/jcb/ and www.lastacts.org), as well as professional organizations (i.e., www.aacn.org and www.nacns.org/) all facilitate the CNS as a lifelong learner.

When implementing new processes in patient care, education is essential for the change to be successful. For example, when the collaborative team developed a Bereavement Program, staff were educated about the program—its goals and its components—before program implementation. Even after the program was established and became a staple of the unit, the need for education continued as new staff joined the unit and as the program evolved.

Ciccarello (2003) observed that, although ICU deaths are not uncommon, nurses do not feel ready to provide end-of-life (EOL) care. A solution offered to better prepare nurses for EOL care included education to address beliefs about death; environments that support palliation and cure; and communication among team members. These can be part of a protocol for EOL.

For continuing certification the CNS must maintain a record of educational programs attended (learning) and a record of programs presented (teaching). A deliberative approach in reviewing this record can help identify ongoing learning about caring practices as well as the integration of this component in teaching.

Collegiality

One only has to scan journal publications and presentations at national meetings to see evidence of the collegiality in disseminating knowledge of caring practices. Over 20 years ago, Guzzetta and Dossey (1984) brought caring practices to the forefront. Their focus on holistic care continues (MacLean et al. 2003; Dossey, 2000b). Opportunities and initiatives to work with colleagues to improve caring practices can occur in all spheres of practice:

1. Supporting a colleague in arranging a family meeting or presenting a patient at rounds
2. Developing a family-support group or an anxiety care plan for your patient population
3. Working with the CNS network to educate staff throughout the organization on relaxation techniques as a means of pain relief
4. Participating in a national initiative focused on caring practices
5. Presenting at a national meeting, sharing expert knowledge about families and family dynamics to acute and critical care nurses

Ethics

Perhaps the most effective way a CNS can make a difference is in role-modeling the behaviors associated with caring practices. The behaviors that support and promote caring practices can be found by reviewing the AACN's mission, vision, values, and the Ethic of Care statements at www.aacn.org. By virtue of the role, the CNS has the opportunity to network with a wide range of individuals and to demonstrate principled behaviors. The ability to speak knowledgeably and to collaborate with a diverse group of individuals in everyday practice are the skills that will enable the CNS to engage patients, families, and clinical staff in discussions of ethical issues in patient care. Honesty in presenting data from a research study and respecting confidential information about colleagues are ways that build the CNS foundation as a principled individual and develop credibility.

Collaboration

Caring practices include collaborative activities with others on the health care team—pastoral care, social work, hospice, discharge planning, and family and friends. More specialists are available in the health care arena—child-life therapists; massage therapists; multicultural health consultants; interpreters; and recreational, art, and music therapists. This level of expertise can be essential to implementing caring practices—relaxation, rest, understanding, and coping within the acute and critical care environment. CNSs can facilitate their success through collaboration. Examples of collaboration are seen in all spheres of practices. The CNS may be instrumental in arranging a patient/family conference with all of the team members present to address issues related to the care of one patient. Halm et al. (2003) described multidisciplinary rounds to review the care of a group of patients. MacLean et al. (2003) reported on collaboration among nurses from seven organizations to examine nurses' practices regarding family presence during CPR and invasive procedures. In addition to generating knowledge, these nurse authors role-model collaboration. Patients and families in their thank-you notes to staff and in their comments on satisfaction surveys acknowledge that many staff members contribute to their recovery and healing. Although they may single out certain individuals who were noteworthy, their comments reflect a belief that their care was a team effort. When patients express dissatisfaction, it is often apparent that there was no collaboration. CNS competencies in collaborative behaviors and then role-modeling, mentoring, and coaching staff are essential to health care delivery. Since CNSs are generally in staff rather than management positions, many become experts at collaboration since it is vital to influencing practice.

Research

Although most clinicians endorse evidence-based practice, clinicians may rely on their own experience and values for caring practices. Examining the evidence is as important in addressing visitation and family presence as it is in monitoring pulmonary artery pressures. In 1992 Hanson & Strawser reported on a midsize community hospital's 9-year experience of permitting family presence during CPR without any ill effects. Eleven years later, in a survey of 3000 emergency department and critical care nurses, 5% of hospitals had policies permitting family presence. Almost half of the hospitals permitted family presence, even though they had not yet formalized the practice with a hospital policy. Families asked nurses to be present during resuscitation (31%) and invasive procedures (61%). Research on family presence during CPR and invasive procedures strengthens the ability to implement caring practices at the bedside (MacLean et al., 2003). AACN's Practice Alert, Family Presence During CPR and Invasive Procedures, provides nurses a ready-to-use tool to implement an evidence-based caring practice protocol (AACN, 2004). Since caring practices include measures to promote rest, comfort, and relaxation, it can be expected that the use of complementary and alternative therapies (CAT) in practice would be beneficial. An examination of nurses' use of CAT revealed that nurses who used CAT for themselves were more likely to use it in patient care (Lindquist, Tracy, and Savik, 2003). A review of the research could lead a CNS interested in promoting CAT to begin by surveying staff use, perhaps by identifying a core group to explore CAT use in patient care. Harnessing nurses' values and experience with the available evidence may lead to further learning and practice innovations in caring.

Resource Utilization

As noted earlier, the CNS role provides opportunities to contribute at the unit and the organizational levels. Because of this, the CNS develops savvy about available resources and how best to access them. For example, most organizations have volunteer departments who can recruit and train volunteers willing to make contributions. Envisioning opportunities for volunteers to contribute generally occurs at the unit level; a receptive unit reinforces volunteers' motivation. The CNS might optimize resource use by proposing roles for volunteers on the unit (i.e., developing role descriptions and working with nursing and volunteer staff as well as the volunteers to implement the role). Caring practices do not have a lot of products associated with them, and resources for patient education or bereavement programs have costs. The CNS must be a good steward of scarce health care resources by integrating on-line resources, use of libraries and resources centers, and other community resources. Family and friends of the patient are often the most available resource. While facilitating family presence is a beginning, matching the desired contribution with the patients' interests and preferences can optimize resource use.

An exemplar for resource use is one developed to prepare children for visits in the ICU. An intervention, the facilitated child-visitation intervention (FCVI) was developed to prepare children to visit parents and grandparents in the ICU and siblings in the neonatal ICU (Montgomery et al., 1997). The FCVI is designed to anticipate what the child would experience during and after the visit. Interventions that are designed to ensure the well-being of the child and the patient are integral to the FCVI program. This child-centered approach elicited positive responses from staff and family. The environment can be a barrier to providing FCVI as can time available for staff to provide the intervention. By developing tools that other institutions can purchase (i.e., video for parents, video for children, and a brochure), the FCVI has the potential to be replicated and evaluated in other ICUs.

SUMMARY

The knowledge nurses and others have generated have led to innovations in practice that promote caring practices. The challenge for the CNS is to ensure that what is known is implemented in practice. The commitment to evidence-based practice permeates practice as does quality (whether known as performance improvement, QI, or assurance) and attention to patient satisfaction (according to the patient and family rather than the staff). One could say that the stars are in alignment for the CNS to be not only part of significant change but champions and leaders of this change.

DISCUSSION

Case Study

Bob Smith, 55 years old, has been hospitalized awaiting a heart transplant for several weeks. His wife Jane has been at his bedside almost continuously during the wait. At times, Bob becomes frustrated and pessimistic about his future, questioning medications, refusing physical therapy or vital signs, or perhaps skipping a meal. When his spirits sink, Jane is able to rally him to find the strength to keep going. Jane recognizes the staff and has written letters to note the excellent care Bob is receiving. Jane keeps track of Bob's progress in a way that has established a warm relationship with the staff.

The longer the wait, the more comfortable Jane seems in the acute care setting and at the bedside. Although she is willing to stay with her husband during tests, some staff members decline her presence and ask her to please wait outside until they are done.

In approaching this situation, the CNS considers the standards of professional performance.

- *Quality*. An element of patient satisfaction is respecting the individual's knowledge of the patient. Jane believes she knows Bob best, and the staff has had the opportunity to see her work with him and help him go through difficult situations.
- *Individual practice*. The clinician doing the procedure may be uncomfortable doing it in front of a family member—perhaps the clinician is acquiring skill in doing the procedure or perhaps family presence has never been requested. If so, would the staff member be more comfortable if a preceptor were there as a buffer?
- *Education*. The clinician declining Jane's presence may believe there are safety reasons to limit access and be unaware of practice in other settings.
- *Collegiality*. The situation may be perceived in different ways. Who has control in this situation? Is taking the side of the spouse seen as opposing the clinician?
- *Ethics*. One could view this as beneficence (the clinician acting for the good of the patient) versus autonomy (the patient and family having the ultimate say in how things go). Is it fair to Jane to permit only those contributions that the staff prefer and not consider her preference? Is it fair to the patient to limit his wife's presence?
- *Collaboration*. Offers opportunities to seek input of all engaged in the decision and develop an outcome that meets their interests. Is the clinician limiting access acting unilaterally? If trust is breached by these events, does it affect the entire health care team or just the clinician who limits access?
- *Research* provides data that can address issues of both the clinician and Bob and Jane. For example, evidence that presence does not increase infection rates or expedite anxiety may be all that is needed to engender the support of the caregiver for family presence. If the clinician usually permits students or orientees to observe at the bedside and does not permit family members, one could question whether the limits are data driven. This occurrence may point to the need for research that addresses issues of concern, as well as the value of presence.
- *Resource utilization*. The CNS could strategize about what resources could be deployed to accommodate this family request (e.g., a chair for Jane to sit by the bed and hold Bob's hand or staff or volunteers to stay with Jane to be sure that she is fine).

DISCUSSION QUESTIONS

1. Does the issue of limiting family presence occur in your unit?
2. Who support this practice? Who question this practice?
3. Who could you engage to address this issue?
4. Do you have patient satisfaction data that address this issue?
5. What are practices on other units in your organization? Outside your organization?
6. Do hospital policies address this issue? Do they support or limit it?
7. Do regulatory standards or professional standards address this issue?
8. How are caring practices addressed in your organization? What are the ways in which they are addressed?

References

American Association of Critical-Care Nurses (2004). Practice Alert: Family presence during CPR and invasive procedures. Retrieved from www.aacn.org, November 2004.

Angus, D.C., Barnato, A.E., Linde-Zwirble, W.T., et al. (2004). Use of intensive care at the end of life in the United States: An epidemiologic study. *Critical Care Medicine, 32*(3), 638-643.

Azoulay, E., Pochard, F., Chevert, S., et al. (2001). Meeting the needs of intensive care unit patient families: A multicenter study. *American Journal of Respiratory & Critical Care Medicine, 163*(1), 135-139.

Benner, P. (2003a). Current controversies in critical care. Reflecting on what we care about. *American Journal of Critical Care, 12*(2), 165-166.

Benner, P. (2003b). Current controversies in critical care. Creating a more responsible public dialogue about the social, ethical, and legal aspects of genomics. *American Journal of Critical Care, 12*(3), 259-261.

Benner, P. (2003c). Current controversies in critical care. Enhancing patient advocacy and social ethics. *American Journal of Critical Care, 12*(4), 374-375.

Benner, P., Kerchner, S., Corless, I.B., et al. (2003). Current controversies in critical care. Attending death as a human passage: Core nursing principles for end-of-life care. *American Journal of Critical Care, 12*(6), 558-561.

Bijttebier, P., Delva, D., Vanoost, S., et al. (2000). Reliability and validity of the critical care family needs inventory in a Dutch-speaking Belgian sample. *Heart & Lung: Journal of Acute & Critical Care, 29*(4), 278-286.

Campbell, M.L., & Thill, M.C. (1996). Impact of patient consciousness on the intensity of the do-not-resuscitate therapeutic plan. *American Journal of Critical Care, 5*(5), 339-445.

Chin, P. (1996). Cultural profile: Chinese Americans. In P.A. Minarik, J.G. Lipson, & S.L. Dibble. *Culture and nursing care: A pocket guide.* San Francisco: UCSF Nursing Press.

Ciccarello, G.P. (2003). Strategies to improve end-of-life care in the intensive care unit. *DCCN: Dimensions of Critical Care Nursing, 22*(5), 216-222.

Dickerson, L., & Lester, B. (2003). *Family liaison: Help for the family while their loved one is in the critical care unit.* Program and Proceedings of the 2003 National Teaching Institute & Critical Care Exposition, p. 205. Aliso Viejo, CA: American Association of Critical Care Nurses.

Dossey, B.M. (2000a). *Florence Nightingale: Mystic, visionary, reformer.* Springhouse, PA: Springhouse Publishing.

Dossey, B.M. (2000b). *Holistic nursing: A handbook for practice.* Boston: Jones & Bartlett Publishers.

Gardner, A., Goodsell, J., Duggan, T., et al. (2001). 'Don't call me sweetie!' Patients differ from nurses in their perceptions of caring. *Collegian: Journal of the Royal College of Nursing, Australia, 8*(3), 32-38.

Gordon, M. (1982). Nursing diagnosis: Process and application. In L.J. Carpenito, (1993). *Nursing diagnosis application to clinical practice* (ed. 5). Philadelphia: J.B. Lippincott.

Guzzetta, C., & Dossey, B. (1984). *Cardiovascular nursing bodymind tapestry.* St. Louis: Mosby.

Halm, M.A., Gagner, S., Goering, M., et al. (2003). Interdisciplinary rounds. Impact on patients, families, and staff. *Clinical Nurse Specialist, 17*(3), 133-142.

Hanson, C., & Strawser, D. (1992). Family presence during cardiopulmonary resuscitation: Foote Hospital emergency department's nine-year perspective. *Journal of Emergency Nursing, 18*(2), 104-106.

Johnson, M., Maas, M., & Moorhead, S. (Eds.). (2000). *Nursing outcomes classification (NOC)* (ed. 2). St. Louis: Mosby.

Kosco, M., & Warren, N.A. (2000). Critical care nurses' perceptions of family needs as met. *Critical Care Nursing Quarterly, 23*(2),: 60-72.

Larson, P.J. (1986). Cancer nurses' perceptions of caring. *Cancer Nursing, 9*(2), 86-91.

Leske, J.S. (1986). The needs of relatives of critically ill patients: A follow-up. *Heart and Lung, 15*, 189-193.

Leung, K.K., Chien, W.T., & Mackenzie, A.E. (2000). Needs of Chinese families of critically ill patients. *Western Journal of Nursing Research, 22*, 826-840.

Lindquist, R., Tracy M.F., & Savik K. (2003). Personal use of complementary and alternative therapies by critical care nurses. *Critical Care Nursing Clinics of North America. 15*(3), 393-399.

MacLean, S.L., Guzzetta, C., White, C., et al. (2003). Family presence during cardiopulmonary resuscitation and invasive procedures: Practices of critical care and emergency nurses. *American Journal of Critical Care, 12*(3), 246-257.

Maloney-Harmon, P. (1999). The Synergy Model: contemporary practice of the clinical nurse specialist. *Critical Care Nurse, 19*(2), 101-104.

Mayer, D.K. (1987). Oncology nurses' versus cancer patients' perceptions of nurse caring behaviors: A replication study. *Oncology Nursing Forum, 14*(3), 48-52.

McCloskey J.C., & Bulechek G.M (Eds.). (2000). *Nursing interventions classification (NIC)* (ed. 3). St. Louis: Mosby.

Mehta, R.H., Montoye, C.K., Gallogly, M., et al. (2002). Improving quality of life for acute myocardial infarction. The guidelines applied in practice (GAP) initiative. *Journal of the American Medical Association, 287*(10), 1269-1276.

Mendonca, D., & Warren, N.A. (1998). Perceived and unmet needs of critical care family members. *Critical Care Nursing Quarterly, 21*(1), 58-67.

Merkel, S.I., Voepel-Lewis, T., Shayevitz, J.R., et al. (1997). Practice applications of research. The FLACC: A behavioral scale for scoring postoperative pain in young children. *Pediatric Nursing, 23*(3), 293-297.

Meyers, T., Eichhorn, D., Guzzetta, C., et al. (2004). Family presence during invasive procedures and resuscitation: The experience of family members, nurses, and physicians. *Topics in Emergency Medicine, 26*(1), 61-73.

Molter, N. C. (1979). Needs of the relatives of critically ill patients: A descriptive study. *Heart and Lung, 8*, 332-339.

Molter, N.C., & Leske, J.S. (1986). Critical care family needs inventory. In Spatt, L., et al. Informational needs of families of intensive care unit patients. *Quality Review Bulletin, 1*, 16-21.

Molter, N.C., & Leske J.S. (1983). Critical care family needs inventory (CCFNI). J.S. Leske, PhD, RN, Associate Professor, School of Nursing, University of Wisconsin-Milwaukee, Milwaukee, WI 53201.

Montgomery, L., Kleiber, C., Nicholson, A., et al. (1997). A research-based sibling visitation program for the neonatal ICU. *Critical Care Nurse, 17*(2), 29-40.

NANDA Nursing diagnoses 2003-2004: Definitions and classification, NANDA Staff, North American Nursing Diagnosis Association, 2003.

Pate, M. & Crider, J. (2003). *Goodnight moon: Helping loved ones cope with the death of a child*. Program and Proceedings of the 2003 National Teaching Institute & Critical Care Exposition. p. 195. Aliso Viejo, Ca: American Association of Critical Care Nurses.

Petlin, A., Becker, C., & Powers, C. (2003). *Completing the circle: A cardiac surgery telephone follow-up program*. Program and Proceedings of the 2003 National Teaching Institute & Critical Care Exposition, p. 205. Aliso Viejo, Ca: American Association of Critical Care Nurses.

Prevost, S. (2002). Clinical nurse specialist outcomes: Vision voice and value. *Clinical Nurse Specialist, 16*(3), 119-124.

Puntillo, K.A., Stannard, D., Miaskowski, C., et al. (2002). Use of a pain assessment and intervention notation (P.A.I.N.) tool in critical care nursing practice: Nurses' evaluations. *Heart & Lung: Journal of Acute & Critical Care, 31*(4),303-314.

Redley, B., & Beanland, C. (2004). Revising the critical care family needs inventory for the emergency department. *Journal of Advanced Nursing, 45*(1), 95-104.

Sackett, D.L., Straus, S.E., Richardson, W.S., et al. (2000). *Evidence-based medicine. How to practice and teach EBM*. (ed. 2). p. 2. Edinburgh: Churchill-Livingstone.

Schwartz, L.P., & Brenner, Z.R. (1979). Critical care unit transfer: Reducing patient stress through nursing interventions. *Heart & Lung: Journal of Acute & Critical Care, 8*(3), 540-546.

Simpson, T. (1991). Critical care patients' perceptions of visits. *Heart & Lung: Journal of Acute & Critical Care, 20*(6), 681-688.

Simpson, T. (1996). Implementation and evaluation of a liberalized visiting policy. *American Journal of Critical Care, 5*(6), 420-426.

Slota, M., Shearn, D., Potersnak, K., et al. (2003). Perspectives on family-centered, flexible visitation in the intensive care unit setting. *Critical Care Medicine, 31*(5):Suppl, S362-365.

Urden, L.D. (2001). Outcome evaluation: An essential component for CNS practice. *Clinical Nurse Specialist, 15*(6), 260-268.

Ward, K. (2001). Practice applications of research. Perceived needs of parents of critically ill infants in a neonatal intensive care unit (NICU). *Pediatric Nursing, 27*(3), 281-286.

Warren, N.A. (2002). Critical care family members' satisfaction with bereavement experiences. *Critical Care Nursing Quarterly, 25*(2), 54-60.

Widmark-Petersson, V., von Essen, L., & Sjoden, P. (1998). Perceptions of caring: Patients' and staff's associations to CARE-Q behaviors. *Journal of Psychosocial Oncology 16*(1), 75-96.

Willis, M.H., Merkel, S.I., Voepel-Lewis, T., et al. (2003). FLACC Behavioral Pain Assessment Scale: A comparison with the child's self-report. *Pediatric Nursing, 29*(3), 195-198.

Response to Diversity

John F. Dixon, Jr.

"Unity does not exclude diversity, nay more, without diversity there can be no true and perfect unity." Farrar (1882)

INTRODUCTION

Definition

Diversity is complex because of the many different characteristics compromising it. For every individual, elements such as socioeconomic status, ethnicity, and gender combine and interact to create a unique set of attributes and needs. To competently provide nursing care within a culturally relevant context, nurses must incorporate these elements into assessments, plans, and interventions. This aspect of practice seems overwhelming, considering the multitude of cultures in the world. In addition, a single cultural group can have many subcultures or variations. A nurse may wonder, "How can I learn everything about all cultures?" The answer is that he or she cannot. The goal of the nurse is to become as knowledgeable and skillful as possible by getting to know and understand the individuals, families, communities, and populations for whom he or she cares. This learning will be an ongoing process, not a one-time event. To fulfill the central premise of patient characteristics driving nurse competencies of the AACN Synergy Model for Patient Care, the nurse's attention and consideration must expand beyond the traditional clinical assessment and incorporate the elements of diversity.

A dictionary definition of diversity includes the terms *different, varied, unlikeness, distinction,* and *variety* (Simpson & Weiner, 1989). The general population's notion of diversity probably revolves around cultural or ethnic differences. Perhaps this mental model was developed or reinforced through workplace programs that focus on only a few traits or lay media reports that spotlight a narrow and repeating set of themes. Diversity is more than culture, ethnicity, race, and gender. The Synergy Model's Response to Diversity lists characteristics such as "individuality, cultural practices, spiritual beliefs, sex, race, ethnicity, disability, family configuration, lifestyle, socioeconomic status, age, values, and alternative care practices" (Curley, 1998), but this roster is not complete. Additional considerations include educational level, housing, residential neighborhoods, language skills, immigration status, acculturation, health beliefs, community resources, and social networks. These characteristics are not isolated components of a person but are dynamic and interactive, creating a unique individual.

Vulnerability, a patient characteristic of the Synergy Model, is related to diversity and is a state of being "susceptible to harm or neglect" (Aday, 2001). Someone with an adequate and stable income, sufficient health insurance, fluent language skills, and a steady and reliable family structure has distinct advantages over someone who does not. Such advantages, or disadvantages, influence the degree of vulnerability and, in turn, risk. For example, an undocumented worker with limited English skills may not seek needed treatment, fearing immigration issues. Another person may not disclose his or her sexual orientation, fearing stereotyping or discrimination by the health care provider. These risk factors may influence morbidity and mortality, and some may be antecedents for the development of yet other risks (Flaskerud & Winslow, 1998). Although all individuals have potential for risk, some persons or groups experience greater levels related to their limited resources (Aday, 2001).

The delivery of culturally competent care requires nurses to broaden our view from the individual patient to include the community in which the patient lives. Aday (2001) uses these two perspectives, individual and community, to evaluate and study health and health care needs of vulnerable populations. Using her framework, nurses can assess the availability of individual versus community resources, exploring whether the interactions have a positive or negative effect. The individual perspective includes resources the patient can use, the degree of susceptibility to harm or risk, and specific health care needs. The community perspective includes the existence of community resources and available networks, the population's risk as a whole, and community health needs influencing health policy. The type and degree of interaction between the individual and the community can increase healthful benefits or risks, determine vulnerability, influence relationships with health care providers, and impact progress along the health care continuum.

Information gained by using Aday's framework may identify factors creating or contributing to the patient's current need for care. The nurse may discover that a patient has a fixed income and is not able to purchase his medications. Another may live in sub-standard housing, aggravating her pulmonary condition. This knowledge can be especially important as the patient and nurse develop discharge plans and interventions to address these needs. The goal, then, is to minimize the chance that the patient will need care again in the near future, thus improving their quality of life.

Population Changes

With the degree and extent that diversity continues to increase in the U.S. population, health care providers' "sensitivity to recognize, appreciate, and incorporate differences into the provision of care" (Curley, 1998) becomes increasingly important. Reports from the U.S. Census 2000 reflect some key trends. The population change between 1990 and 2000 was the largest increase recorded in a sequential census-to-census comparison (Perry & Mackun, 2001).

Populations in counties along the Mexican border grew by 21%. The foreign-born population increased by 57%, with over one half born in Latin America (Malone, Baluja, Costanzo, & Davis, 2003). Mexico was the primary country of origin. The number of homes in which languages other than English was spoken also increased during this time period (Shin & Bruno, 2003). Primarily in the South and West, Spanish was the most prevalent language, followed distantly by Chinese and then French. The number of households in which no person age 14 or over speaks English at least "very well" rose significantly. Language issues such as these can create communication challenges between patients and providers.

As the diversity of the U.S. population is changing, it is also aging just as median ages are rising worldwide (McDevitt & Rowe, 2002). The impact on health care is that the number of working adults may not be sufficient to support the number of elderly. All of these changes and more are creating new and greater demands on nurses and health care systems.

Along with these patient population changes, nurses and other health care providers are beginning to reflect an increase in diversity. Today's workforce is more mobile and global compared with years ago. It is not unusual to have a nurse practicing outside of her home country or an international worker receiving nursing care outside of his native country.

In the United States nursing is slowly changing. Of the top 10 professions employing the most women in the United States in 2000, nursing was third (Fronczek & Johnson, 2003). Minority representation in nursing is rising and accounts for 12% of the profession, but this still does not reflect the general population at over 30% (Spratley, Johnson, Sochalski, Fritz, & Spencer, 2000). Among advanced practice nurses, minority representation is nearly 10%, with the majority in the nurse practitioner role. First-year enrollments in medical schools also reflect this under-representation of minorities (Barzansky & Etzel, 2003). The blend of patients requiring care and those delivering care continues to evolve, representing a growing variety of patient characteristics and needed nursing competencies.

Outcomes

In the 2003 National Healthcare Disparities Report (AHRQ, 2003), differences in access to health care and quality were associated with race, ethnicity, income, education, and place of residence. Increasing attention has been directed at ways to reduce these disparities. Governmental agencies have launched various initiatives (CDC, 2004; U.S. DHHS, 2000). The Office of Minority Health, U.S. Department of Health and Human Services, finalized and published the culturally and linguistically appropriate services (CLAS) standards in December, 2000 (Ross, 2001). This document is a "blueprint to follow for building culturally competent health care organizations and workers" (Ross, 2001). These 14 standards address three major themes: culturally competent care, language access services, and organizational supports for cultural competence.

The 2004 Comprehensive Accreditation Manual for Hospitals (Joint Commission on Accreditation of Healthcare Organizations, 2004) has various standards and expectations addressing culture or diversity for staff orientation, environmental design and planning, ethics, food preparation, and patient care. In an ever-changing environment, the ability to respond to differences is a requisite to reduce and eliminate existing disparities and prevent

the development of future ones. Nurses need to develop cultural competence because without it they will struggle to achieve synergy and make our optimal contribution.

CNS Level of Expertise

Education
Response to diversity requires knowledge and skills beyond a traditional clinically focused education. Such content may or may not have been a part of the academic preparation of clinical nurse specialists (CNSs), depending on the school's curriculum and framework, the program's study focus, or specialty pathway selected. Adding a population perspective to a traditional clinical focus may be a new undertaking. The CNS needs to know who makes up a particular clinical group and how to identify and accommodate needs and differences represented not only by the population but also by its various sub-populations. This requires the CNS to explore and learn about key diversity elements within these primary populations for whom they are responsible. Acquiring this knowledge is not always easy. Available relevant research that is plentiful for one group may be extremely limited for another, even though both share a common clinical condition. For example, a CINAHL or MEDLINE search for congestive heart failure returns thousands of citations. If this search is then narrowed to Hispanics, the result is only a small number of articles.

Environmental Assessment
The greater the knowledge about the patient, family, and nursing personnel, the better the CNS can evaluate organizational systems. The CNS has opportunities to talk with the health care team members one-on-one and in group settings and to observe their interactions with patients, families, and each other. This information may give insight into staff strengths or concerns and provide feedback on how well the nurse's competencies complement the patient's needs. Knowledge gained from these observations and perspectives may identify

needed organizational changes (e.g., change in visitation policy, increased number of translators, better understanding of certain religious practices) or provide rationale for developing and championing new programs (e.g., population-specific content during new staff orientation, transcultural nursing seminars).

Information learned through these activities contribute to setting priorities for organizational initiatives and developing programs to decrease the gaps between the patient's needs and the nurse's competencies. Printed materials such as education brochures may need to be translated into other languages, to be provided in large-print options or pictographs, or to include photographs updated to reflect the diversity of the patient population. New-hire orientation or annual updates for incumbent staff may need content changes or additions. Research into staff perceptions may give insight into how best to approach a broadening spectrum of patient needs. Although the journey to building cultural competence may be varied, the commitment is long-term, learning ongoing, and role modeling a requisite (Frusti, Niesen, & Campion, 2003).

Communication

Formal and informal communication channels are means to collect a rich amount of information. Chart documents such as an admission inventory or patient history are a traditional formal source. Items found on such a form may include the patient's religious preferences, dietary habits, cultural practices, ways of coping, significant others, current concerns or worries, and age-related physical limitations or safety risks. Certain responses can serve as automatic triggers for needed interventions such as dietary consults, physical therapy assessments, financial assistance referrals, or chaplain notification. The CNS should evaluate currently used forms to ensure they adequately capture patient characteristics.

Another formal communication mechanism is interdisciplinary rounds during which goals of care can be discussed. An established communication system ensures that the whole health care team remains current on information learned during rounds and updates shared with the patient and family. The method may be a permanent chart document such as an interdisciplinary record or a temporary form such as a rounds log. Interactions with the patient and family through casual conversations or formal solicitation of feedback and input may provide further insight into current needs or identify new ones. Some discussions may reveal potential obstacles to reaching optimal outcomes (e.g., patient is thinking about replacing current medical treatment with alternative measures), whereas others may support overall care initiatives (e.g., patient believes that praying supplements the healing process).

The collection of assessment data is an ongoing process requiring good dialogue skills. Communication is a common thread throughout these processes but can be challenging when all parties do not share a common language. The flow of information is vital to maintaining and developing responsiveness to diversity issues.

Transcultural Caring

The CNS has a key role in elevating diversity awareness by sharing knowledge, research, and personal experience. Some health care team members may be too involved with a situation or limit their assessment to the clinical condition, resulting in a narrow view. Although not incorrect since a primary objective is to provide clinical care, a limited scope creates an incomplete patient evaluation and thus can impact care delivery and regimens.

Patient diversity creates a need for cultural competency in nurses and the environments in which they practice. To support culturally relevant care delivery, several nursing leaders have proposed culture care theories, models, and frameworks (Table 12-1).

Through established relationships, the CNS can engage health care team members to think of diversity considerations and

TABLE 12-1

Transcultural Care Theories, Models, and Frameworks

Nurse Leader	Key Points
Madeleine Leininger, PhD, LHD, DS, CTN, FAAN, FRCNA	Culture Care Diversity and Universality Theory • Introduced in the mid-1950s • Oldest and most comprehensive • Sunrise Model used with the theory • Focuses on differences and commonalities • Addresses folk care and professional practice (Leininger, 2002)
Larry Purnell, PhD, RN, FAAN	Purnell Model for Cultural Competence • Introduced in 1998 • Uses 12 domains to address various concepts related to assessment, planning, and intervention (Purnell, 2002)
Joyce Newman Giger, EdD, RN, CS, FAAN	Giger and Davidhizar Transcultural Assessment Model • Introduced in 1998
Ruth Davidhizar, DNS, RN, CS, FAAN	• Uses six cultural phenomena as an assessment frame work (Giger & Davidhizar, 2002)
Josepha Campinha-Bacote, PhD, RN, CNS, BC, CTN, FAAN	Campinha-Bacote's Model of Cultural Competence in Health Care Delivery • Development began in 1969 • Five major cultural constructs that intersect to create the process of cultural competence (Campinha-Bacote, 2002)
Rachel E. Spector, PhD, RN, CTN, FAAN	• Uses three different theories and models • Promotes the role of the nurse as patient advocate (Spector, 2002)

interventions in reference to the Synergy Model's eight patient characteristics (Table 12-2). CNSs have the advantage in that the health care team already views their advanced practice role as an established clinical expert and reliable resource. Using this influence, the CNS can act as a role model, change agent, teacher, coach, and mentor, ensuring that key diversity factors are identified and integrated into the provision of care. Knowledge and expertise shared through these roles support a primary focus on the total patient, assist with care customization, and foster matching of nurse competencies to patient needs.

IMPLEMENTATION WITHIN THE RESPONSE TO DIVERSITY

Case Study

Mrs. A., a 75-year-old Russian woman with acute exacerbation of congestive heart failure, was admitted from the emergency department to a critical care unit. Her condition required intubation and ventilatory support. According to her family, her activity level had been diminishing over the last week, and she required more frequent periods of rest. Despite their concerns and questions, she insisted she was fine.

TABLE 12-2

Synergy Model Patient Characteristics and Diversity

Patient Characteristics	Diversity Considerations	Implementation Examples
Resiliency	Personal belief/value systems Religion and religious symbols Community resources	Allocate time for prayer or meditation. Encourage use of religious artifacts and icons in the patient's room. Contact clergy to visit as requested by patient. Evaluate patient's need for supporting community services as discharge plans are formulated.
Vulnerability	Age-related limitations or risks Disability Family support Other support networks Group membership	Create safety-oriented environments by accommodating for age-related deficits. Determine who, if anyone, will be available to the patient after discharge. Explore degree of family support and interaction.
Stability	Alternative care practices Cultural practices Health care beliefs	Assess how traditional medical interventions and alternative care practices can be integrated. What would the patient/family like to see present to aid progress (e.g., placement of crystals, following certain rituals, involvement of a local healer)?
Complexity	Family systems Family member roles Family dynamics	Assess family roles and responsibilities. Determine if there are identified leaders such as a patriarch or matriarch.
Resource availability	Socioeconomic status Housing	Consult with nurse case manager, social worker, or facility's financial counselor.
Participation in care	Insurance status Definition of the sick role Family member obligations or roles in the care of other family members Medical bureaucracies	Incorporate family members in the provision of care. Customize visitation times as needed by the patient/family. Regularly seek input from the patient/family related to caring practices.
Participation in decision making	Passive versus active role Trust or mistrust of health care Gender roles Locus of control	Consult often with the patient/family for input regarding needed decisions. Answer questions honestly. Keep promises. Fulfill commitment. Demonstrate respect. Value the patient/family contribution.
Predictability	Immigration Ethnicity/Race Discrimination/Prejudice	Validate patient/family understanding and rationale for care processes. Provide consistent core messages by all health care team members. Use a common language. Inquire into patient/family satisfaction with care practices.

Assessment

Patient/family: Due to her condition, Mrs. A. was unable to provide background information. Her grown son and daughter answered questions as best they could. The staff learned that Mrs. A. is a deeply spiritual person and depends on her faith as a strong ally. She graduated from high school in Russia and her ability to communicate in English is extremely limited. She lives alone in a house one mile from her daughter. Not wanting to be a burden on her family, she prides herself on being as independent as possible. The family frequently visits and assists her with errands such as grocery shopping. She has been a widow for a number of years. Besides her family, her social circle primarily includes ladies from her church who are also Russian immigrants. She has a limited, fixed income. Her health insurance is a policy originated by her husband, but coverage is limited. Her family provides additional assistance as necessary.

Nursing personnel: None of the nursing staff speak Russian. One nurse has expressed great frustration in not being able to communicate with Mrs. A. and has asked to not be assigned to her.

Organizational systems: The hospital has translators available but not on site. A call is placed to the service, and a translator can provide services over the phone or come to the hospital as required. Visiting hours for the unit are very restricted.

Diagnosis

The use of existing nursing diagnoses in an increasingly transcultural context has generated discussion about congruence and applicability. The recurring issue is the presence of embedded cultural bias that requires the nurse to reexamine how well the definition matches with the patient and assessment data (Dennis & Small, 2003). For example, the nurse may make diagnosis selections based on his or her personal values or cultural perspective without consideration for the patient. Walsh (2004) identifies two major

challenges for the nurse. The first is to increase knowledge related to cultural care, especially related to concepts such as illness and wellness. Nursing diagnoses with a particular potential for such bias are those addressing behavior. In these cases, behavior may be the expression of a person's culture. Second, the nurse must be self-aware of stereotyping or judgmental decisions when developing diagnoses and plans of care.

If the nurse selects the nursing diagnosis Impaired Verbal Communication, questions related to its application to Mrs. A. include: "What is the definition of this diagnosis?", "Does the definition address any unique cultural patterns of communication?", and "Does the definition recognize nonphysiological etiologies of communication impairment such as the mismatch between the patient's primary language and that of the health care system?"

Outcome Identification

Patient/family: Return Mrs. A. to her prehospital state, chronic and stable. Educate Mrs. A. and her family to minimize her risk for readmission. Validate patient and family understanding of self-monitoring and medications. Accommodate as best as possible any patient/family differences that may impact adherence to the plan of care.

Nursing personnel: Establish a strong connection with Mrs. A. in spite of the language difference.

Organizational systems: Establish good communication options. Tailor and organize care to meet the needs of patients and their families.

Planning

Patient/family: Have family members bring in religious items of significance to Mrs. A. Notify her priest of her admission. Involve family members in the delivery of care if they so desire and as appropriate or allowable. Use these opportunities to teach and reinforce or validate prior teaching.

Nursing personnel: Have the son and daughter work with staff related to some key Russian words.

Organizational systems: Accommodate the schedules of family and visitors who speak Russian. Conduct a multidisciplinary conference with the family to assess Mrs. A.'s environment at home, identify any potential risks for readmission, answer any questions, agree to a plan of care, and set goals.

Implementation

Patient/family: Mrs. A.'s bible, a cross, and a religious icon were placed on a bedside table where she could see and touch them. The priest made arrangements for himself or one of the ladies from the church to come and visit with Mrs. A. on a daily basis.

Nursing personnel: Mrs. A.'s children helped the nurses with several key words in Russian such as "pain," "where," "hot," and "cold." These were written phonetically on a reference card for all staff to use. In addition to the hospital's contracted translator service, the staff optimized use of the family, priest, and ladies from the church to communicate with the patient.

Organizational systems: The unit's visitation policy was liberalized to accommodate the availability and work schedules of families and visitors.

Evaluation

Patient/family: Mrs. A. was on the ventilator less than 24 hours. She was ready for discharge on her fifth hospital day. During the stay the CNS learned the patient had begun to ration her medications because of financial concerns, which resulted in her acute exacerbation. A consultation with the nurse case manager and the hospital's financial counselor helped Mrs. A. to explore some additional financial resources. Mrs. A.'s family was unaware of her rationing, and, being proud, she was reluctant to tell them. Once they learned of this, they said they too would help out financially as best as they could. The CNS knew the patient education materials were only available in English and Spanish, so she worked with the family to create an abbreviated version in

Russian, using many pictures representing daily monitoring and medication management.

Nursing personnel: Staff became more familiar with the key Russian words. By incorporating family and other key individuals in Mrs. A.'s care delivery, communication was enhanced. Through the staff's striving to speak Russian, a stronger bond grew between the staff and Mrs. A. She told her family she felt very respected because the nurses were taking the time and making the effort to communicate in her native language. Mrs. A.'s family had developed similar opinions of the staff and they shared these with the nurse manager.

Organizational systems: In talking with colleagues, the CNS discovered that the number of Russian-speaking patients seemed to be increasing. Further investigation revealed a small but growing Russian immigrant community in the city. An analysis of admissions over the past year showed these to be primarily in the cardiovascular service line. Priorities for translating patient education materials into Russian were set based on the frequency of diagnoses admitted. The education council collaborated with the local community through the priest to develop for the nursing staff an expanded, quick-reference Russian language sheet similar to the one used with Mrs. A. During these working sessions the education council learned more about Russian customs and heritage. Open visitation was successful. Families besides Mrs. A.'s commented on how it helped to reduce their anxiety, and they thought it enhanced communication. The staff reported that their anticipatory worries about making this change did not become a reality. The CNS was able to engage the staff's interest in a research project evaluating the impact on patient and family satisfaction related to the visitation policy change.

INTEGRATION OF THE STANDARDS OF PROFESSIONAL PERFORMANCE

Quality Care and Research

A key focus for quality of care is carefully monitoring for health care disparities. When participating in quality of care activities, be sensitive to care issues or outcome variations possibly related to diversity such as miscommunication and lack of patient/family education options. An analysis of these data may lead to more frequent or detailed monitoring. New audit criteria may need to be implemented; and nursing practices, care paths or other forms, and care delivery altered to meet the needs of both the patient and family. Although the primary focus of this monitoring is the patient, it is important to include measures about and feedback from the family through mechanisms such as care conferences, satisfaction questionnaires, or needs assessments.

Opportunities exist for using and doing transcultural research. The CNS is in a key role to advocate for inclusion of cultural research when hospital policies, procedures, and programs are revised. Another area of research is to challenge traditional notions or practices. Some questions to be asked from a diversity framework might include: "Are the needs of all families the same?", "What is the image of nursing in various cultures?", "What are the best ways to educate individuals?", and "How is caring defined?" Studies have shown that some generalizations to the population as a whole have not held true when examined from a cultural context (Kumpfer, Alvarado, Smith, & Bellamy, 2002; Waters 1999).

Individual Practice Evaluation

A first step on the journey of cultural competence is for the CNS is to explore and understand his or her own cultural frame of reference. One means to do this is through a cultural rooting exercise (Zoucha, 2000). By understanding his or her own cultural self, the CNS is better prepared to understand, work with, and assist others in a cultural context. Zoucha (2000) suggests four rules for incorporating cultural knowledge into care processes:

1. *Be aware of your own culture.* This will help you in your interactions and actions with culturally diverse patients.
2. *Be open.* Your patient will be more likely to share information about his or her

health and nursing care needs if they perceive you as open with them.
3. *Be honest with yourself.* What are your beliefs about people from different cultures? Do you have any racist or prejudicial feelings? Educate yourself about cultures. You can then understand what is the most appropriate manner of caring for an individual or family. People often sense prejudice, even if these feelings aren't expressed verbally.
4. *Be real* (i.e., recognize that the other person's culture is different from your own but equally valid) *in your use of respect and concern for culturally different patients.* How would you like to be treated? What have you learned in the process of being open and honest toward culturally different patients?" (Zoucha, 2000, p. 24HH).

Education

Transcultural education is an ongoing process because our knowledge and nursing models in this arena is expanding. The number of resources, research, and manuscripts in transcultural nursing continues to increase. The Transcultural Nursing Society (www.tcns.org) and the *Journal of Transcultural Nursing* are primary references. The U.S. Department of Health and Human Services established The Office of Minority Health Resource Center (www.omhrc. gov) in 1985 with a mission to "improve and protect the health of racial and ethnic minority populations through the development of health policies and programs that will eliminate health disparities." The OMHRC website is a key source for information such as statistics, publications, and conferences and includes the National Standards on Culturally and Linguistically Appropriate Services (CLAS) in Health Care under the Cultural Competency program. When researching clinical issues of target populations, searches can be further restricted by adding cultural qualifiers to find publications addressing unique needs of particular groups.

Collegiality, Collaboration, and Resource Utilization

Open communication and role modeling of desired practices and behaviors are important to increasing awareness of the need for cultural competence. The Internet affords CNSs an opportunity to make contact with individuals far beyond their own geographical area and cultural domain. Establishing on-line professional collaborations with hospitals and nurses in other countries is a good means for expanding cultural knowledge and care practices. Such exchanges can benefit practitioners and patients at both locations.

Interdisciplinary team discussions need to include not only the goals of care but also an evaluation of the goals from a cultural context (e.g., How does the treatment regimen fit or conflict with the patient's and family's belief system and what community resources are available to meet their needs?). Identifying and establishing community networks may have positive impacts on length of stay, charges, or readmission rates by being able to match their services with the needs of patients.

Ethics

The threads of culturally competent care and advocacy are present in ethical codes for nurses. The American Nurses Association Code of Ethics for Nurses (2001), Provision 1, addresses nursing practice based on respect for the uniqueness of the patient without influence of characteristics such as socioeconomic status. Similarly, the International Council of Nurses Code of Ethics for Nurses (2000) discusses providing care in consideration of the patient's diversity. To ensure that nursing practice is consistent with these tenets, nurses must be sensitive to patient needs that arise from diversity.

The nurse is in a primary role to serve as the patient's advocate, ensuring that needs are addressed and that care is not delivered in a manner of "one size fits all." Research of diverse and vulnerable populations is a good example of this need for advocacy. The characteristics of some patients make them doubly vulnerable and can further reduce their autonomy (Moore & Miller, 1999). For a researcher, exclusion of such subjects from a study would pose fewer challenges, but the study would lose valuable information on the unique needs of such a population that can only be answered by that population. Carefully monitoring for sound ethical research strategies when involving such populations is an important advocacy role. Established notions of wellness, illness, and compliance may need to be reevaluated within an ethical framework and may possibly include alternative or complementary care practices. Advocating for identification of new resources, development of broader perspectives, and a more diligent focus from a cultural viewpoint is important to meeting the needs of this population.

DISCUSSION QUESTIONS

1. Does your organization's mission or philosophy of care address cultural sensitivity and competence?
2. How and when do new hires and incumbent staff receive information on culturally competent care?
3. How well do the current forms in your organization capture culturally relevant data? How is that information used to plan care? How does your organization ensure that culturally sensitive interventions are part of care delivery?
4. Has your organization identified any trends in patient admissions or discharges signaling demographic shifts in your target patient populations?
5. What supporting structures and resources are present in your organization to meet the unique needs of your culturally diverse population?
6. Does your organization assess for the presence of health care disparities in patient outcomes?
7. In research studies, how well do study populations reflect the demographics of the local community?

References

Aday, L.A. (2001). *At risk in America: The health and health care needs of vulnerable populations in the United States* (ed. 2). San Francisco, CA: Josey-Bass.

Agency for Healthcare Research and Quality (AHRQ). (2003, July). *National healthcare disparities report*. Rockville, MD: AHRQ.

American Nurses Association (2001). Code of Ethics for Nurses with Interpretive Statements. Retrieved August 30, 2004, from American Nurses Association website: http://www.nursing-world.org/ethics/code/ethicscode150.htm.

Barzansky, B., & Etzel, S.I. (2003). Educational programs in U.S. medical schools, 2002-2003. *Journal of the American Medical Association, 290*(9), 1190-1196.

Campinha-Bacote, J. (2002). The process of cultural competence in the delivery of healthcare services: A model of care. *Journal of Transcultural Nursing, 13*(3), 181-184.

Centers for Disease Control and Prevention (CDC). (2004). *Racial and ethnic approaches to community health (REACH) 2010: Addressing disparities in health 2004*. Atlanta, GA: CDC.

Curley, M. (1998). Patient-nurse synergy: Optimizing patients' outcomes. *American Journal of Critical Care, 7*(1), xxx.

Dennis, B.P., & Small, E.B. (2003). Incorporating cultural diversity in nursing care: An action plan. *The Association of Black Nursing Faculty Journal, 14*(1), 17-25.

Flaskerud, J.H., & Winslow, B.J. (1998). Conceptualizing vulnerable populations health-related research. *Nursing Research, 47*(2), 69-78.

Fronczek, P., & Johnson, P. (2003, August). *Census 2000 brief: Occupations: 2000*. Washington, D.C., U.S. Census Bureau, U.S. Department of Commerce, Economics and Statistics Administration.

Frusti, D.K., Niesen, K.M., & Campion, J.K. (2003). Creating a culturally competent organization: Use of the diversity competence model. *Journal of Nursing Administration, 33*(1), 31-38.

Giger, J.N. & Davidhizar, R. (2002). The Giger and Davidhizar transcultural assessment model. *Journal of transcultural Nursing, 13*(3), 185-188.

Joint Commission on Accreditation of Healthcare Organizations: *2004 Comprehensive Accreditation Manual for Hospitals*. Oakbrook Terrace, IL: Joint Commission Resources.

Kumpfer, K., Alvarado, R., Smith, P, & Bellamy, N. (2002). Cultural sensitivity and adaptation in family-based prevention interventions. *Prevention Science, 3*(3), 241-246.

Leininger, M. (2002). Culture care theory: A major contribution to advance transcultural nursing knowledge and practices. *Journal of Transcultural Nursing, 13*(3), 189-192.

Malone, N., Baluja, K., Costanzo, J.M., & Davis, C.J. (2003, December). Census 2000 Brief: The foreign-born population: 2000. Washington, D.C., U.S. Census Bureau, U.S. Department of Commerce, Economics and Statistics Administration.

McDevitt, T.M., & Rowe, P. (2002, February). Census 2000 Brief: The United States in international context: 2000. Washington, D.C., U.S. Census Bureau, U.S. Department of Commerce, Economics and Statistics Administration.

Moore, L.W. & Miller, M. (1999). Initiating research with doubly vulnerable populations. *Journal of Advanced Nursing, 30*(5), 1034-1040.

Perry, M.J., & Mackun, P.J. (2001, April). Census 2000 Brief: Population change and distribution: 1990-2000. Washington, D.C., U.S. Census Bureau, U.S. Department of Commerce, Economics and Statistics Administration.

Purnell, L. (2002). The Purnell model for cultural competence. *Journal of Transcultural Nursing, 13*(3), 193-196.

Ross, H. (2001, February/March). Office of Minority Health publishes final standards for cultural and linguistic competence. *Closing the Gap*, 1-3, 10. http://www.omhrc.gov/CLAS.

Shin, H.B., & Bruno, R. (2003, October). Census 2000 Brief: Language use and English-speaking ability: 2000. Washington, D.C., U.S. Census Bureau, U.S. Department of Commerce, Economics and Statistics Administration.

Simpson, J.A., & Weiner, E.S. (Eds.). (1989). *Oxford English dictionary on-line* (ed. 2). Oxford, UK: Oxford University Press.

Spector, R.E. (2002). Cultural diversity in health and illness. *Journal of Transcultural Nursing, 13*(3), 197-199.

Spratley, E., Johnson, A., Sochalski, J., Fritz, M., & Spencer, W. (2000, March). *The registered nurse population: Findings from the national sample survey of registered nurses*. Washington, D.C., U.S. Department of Health and Human Services, Health Resources and Service Administration, Bureau of Health Professions, Division of Nursing.

The International Council of Nurses (2000). The ICN Code of Ethics for Nurses. Retrieved August 30, 2004, from The International Council of Nurses website: http://www.icn.ch/icncode.pdf.

U.S. Department of Health and Human Services. (2000, November). *Healthy people 2010: Understanding and improving health* (ed. 2). Washington, D.C.: USDHHS.

Walsh, S. (2004). Formulation of a plan of care for culturally diverse patients. *International Journal of Nursing Terminologies and Classifications, 15*(1), 17-26.

Waters, C. (1999). Professional nursing support for culturally diverse family members of critically ill adults. *Research in Nursing & Health, 22,* 107-117.

Zoucha, R. (2000). The keys to culturally sensitive care. *American Journal of Nursing, 100*(2), 24GG-24II.

Professional Development of the Clinical Nurse Specialist

Mary Lou Sole

INTRODUCTION

Graduates of master's programs in nursing are expected to be contributing members of the profession and leaders within nursing and health care systems to advanced nursing practice (American Association of Colleges of Nursing, 1996). Curricula for advanced practice nursing roles, including the clinical nurse specialist (CNS), include essential content such as research, policy, and professional role development. Little has been written about professional role development for advanced practice nurses (APNs), and the scope of content related to professional role development is very general. It is recommended that graduate students have content in advanced practice roles and issues related to advanced practice (American Association of Colleges of Nursing, 1996).

The American Nurses Credentialing Center, which offers several CNS certification examinations, notes that the CNS is engaged in education, case management, expert clinical practice, consultation, research, administration, and practice (http://nursingworld.org/ancc/certification/cert/certs/advprac/cns.html; accessed 06/06/05). These traditional roles of the CNS provide outstanding opportunities for the CNS to participate in professional development opportunities.

The National Association of Clinical Nurse Specialists (NACNS) *Statement on Clinical Nurse Specialist Practice and Education* notes that CNS competencies advance nursing practice (NACNS, 2004). Although not explicit, several of the CNS core competencies can include professional involvement:

- Serve as a leader/consultant/mentor/change agent in advancing the practice of nursing.
- Advance nursing practice through innovative evidence-based interventions
- Lead multidisciplinary groups.
- Expand the practice of nursing through ongoing generation . . . of scientific knowledge and skills (NACNS, 2004, p. 26).

The American Association of Critical-Care Nurses *Standards of Practice and Professional Performance for the Acute and Critical Care Clinical Nurse Specialist* discuss several broad elements of CNS practice that are related to professional role development (AACN, 2002):

- Use research-based evidence to design, revise, and evaluate innovations.

- Facilitate learning for patients, families, peers, health care providers, and communities.
- Collaborate to facilitate best practices.

According to the standards, the CNS uses collegiality to contribute to the professional development of peers, colleagues, and others. The standards also state that the APN serves as a resource to influence health care delivery and policy (AACN, 2002).

The critical care CNS applies the AACN Synergy Model for Patient Care as a framework for practice. This model notes that optimal outcomes result when the nurse's competencies match the needs of the patients and families (Hardin, 2005). Several of the nurse characteristics described in the Synergy Model can serve to stimulate participation in professional development activities: collaboration to promote optimal outcomes, systems thinking, clinical inquiry, and facilitator of learning.

The CNS also practices within three spheres of influence: patient/family, nurse, and the health care system (AACN, 2002; Hardin, 2005). Although the majority of professional activities relate to the nursing sphere of influence (e.g., writing nursing articles, presenting at professional meetings), activities can influence all three spheres. For example, the CNS influences the patient/family by serving as a leader in lay groups or giving a talk to the public on a health-related topic. The CNS may influence the health care system sphere by evaluating and disseminating outcomes of evidence-based practice.

Participation in professional activities involves time, energy, and commitment. However, involvement provides a source of job satisfaction and professional enrichment for the CNS. Activities are usually fun and provide valuable opportunities to collaborate and network with colleagues. Professional involvement of the CNS also benefits the institution by showcasing the expertise and innovations of its CNS staff and nursing department locally and nationally. It demonstrates to others the facility's commitment to supporting CNS practice and dissemination of outcomes, which may assist in recruitment and retention of staff nurses, managers, and other APNs.

This chapter discusses a variety of professional development opportunities for the CNS. Activities for and about professional development should be included during the educational preparation of CNS students. CNS graduates will then be prepared for organizational involvement, peer review activities, professional presentations, and authorship as expected in the CNS role. When a CNS takes a position, he or she must incorporate professional development activities into the role, make an action plan, and strive to maintain a high level of professional competence.

GETTING STARTED

The CNS must be self-directed in seeking professional development activities and must also take advantage of opportunities as they arise. It is important to include professional activities into the CNS job description so that involvement is an expectation and supported and rewarded by the hiring institution. Both annual and long-term goals for the CNS position must include professional activities (Box 13-1). Activities include active involvement in professional organizations; reviewing and writing manuscripts for publication; and presenting sessions at local, state, and national conferences. (Activities specific to clinical inquiry and research are addressed in other chapters in this text.) Support for professional activities from nursing administration is essential to CNS success. Sharing the benefits of involvement with the organization is one strategy for gaining support for professional activities.

Successful professional involvement and expertise in activities is developmental in implementation of the CNS role. Novice-to-expert skill acquisition models have been used to explain role development of nurses, including those in advanced practice (Dreyfus and Dreyfus, 1986; Brykczynski, 2000; Benner, 2001).

BOX 13-1

Sample Goals Related to Professional Development Activities

1. Run for office in local chapter of American Association of Critical-Care Nurses.
2. Submit at least one article per year related to a clinical topic or innovative practice to a peer-reviewed journal.
3. Serve as a peer reviewer for *Critical Care Nurse*.
4. Submit at least one abstract for presentation at the National Teaching Institute (NTI) each year. If beginning, consider participating in a mentoring process, such as the Learning Connections opportunities.
5. Submit at least one abstract for poster presentation at local, regional, or national meeting. The Creative Solutions opportunity available at the NTI is a wonderful way to get started.
6. Partner with a faculty member at *local university* to begin involvement in a clinical research study.

Professional expectations and accomplishments of the CNS are also developmental. Using a similar novice-to-expert model, Table 13-1 provides examples of professional development activities for the CNS.

Strategies for beginning professional development include reading about opportunities for involvement. Printed and electronic newsletters from professional organizations often include volunteer opportunities at local, state, and national levels. Familiarity with general nursing and specialty journals increases awareness of current topics and issues. Identifying knowledge gaps in the literature provides an opportunity for the CNS to develop ideas for presentations and publications on clinical topics and issues relevant in practice.

Another strategy for success is to make a 3- to 5-year plan that includes professional activities. Start with small goals (local activities) and proceed to local, state, and national activities. Concurrently the CNS job description can be updated to reflect the professional role activities and expectations.

Professional Organization Involvement

One of the easiest ways to develop professionally is involvement in professional organizations. Volunteer involvement ensures that the APN is aware of current issues affecting the profession and/or specialty. Involvement also helps to develop leadership skills, apply the change process, and collaborate with local and national colleagues.

Organizations include groups that represent nurses globally, such as the American Nurses Association (ANA) or Sigma Theta Tau International—these groups have opportunities at both local/state and national levels. The NACNS has periodic calls for volunteers to serve as NACNS representatives on national committees and work groups. Specialty organizations such as the American Association of Critical-Care Nurses (AACN) and the Society for Critical Care Medicine also provide numerous opportunities for involvement. Opportunities to participate in general health-related or community organizations such as the American Heart Association or American Lung Association also exist. Involvement with most groups begins at the local level and progresses to state/regional and national volunteer activities.

Every organization needs volunteers to achieve its goals, and it is easy to get into "volunteer overload." It is important for the CNS to determine on which group(s) to focus active involvement. A strategy is to volunteer in one general organization, one specialty organization, and one lay group. Others may choose to work with a specialty group and volunteer with other groups as time permits. The time commitment for volunteer activities varies widely and includes attending meetings, recruiting staff members for membership, participating in projects, and/or serving as a committee member or chairperson or elected officer.

Being aware of volunteer opportunities as they become available is an important aspect of the CNS professional development role. Materials may be disseminated via print or online requests for participation. Organizations post periodic

TABLE 13-1			
Skill Acquisition Related to Professional Activities			
Activity	**Novice/Beginner**	**Competent/Proficient**	**Expert**
Professional organization involvement	Active member of local and district chapters of professional organizations Leadership role (officer or committee) in professional organizations at local and district level	Leadership role in professional organizations at state and regional levels	Leadership role in professional organizations at national and international levels National office or other leadership positions Liaison to professional groups
Peer review	Become familiar with content and style of selected journals in specialty area Submit letter of interest in serving as peer reviewer	Peer reviewer Section editors Advisory boards	Editorial board member Editor
Writing for publication	Author short articles for organizational newsletters or workplace Summarize research reports for utilization Collaborate with colleagues on joint publications	Author journal article Lead author of writing team Author textbook chapters Edit newsletter	Journal article authorship Mentor to other authors Textbook writer and editor
Professional presentations	Present within an organization and/or local chapter of professional organizations Present to lay groups on topics of expertise Observe best presentation practices at national meetings Poster presentations at local, state, national meetings on best practices, innovative ideas, etc.	Speak at regional or national meetings on topics of expertise Serve as panelist related to expertise Coordinate symposia and workshops	Mentor new speakers Coordinate symposia and workshops Participate in national speakers' bureaus Accept international speaking invitations
Consultation	Begin networking with consultants to identify areas of expertise	Consult with local organizations on selected projects in area of expertise	Consult with organizations and companies on a variety of projects; scope may be national or international

notices for individuals to volunteer to serve as an officer, committee member, task force member, or a similar position. Some positions are appointed, whereas others (usually officers) are elected. For example, AACN has an annual call for individuals to run for national office in the organization and for the AACN Certification Corporation. An annual call for volunteers is also conducted, along with solicitation for volunteers on an "as needed" basis when new task forces, review panels, item writers, or other volunteers are needed. Information about volunteer opportunities and procedures for applying for AACN volunteer opportunities is available on the AACN website (www.aacn.org). To apply for volunteer positions, individuals must submit an application or letter of interest, along with an updated curriculum vitae (CV), biosketch, or resumé (Box 13-2). It is important to keep an electronic file with an updated CV that can be readily modified and submitted when needed. Self-nomination for most positions is solicited and encouraged.

Another volunteer opportunity is serving on review panels for research grants, conferences (e.g., AACN National Teaching Institute), or award selection committees. Serving on a review panel is an excellent way to learn the selection and review processes and often serves as an impetus to submit abstracts and proposals. Professional organizations publish a call for reviewers on a periodic basis. The process usually requires a letter of interest or completion of an application and a CV.

Many organizations have awards programs to honor members for their involvement and expertise. Nominating colleagues and oneself is another way to be involved in professional organizations. For example, AACN solicits annual nominations for individuals to receive "Circle of Excellence" awards in numerous categories, including teaching, management, caring practices, research, and clinical nurse specialist. It is an honor to both the individual and the organization when one is recognized with a local, state, or national award.

Professional Presentations

The CNS has many opportunities to provide presentations to professionals and the public. Presentations may be formal or informal, traditional lectures, or posters. A comparison of verbal versus poster presentations is shown in Table 13-2.

In the educator role the CNS provides poster and traditional presentations on a routine basis to staff members, administrators, and patients. Developing a poster for the workplace is an easy activity to build confidence in presentation skills. A single poster or multiple posters on a clinical topic can relay important information to multidisciplinary staff members (Miracle, 2003a). Staff development programs and institution-based conferences and workshops provide many opportunities to develop expertise in verbal presentation skills.

Presentations may result from informal invitations such as, "Would you speak to the local AACN chapter on care of cardiac surgery patients?" or "Would you present a short presentation to our organization on reducing risks of a heart attack?" Formal invitations to serve as a keynote speaker at local, state, national, or international conferences are offered as the CNS develops his or her expertise. The best way for a

---

BOX 13-2

Comparison of Curriculum Vitae, Biosketch, and Resumé

Curriculum Vitae (CV): Summary of academic and professional activities. The CV includes education/degrees; professional licensure/certification; academic and clinical experiences; research/scholarly activities (e.g., publications, presentations); grants, membership, and service in professional organizations; volunteer activities, and consultation. Pages are not limited; the CV should be a thorough history of professional activities.

Biosketch: Brief (1- to 4-page) summary of academic and professional activities generally submitted in a standard format when grants are submitted (e.g., National Institutes of Health http://grants.nih.gov/grants/funding/phs398/biosketchsample.pdf; accessed June 7, 2005).

Resumé: A brief (1- to 2-page) summary of an individual's education, work experience, and accomplishments, usually for the purpose of finding a job. The resumé usually includes a goal statement and is more job-related experiences, and skills are more detailed than the CV or biosketch.

Note: Many websites have examples of CV and resumés.

TABLE 13-2

Comparison of Verbal and Poster Presentations

	Presentation	Poster
Format	Traditional lecture	Ability to showcase project in creative format
Atmosphere	Formal	Informal
Speaking ability	Must develop good presentation skills and be able to develop related audiovisual materials	Opportunity to speak to many people in an informal atmosphere
Time	Designated time for presentation; may be very short time to convey difficult concepts	Designated time for attendees to view content; presenter expected to be at poster for certain times during a conference
Guidelines	Presentation developed by presenter, often using an outline format as required by the conference sponsor	Specific guidelines for developing the poster are provided by the conference organizers; poster must be developed according to these guidelines (e.g., free-standing poster, bulletin board)
Creativity	Encourages creativity in delivering the content	Encourages creativity in developing the poster content; can focus on one main idea or several, depending on the topic and concept to be emphasized
Cost	Electronic presentations (e.g., PowerPoint) becoming common, reducing costs associated with producing a presentation	Posters can be costly to produce; however, many institutions that have departments provide assistance and reasonable production costs
Networking	Provides networking with participants during question periods or after the session is over	Provides one-on-one networking with attendees who are interested in the topic; facilitates dialogue

CNS to get invited to serve as a speaker is to become an expert on a specific topic, publish on the topic, and network with others to let them know of his or her interest and availability.

Other presentations are selected based on submission of an abstract or proposal and a peer review process. Topics may be related to clinical topics or research presentations, depending on the conference. Professional groups regularly publish a "Call for Papers" for presentations at meetings. For example, AACN annually has a call for speaker proposals for the National Teaching Institute, and many CNSs regularly speak at the conference.

It is a good idea to mark abstract deadlines on a calendar as a reminder to write and submit abstracts for conferences of interest. Potential presenters are asked to submit an abstract and/or content outline for consideration. A well-written abstract or proposal is creative and presents new information. Abstracts must be written in the format requested by the conference sponsor and be submitted by posted deadlines for consideration. Many groups require online submission of abstracts and proposals, and all directions for submission must be followed carefully. Once submitted, many organizations use a blind peer review process to review abstracts and make final selections. Names are deleted from the abstract, and a panel of volunteers rates the abstract on specific criteria such as topic, congruence of presentation with conference theme, and clarity of written abstract.

Once the CNS agrees to be a speaker (verbal or poster) at a meeting, it is essential to develop presentation skills. Various books, journal articles, and websites provide guidance in mastering verbal and poster presentation skills. Regardless of format, an outline is a must to organize thoughts and content to be covered. Knowledge of the characteristics of the audience helps to plan the content to meet their learning needs (McConnell, 2002). Effective planning, appealing audiovisual materials, and public speaking practice ensure that the presentation will be of high quality. The CNS must coordinate audiovisual needs with the conference planners during early preparation for the session. Most individuals use PowerPoint presentations that require a laptop connected to a projector. The speaker may be expected to bring his or her own computer or provide presentation files ahead of time. Most groups provide formal or informal feedback after the conference that should be used constructively for ongoing skill development in presentations.

Journal Peer Review

Publishing is an important way to share knowledge and expertise with others. Serving as a peer reviewer is one of the best ways to get involved and learn the publishing process. Articles submitted to peer-reviewed journals (also known as referee journals) are critiqued by a panel of individuals with knowledge and expertise in the topical area. By serving as a peer reviewer, the CNS observes the process of how articles are submitted, reviewed, and revised before publication. Serving as a peer reviewer also provides the impetus for publishing since the

CNS often notes, "I could have written that article—and, I would have written it better!"

All peer-reviewed journals have a list of potential reviewers for manuscripts that are submitted for publication. Since article topics vary, each journal needs a large database of potential reviewers. Periodically editors solicit new reviewers; however, the CNS does not need to wait for this solicitation. Box 13-3 describes the process to become a peer reviewer.

The editor sends manuscripts to peer reviewers with knowledge and expertise on the topic of the potential article. Peer reviewers are responsible for reading a manuscript that has been submitted for publication for a variety of criteria: accuracy, relevance, appropriateness for journal's audience, organization of content, and format, including figures and tables. Most journals have a checklist for reviewers to complete, making the review process easier. After the manuscript is reviewed, the peer reviewer makes a recommendation about the manuscript: accept for publication, revise and resubmit, or reject. If the recommendation is revision or rejection, the reviewer should provide specific recommendations that need to be addressed by

---

BOX 13-3

Becoming a Journal Peer Reviewer

- Select one or two journals that you read on a regular basis. Become familiar with the level of content and how typical articles are written.
- Review author guidelines for the journal(s).
- Submit a letter of interest along with curriculum vitae to the journal editor or editorial office. Include the manuscript content in your area of expertise (e.g., cardiac, psychosocial). Contact names and address are listed in the author guidelines.
- The editor follows up with potential reviewers. You may be asked to complete a reviewer profile for the database.
- You will receive periodic manuscripts for review, often with a specific format or checklist to complete. Follow the guidelines for review and meet established deadlines for completing the review.

the author to improve the manuscript. Reviewers are expected to be prompt in meeting deadlines for the review; be objective, specific, and constructive in comments; fill out the review form legibly and completely; and spot check references for accuracy (Alspach, 2004).

Writing for Publication

Writing for publication is a professional responsibility for those in advanced practice roles. CNSs can assist in identifying gaps in the literature, disseminate new knowledge, or share pointers with others to improve nursing care delivery and patient outcomes. Writing also opens doors to other opportunities such as speaking, collaborating, and consulting (Tonges, 2000).

Most writing is done without remuneration. However, payment or other incentives (e.g., free reprints, coupon for books) may be rendered for some proprietary publications, continuing education articles, solicited manuscripts for topical journals (e.g., *AACN Advanced Critical Care*), and authoring book chapters or study guides. Publications also provide professional exposure to the author, who may subsequently be contacted to speak, consult, or write a follow-up article.

Unless the CNS has an academic appointment, writing is often not valued or rewarded. It is thus important to have an innate desire to succeed as an author and have support and encouragement from others. Individuals note numerous excuses for not writing: low confidence, procrastination, lack of time, fear of rejection, and lack of support (Miracle, 2003b). Seeking help, setting goals and deadlines, and collaborating with colleagues in the writing process assist in overcoming these barriers. Including publication goals in annually and 3- to 5-year plans helps to ensure success. It is a good idea to keep an ongoing list of publication ideas and set a timetable for writing. Other tips and strategies for writing are discussed in the periodical, *Nurse Author & Editor*, published by CINAHL (www.cinahl.com).

Authorship ranges from writing newsletter articles to editing textbooks. Most opportunities involve authoring peer-reviewed publications. Numerous journals are published in either traditional print copy or electronic media (Internet publications). Journals may be targeted to a variety of audiences such as the CNS *(Clinical Nurse Specialist)*, general nursing audiences *(American Journal of Nursing)*, or specialty groups *(Critical Care Nurse, MedSurg Nursing, American Journal of Critical Care)*. The numbers of peer-reviewed journals have expanded dramatically in recent years, including online publications. In addition, many free magazines are disseminated on a frequent basis (e.g., *Advance, Nursing Spectrum, Vital Signs*). All of these journals seek high-quality articles; thus opportunities to publish abound.

A systematic approach is necessary in the writing process. The steps of the publication process and helpful hints are summarized in Boxes 13-4 and 13-5. When beginning to think about writing, *identify a topic of interest*. Topics may include a clinical area of expertise, new or

---

BOX 13-4

Steps in the Publishing Process

- Identify journal
- Review author guidelines
- Look for calls for papers on specific topics
- Query editor about your specific ideas
- Conduct literature search on topic
- Outline content
- Write article
- Reference adequately
- Obtain permission to use copyrighted material
- Revise, rewrite
- Have colleague conduct peer review
- Revise
- Submit to editor
- Peer review by journal board
- Revise if requested by reviewers
- Resubmit
- Get acceptance letter
- Review page proofs
- Publish article in journal
- Respond to "Letters to Editor"
- Respond to reprint requests

BOX 13-5

A to Z Hints for Publishing

- *Assess* journal; author guidelines
- *Begin* with an idea
- *Collaborate*
- *Develop* effective writing
- *Don't* send in school papers
- *Determine* co-authors' roles and order of authorship
- *Expect* revisions
- *Follow* directions
- *Get* hooked on writing
- *Headings* are essential
- Incorporate figures/tables
- *Juggle* your time
- *Keep* lists of ideas
- *Keep* copies of everything in an organized file
- *Library* searches are a must
- *Motivate* and mentor others
- *Never* give up
- *Organize* thoughts via an outline
- *Participate* as a peer reviewer
- *Query* the editor
- Revise, revise, revise
- *Reference* appropriately
- *Spell* check
- *Timetables* assist in completion of projects
- *Unique* slant makes quality manuscript
- *Value* writing
- *Work* with supportive editor
- *Xerox*
- Yes, you can!
- *Zero* in on main topic

emerging technology or treatment, a clinical case study, innovations in practice, and creative solutions to nursing education or clinical practice. If articles on a specific topic are limited or targeted to another field (e.g., medicine), an opportunity to disseminate information to a nursing audience exists.

Next, *identify the target audience* for the publication. The audience may include staff nurses, managers, educators, or the public.

Determine the *type of publication* in which to write. Publications include letters to the editor, newsletter articles, book and software reviews, journal articles (print and electronic), book chapters, and books. Some journals are peer reviewed, whereas others are editor reviewed. More prestige is associated with peer-reviewed publications; however, sometimes writing manuscripts that are not peer reviewed is a good strategy to get started and develop a successful track record in publishing. Writing book chapters takes much more time to develop and write than writing journal articles and should not be the CNS's first attempt at professional writing unless it is done collaboratively with an experienced colleague. Careful consideration of content, writing expectations, and deadlines must be considered if given the opportunity to write a chapter (Tamburri, Hix, Sole, 2002).

Once an idea has developed into a topic for publication, identify the journal that best suits the goal for the article. Several factors should be considered. Look at several journals to determine their purpose and focus. Review what has been published recently on the topic in several journals. Identify whether the journal is peer reviewed or editor reviewed. Review the author guidelines carefully. The journal editor may provide you with information about the acceptance rate for submissions. Identify how much editing will be done with the manuscript once it is accepted for publication. Finally consider the time lag between acceptance and publication. Some editors ask that a query letter be written (or submitted electronically) to determine interest in a specific topic or if an article on the subject is needed or a similar manuscript has already been accepted for publication. An excellent resource that links authors to editors, journals, and author guidelines is the ONLINE Nursing Editors website sponsored by Nurse Author and Editor (www.nurseauthor.com; accessed June 7, 2005) (Levy, 2004).

Writing is the next part of the publication process. This is the most time-consuming part of the process. Most sources recommend starting with an extensive literature search, followed by an outline (Wink, 2002; Schulmeister and Vrabel, 2002; Miracle, 2003a). The article should have a unique focus for the targeted audience. Headings, key points, tables, and figures are included to enhance readability of the manuscript. It is important to reference information during the writing process. Bibliographic software such as EndNote can assist in referencing. Setting deadlines for completing the writing process helps to achieve target goals for submission.

Some individuals choose to *partner* with colleagues to write for publication. Collaboration is a great way to publish. However, someone must assume the leadership role for completing the writing and submitting the manuscript. At the onset, identification of order of authorship helps to prevent issues later. Everyone whose name is listed as an author has the ethical responsibility of contributing substantially to the project (Erlen, 2002).

Manuscripts have a greater chance of acceptance if a colleague experienced in publication reviews the manuscript before submission. Papers written for school must be revised to suit the journal's style before submission (Johnson, 1991). Never send in a school paper without revising it, even if it was an exceptional paper for a course.

Submit the manuscript according to the author guidelines once the manuscript is completed. Many journals have checklists to ensure that authors submit the appropriate number of copies, tables, and figures. Many journals request electronic submission of files and specify formats for saving electronic files. A copyright release is submitted with the manuscript. This release acknowledges that the work is original and is being submitted to only one journal for consideration. All authors usually sign the release, acknowledging their contribution to the manuscript.

Keep a file of the manuscript, figures, and all references used to write the manuscript. This will be very helpful if changes need to be made after the peer review is completed. If permissions were obtained to use material such as a figure or table from another source, also keep that documentation in the manuscript file.

Await outcomes of the *peer review process.* If the article is submitted to a peer-reviewed journal, a panel of two to three colleagues will review the manuscript on a variety of items: accuracy of content and references, timeliness and uniqueness of the topic, suitability for the readership of the journal, organization (logical, headings, well-written), style, and evaluation of tables and figures. The peer review process generally takes 2 to 3 months. If no feedback is received by that time, it is important to contact the editor to determine the status of the review process.

Most of the time the reviewers will ask that content be revised before accepting the manuscript for publication. Do not view getting feedback for revision as a negative process; view it as an opportunity to improve the manuscript. If revisions are recommended, make a plan to *revise the manuscript* according to the reviewers' suggestions and set a short deadline for making the revisions. It is helpful to include a summary of changes made when resubmitting the manuscript to the editor. If changes recommended by the reviewer are not made, discuss why those changes were not incorporated into the revision. Depending on the scope of the revision, the editor may send the manuscript out for a second round of peer review after the revision, or the editor may review the changes and determine acceptability of the manuscript for publication.

The last step before publication is careful *review of page proofs* for accuracy. A copyeditor at the publisher will edit the manuscript to suit the style of the journal and query the author about changes and/or items that need clarification. Good attention to detail is essential when reviewing page proofs, and it may be helpful to have a colleague review them as well to identify and correct potential errors. A very short timeline is given for review of page proofs.

After publication, *celebrate success.* Post the article for others to see. Share a copy of the article with peers, immediate supervisor, and other administrators in the organization.

If readers write any letters to the editor, the author might have to respond to the comments. Replies should be objective and address any issues that readers may have expressed in the letter to the editor. Authors may also be contacted for reprints of the article, especially from international colleagues. With the increased availability of electronic mail, authors also get questions and feedback electronically from colleagues on publication of an article.

If the manuscript is rejected by the journal, it is important to evaluate the feedback received during the peer review process. Assess the reasons for rejection such as writing style, content, or article not suited for the journal. The article may be able to updated and submitted to a different journal.

ONGOING STRATEGIES FOR SUCCESS

Professional development activities are essential to self-fulfillment and growth in the CNS job role. Building expectations into the job description, establishing goals, and designating time for activities assist the CNS in successful role development. Keeping lists of potential projects, deadlines for abstract submissions, and publication ideas are key motivators—especially when written with target dates for completion. Support from supervisors for activities is also essential and includes time for activities during the work week; time off for attending meetings; financial support to attend meetings; and resources such as library support, secretarial assistance, and media development for presentations and posters.

Collaborate on projects with fellow CNSs, staff members, and supervisors on professional development activities. The right team gets much more done, and more people can celebrate achievements. Collaboration also encourages institutional support as everyone is acknowledged for accomplishments.

Keep a file of accomplishments and *update the CV* on a regular basis. It is helpful to keep letters of thanks, electronic letters of support, and other correspondence in paper and/or electronic files. Also keep a file of all publications and evaluations of presentations. These materials help during the periodic review and evaluation (self and supervisor). The file/portfolio also

assists in preparing and submitting award applications. Call the file the "kudo" file!

Network with others to achieve ongoing success. Make contacts with colleagues and companies during professional meetings. Keep a supply of professional business cards readily available to give to others during meetings. Follow up with contacts soon after meetings. Electronic messaging is a good way to acknowledge meetings and discussions. Subscribing to listservs in your area(s) of interest and being an active participant are other ways to network with colleagues nationally and internationally.

SUMMARY

Professional development activities are expected of the CNS. A variety of activities need to be completed on an ongoing basis. These activities are just as important as the other expectations of the advanced practice role. Having a plan and acting on it ensure success and growth in professional development activities.

References

Alspach, G. (2004). *Critical Care Nurse* guidelines for reviewers. Retrieved from http://www.aacn.org/ccn/ccnjrnl.nsf/Files/RwGuide/$file/RwGuide.pdf. Accessed June 7, 2005.

American Association of Colleges of Nursing. (1996). *The essentials of master's education for advanced practice nursing.* Washington, D.C.: Author.

American Association of Critical-Care Nurses. (2002). *Scope of practice and standards of professional performance for the acute and critical care clinical nurse specialist.* Aliso Viejo, CA: Author.

Benner, P. (2001). *From novice to expert: Excellence and power in clinical nursing practice.* Upper Saddle River, NJ: Prentice-Hall.

Brykczynski, K.A. (2000). Role development of the advanced practice nurse. In A.B. Hamric, J.A. Spross, & C.M. Hanson. *Advanced nursing practice: An integrative approach* (ed. 2). Philadelphia: Saunders.

Dreyfus, H.L., & Dreyfus, S.E. (1986). *Mind over machine: The power of human intuition and expertise in the era of the computer.* New York: Free Press.

Erlen, J.A. (2002). Writing for publication: Ethical considerations. *Orthopaedic Nursing, 21*(6), 68-71.

Hardin, S. (2005). Introduction to the AACN Synergy Model for patient care. In S.R. Hardin & R. Kaplow. *Synergy for clinical excellence: The AACN Synergy Model for Patient Care*. Boston: Jones and Bartlett.

Johnson, S.H. (1991). Avoiding the "school paper style" rejection. *Nurse Author & Editor, 1*(3), 1-6.

Levy, J. (2004). *ONLINE Nursing Editors*. www.nurseauthor.com. Accessed June 7, 2005.

McConnell, E.A. (2002). Making outstandingly good presentations. *Dimensions in Critical Care Nursing, 21*(1), 28-30.

Miracle, V.A. (2003a). How to do an effective poster presentation in the workplace. *Dimensions in Critical Care Nursing, 22*(4), 171-172.

Miracle, V.A. (2003b). Writing for Publication. *Dimensions of Critical Care Nursing, 22*(1), 31-34.

National Association of Clinical Nurse Specialists. (2004). *NACNS statement on clinical nurse specialist practice and education* (ed. 2). Chicago: Author.

Schulmeister, L., & Vrabel, M. (2002). Searching for information for presentations and publications. *Clinical Nurse Specialist: The Journal for Advanced Nursing Practice, 16*(2), 79-84.

Tamburri, L.M., Hix, C.D., & Sole, M.L. (2002). Revising a book chapter written by a previous author. *Nurse Author & Editor, 12*(3), 7-9.

Tonges, M.C. (2000). Publishing as a career development tool: Don't forget to write. *Seminars in Nursing Management, 8*(4), 212-214.

Wink, D.M. (2002). Writing to get published. *Nephrology Nursing Journal 29*(5), 461-467.

Expanded Opportunities: The Clinical Nurse Specialist as Entrepreneur

Marcia Bixby
Karen Giuliano

INTRODUCTION

The National Association of Clinical Nurse Specialists (NACNS) statement on clinical nurse specialist (CNS) practice and education embodies the essential characteristics and skills that a CNS must have to be successful in all the dimensions required of CNS practice (NACNS, 2004). One of the hallmarks of expert CNS practice is advanced knowledge and specialization in a specific clinical domain, encompassing the theoretical knowledge as well as the basic science and nursing science relevant to that clinical domain. However, equally important for expert CNS practice is the ability to share this knowledge by influencing the clinical practice of others, which requires a completely different set of competencies. To be successful, CNS practice requires a blend of competencies, which at any moment may be called into action. These include leader, consultant, teacher, mentor, informatics expert, and collaborator, just to name a few. In addition, requisite personal characteristics include expert interpersonal skills,

self-awareness, positive attitude, honesty, integrity, ability for self-reflection, and, perhaps most important, a willingness to take risks. In one study CNSs reported (listed from most frequently to least frequently) spending the most time in the roles of expert practitioner, educator, consultant, administrator, and researcher (Giuliano and Adams, 2000).

Inherent in the execution of these diverse role responsibilities is the need to frequently adapt to the changing needs of patients, families, nurses, physicians, and institutions. This need serves as the basic tenet and core concept of the AACN Synergy Model for Patient Care (AACN, 2005). According to AACN (2005), synergy is the result of a convergence of patient, clinical, or system needs and nurse competencies. AACN has identified several nurse competencies that must be present for true synergy to occur, and each of these competencies includes a detailed operational definition. The AACN synergy competencies are: clinical judgment, advocacy and moral agency, caring practices, collaboration, systems thinking, response to diversity, facilitation of learning, and clinical inquiry. To be successful as an expert CNS, proficiency in each of these competency domains is necessary.

Thus even a quick review of the competencies and personal characteristics necessary for success as a CNS from the perspective of the NACNS list of CNS competencies and the AACN Synergy Model makes it simple to see why there are so many opportunities for the successful CNS outside of the realm of traditional expert clinical practice.

THE CNS AS ENTREPRENEUR

Because of the diverse skill set intrinsic to the CNS, perhaps the most natural role outside of a traditional hospital environment is that of an entrepreneur. Even a brief review of the literature of CNS entrepreneurship quickly yields over 400 articles and websites related to nurse entrepreneurs. A few examples include Marie Tobin's business on helping women become entrepreneurs and as a founder of the organization "Entrepreneurial Networking Group for Nurses" (ENGN, 2006). Barbara McLean is an international speaker on critical care topics (McLean, 2006). Claudia Ellis has a business designing websites for nursing organizations (ENGN, 2006). Kathleen Vollman is known both as the inventor of the Vollman Pronator and as a widely recognized nurse expert and consultant (Vollman, 2004). Marcia Bixby provides education to facilities that do not have full time critical care CNS support and also offers critical care education to pre-hospital providers (Bixby, 2004). Bixby also provides consultation to industry partners in product design and development. A quick search of the Internet will easily reveal numerous links to nurse entrepreneurs who teach classes and seminars, provide books and information on starting your own nursing business, and many other entrepreneurial endeavors.

Nurses as entrepreneurs has its roots in the 1980s as opportunities began to evolve that allowed nurses to take their skills outside of the traditional hospital boundaries. CNSs as entrepreneurs rapidly evolved as the health care system began the restructure/redesign craze. According to the American Hospital Association (AHA), in the late 1980s and 1990s an unprecedented number of United States hospitals sought to maintain a competitive, cost-effective position by restructuring (Walston, Burns, & Kimberly, 2000). Changes in resource allocation prompted hospitals and other health care providers to do everything possible to reduce their operating costs, which most often included the shortsighted act of eliminating CNS positions in many hospitals and health care systems. This resulted in a large number of CNSs becoming available to apply their vast knowledge and skills outside of the traditional realm of CNS practice; many of these talented individuals never looked back.

One of the distinct advantages of this movement out of the traditional CNS environment was that the often-restrictive rules and regulations inherent in the hospital or medical center environment were left behind as CNSs took their skills and applied them to the community and business world. Nurses as entrepreneurs have flourished as health care facilities have downsized, the workforce has continued to age, and nurses have sought alternative modalities for providing health care. CNSs are adept at looking at the patient as a whole entity and incorporating holistic and alternative therapeutic approaches to patient care and well-being, a perspective that is increasingly valued by patients and other health care consumers. As health care continues to become more and more related to cost effectiveness and utilization of resources and more outcome based, CNS entrepreneurs are able to use their expertise on an independent and consultive basis. The entrepreneurial opportunities for the CNS are truly limited only by imagination, the ability to finance his or her ideas, and the initiative to get started. In addition, passage of Medicare laws in 1997 enabled CNSs to apply for reimbursement as independent practitioners, making independent entrepreneurship even easier (Ieong, 2005).

The CNS as an entrepreneur can work for a health care facility (Dayhoff & Moore, 2003). The irony is that the very same health care facilities that previously eliminated CNS positions are often the same ones that use the CNS as an independent consultant. Because of their skill set and vast understanding of the health care system, CNSs are in a unique position to offer creative solutions for the delivery of patient care. Many CNSs have also worked successfully in the community as business owners, by offering services that incorporate specific advanced nursing expertise. CNS entrepreneurs have a distinct advantage in that CNS services are broadly applicable, are optimized to improve the delivery of health care and have the capacity to improve outcomes for both patients and health care providers. For the individual CNS, flexible hours, creative license, control of one's business, the ability to use problem identification and problem solving, and the choice to develop the program as fast or slow as you desire are all great incentives for becoming an entrepreneur. Other advantages include being your own boss, acting on your wishes and dreams, and being respected for your knowledge and expertise. There are also some disadvantages that should be considered before embarking on an independent career as a CNS entrepreneur, including the cost of starting a business, the cost of malpractice insurance, and competition for the services rendered. Office space and supplies and technical support or staff can be a limiting factor, especially during start up of your business. Managing workflow, taking on too many jobs, and handling cash flow should also be considered before deciding to become an entrepreneur.

THE CURRENT HEALTH CARE ENVIRONMENT

The current climate of health care has probably never been better for anyone who is willing to do his or her homework in order to have the greatest chance of success as an entrepreneur. When thinking about becoming an entrepreneur, one first needs to envision where health care will be in 5, 10, and even 20 years from now.

This is necessary for long-term success because it positions the CNS and his or her business to be on the cutting edge of health care and to anticipate upcoming needs. Some of the most important trends that the CNS entrepreneur should be aware of are highlighted in the following paragraphs.

Increasing Patient Acuity

- Medical advancements now allow people to live longer. An increasing number of patients are presenting with co-morbidities, meaning that patients have a higher acuity and prolonged recovery.
- There is increased need and requirement for "step-down" units to cater for the sicker patients.

Reduced Health Care Spending

- This phenomenon will not be reversed any time in the near future. Worldwide governments are struggling to find solutions that enable a high standard of care without the huge costs associated with caring for patients.

Shortage of Clinicians

- The Joint Commission on Accreditation of Healthcare Organizations (JCAHO) estimates 126,000 nursing positions in hospitals within the United States alone are currently unfilled (JCAHO, 2005). According to the U.S. Bureau of Labor Statistics, by 2012 over one million new and replacement nurses will be needed (Hecker, 2004).
- The United States is recruiting clinicians from overseas and setting up nursing schools for example in Mexico, the Philippines, and Africa. This is draining nursing expertise from third-world countries (Bryant, 2004).
- Globalization of nursing introduces different levels of competencies, language barriers, and cultural differences that ultimately affect the standard of care provided to patients.

- Many critical care areas with inexperienced/unqualified staff are expected to "learn on the job," adding to the responsibilities of already stressed experienced clinicians.
- Many critical care areas still use "nurse extender" type staff to supplement for lack of nurses.
- There are patient safety concerns.
- One in 25 patients is injured as a result of medical error (Kohn, Corrigan, & Donaldson, 2000).
- Patient safety is a top agenda item for all the major quality and regulatory agencies in the United States, including the National Patient Safety Foundation, JCAHO, Leapfrog, Institute of Medicine, Agency for Health Care Research and Quality (AHRQ), and the Institute for Health Care Improvement (IHI). In today's health care environment, addressing patient safety in tangible ways is a requirement.

Rising Costs of Health Care

- Forty-six percent of respondents to the 2004 Kaiser health poll report named the rising cost of health care as the most important government issue in the United States (Ginsburg, 2004).
- Of the 2004 United States gross domestic product, 13.6% was spent on health care. This figure is expected to rise to 16% by the year 2010 (Thompson Business Intelligence, 2005).
- A Harris poll of 2114 Americans asking about the most important health care issue to them revealed that 86% (listed as issue No. 1) of Americans cared a great deal about the total cost of health care and 85% (listed as issue No. 7) of Americans cared a great deal about the quality of health care (Harris Interactive, 2004).
- Over the next 20 years, the fastest growing segment of the United States population will be those ages 55 and older. By 2023 Americans ages 55 or older will constitute nearly 30% of the United States population,

further driving increases in the rising costs of health care, since the elderly are the principal consumers of health care (Thompson Business Intelligence, 2005).
- More than 44 million Americans are uninsured, which is about 15% of the population (Ayanian, Weissman, Schneider, Ginsburg, & Zaslavsky, 2000).
- Health care pressures will continue to worsen, forcing providers to look for evermore creative ways to save money and streamline care.

Increasing Pressure to Provide Quality Health Care (Coile, 2005)

- Hospitals and other health care systems are reacting to and scrambling to get ahead of a variety of trends that are reshaping U.S. health care.
- Organizations that provide a quality product that exceeds expectations and excels at accommodating consumer preferences will be at a distinct advantage.
- Preference will be given to health care that addresses patient safety or improving clinical outcomes. These investments will also need to be cost effective.
- Quality will be an ever-increasing differentiator among health care providers as payers continue to launch and broaden pay-for-performance initiatives that will shift resources from some hospitals to others.

Targeted Improvements for Health Care in the 21st Century (Wolfe, 2001)

- The six aims that should be targeted to improve health care for the 21st century include care that is:
  1. Safe
  2. Effective
  3. Patient-centered
  4. Timely
  5. Efficient
  6. Equitable

EXPANDED CNS OPPORTUNITIES

Specific environments where the CNSs can easily apply their unique skill set include contracting services with health care institutions for patient care, health maintenance organizations (HMOs), outpatient facilities and clinics, primary care and long-term facilities. Nurse entrepreneurs are education consultants, inventors, professional consultants, legal nurse consultants, and providers of holistic and alternative therapies. Many nurses have started agencies for staffing, education, and consultation for professional growth. From the list of current health care trends, it is easy to see that the types of services that are already being provided by CNS entrepreneurs address and will continue to address many of the current needs in health care.

In addition, nurses are being used more and more by industries that develop equipment and provide services in which nurses are the end users. Rewarding careers for nurses who are outside the traditional role of CNS exist in sales for both the medical device industry and pharmaceuticals. Another way to put the CNS skills to good use is in medical product development and research (Giuliano & Adams, 2000). For example, Karen Giuliano is employed as a clinical research scientist for Philips Medical Systems. In her current role, Karen's CNS skills are put to good use for both clinical research on existing products and development of future products. A brief review of any major job search website can reveal many interesting possibilities for applying the CNS skill set in a creative and nontraditional manner in an industry setting. Furthermore, by branching out into these nontraditional roles, CNSs can showcase their value to industries that might not otherwise be aware of the valuable services that a CNS can provide outside of the hospital setting.

GETTING STARTED

A good place to start when considering a move into the world of nurse entrepreneurship is simply to take a look around your current work environment, identify your frustrations, and imagine a list of potential solutions. Most work environments have some areas in obvious need of improvement, and a hospital or health care system is no exception. In fact, because of rapid changes in health care related to cost constraints, quality reporting, and the ever-increasing complexity related to the delivery of health care, most providers, particularly hospitals, are in desperate need of numerous and significant improvements and changes. Easily identifiable are system issues, supply issues, educational issues, equipment issues, or management deficits. Once issues are identified in the CNS's own work environment, it is very likely that nurses in similar work environments in your area or around the country are experiencing the same kinds of problems.

Another necessary step in the path to nurse entrepreneurship is for CNSs to identify what helps them derive the most satisfaction from their professional role as a CNS. Once the specific dimensions of the CNS role that are most consistent with the CNS's interests and expertise have been determined, he or she can begin to engage his or her vision regarding the best strategy to provide a unique, efficacious, and cost-effective service or solution. It is also a good idea to contact other nurses who have started businesses, and networking is an important part of the planning process. Talking to other nurses who have started a business can help to more successfully develop plans and avoid their pitfalls. Because of the nature of nursing, nurses are often very generous in helping to discuss plans and giving advice. Planning should also include reading books written by successful nurse entrepreneurs.

GOING FROM NOVICE TO EXPERT

Nurses are skilled at identifying a vision because the process is so similar to the nursing process (i.e., identifying or assessing the problem, diagnosing or determining all aspects of the problem, implementing the correct interventions, and continually reassessing and evaluating the response to the interventions). Nurses do this with every patient, so this part generally comes naturally. Just as nurses use Benner's model of novice to expert as they gain knowledge and experience, they can also apply this model to their role as nurse entrepreneurs (Benner, 1982; Ieong, 2005). Novice nurses tend to focus on the immediate needs of the patient and believe that patient care can be largely guided by rules, orders, and protocols. They tend to be aware of their lack of a comprehensive understanding of the care required by their patients, are uncomfortable in making autonomous decisions, and will defer to more experienced nurses for assistance when a clinical judgment is required. The novice or amateur CNS entrepreneur shares many of these same traits and can often be too task oriented as he or she strives to gain an understanding of the complexities that often surround a fledgling idea or business. The amateur tends to think in smaller spheres, is subject to making hasty decisions, and is more likely to make some mistakes with their initial business decisions.

In practice, once nurses become more competent, they are better able to use independent clinical judgment and question some of the judgments of the more experienced nurses who surround them. Although the competent nurse is able to see the need for clinical judgment, he or she lacks to ability to understand the relative importance of multiple clinical cues and tends to be hypervigilant, be critically self-reflective, be lacking in confidence, and have an unrealistic sense of responsibility for patient care. This is also true for the competent nurse entrepreneur.

Proficiency for both practicing nurses and successful nurse entrepreneurs is marked by an ever-increasing skill in understanding and articulating the importance of various relevant cues. Proficient nurses and CNSs feel more comfortable not following rules and protocols and can shift priorities based on changing needs. More confidence is exhibited in their practice, and proficiency nurses are less concerned with "forgetting" something important.

Finally, expert nurses and CNS entrepreneurs understand complex situations, are not concerned with irrelevant facts, easily recognize familiar patterns, know they practice at a different level than nurses who are not expert, and openly articulate and seek guidance for situations in which they are uncomfortable. Experts show great skill in managing complex, difficult, and rapidly changing clinical situations. As the CNSs become expert, they gain a better understanding of the product or service they provide and are comfortable being the inventor, creator, and consultant in a more complex environment.

PUTTING A PLAN INTO ACTION

Another important part of being a nurse entrepreneur is to assess your own comfort level with risk taking. Because risk taking is an important part of the CNS role, this aspect of nurse entrepreneurship is generally not too foreign to most CNSs. However, it helps to have a healthy level of skepticism without being too intimidated by the unknown. Thorough preparation and homework before beginning a business can help to minimize the unknowns. Starting gradually on a part-time basis is also a good strategy for most nurse entrepreneurs. Once the CNS decides on a plan of action, he or she should use as much self-confidence as can be mustered and be sure to have adequate support services in the beginning phases. The CNS should not be afraid to use any expertise that may exist in family and among trusted co-workers and friends to test your ideas. Their thoughts, ideas, and comments should be considered carefully.

The next step on the journey is to talk to business and financial organizations. To optimize the chances of success, a thorough business plan is necessary. Many resources can help with this, including books on business, reputable on-line sites, and professional business or specialty organizations or agencies. Attending workshops and classes on business topics and contacting state and local organizations for assistance and guidance are helpful. Some federal and state organizations provide services for free or for a nominal fee. A good business plan should include such things as a detailed description of the product or service, why the CNS thinks it is a needed service, and the targeted audience. A sample is provided in Box 14-1. In addition, the American Nurses Association (ANA) has published information and the National Nurses Business Association also has a very comprehensive website. There are also federal and state programs such as SCORE (Service Corp of Retired Executives) and SBA (Small Business Association) that help develop ideas and provide some financial support. Many professional businesses and professional women's organizations can also be used as great resources, and financial support may be available if the business plan has been prepared well.

BOX 14-1

Sample of a Comprehensive Business Plan

1. Executive summary
   Brief project summary
2. Proposal summary
   a. Definition and description of product or service
   b. Explanation of why this is the best/most feasible solution to strategic needs
3. Strategic fit
   a. Overview of the underlying strategy that the product or service supports
   b. Explanation of why this is the best/most feasible solution to strategic needs
4. Alternative considerations
   Explanation of why the proposal is the best alternative
5. Target market overview
   a. Key market trends and drivers
      (1) Who are the customers?
      (2) What are the external influences?
   b. Key market descriptors/metrics
      (1) Describe the relevant market
      (2) Size and future growth
      (3) What is the total market for your product or service?
      (4) Likely impact of product or service on total market: How much market share do you expect to get each year?
   c. Competitive situation
6. Partnerships
   a. Need for a partner
   b. If so, partner business description
   c. Company structure
   d. Company's business model
   e. Partner's core competencies
   f. Differentiation of the targeted partner company from its competitors
7. Financial impact of project
   a. Market opportunity model
      (1) Identify the total economic opportunity (based on market research if available)
      (2) Assess the timing of current and future market development
      (3) Identify the addressable opportunity
      (4) Identify how much and how value will be captured
   b. Economic model for capturing value
      (1) Decide how the product or service will be sold (e.g., embedded in a device such as software, service, or a new product)

Continued

BOX 14-1

Sample of a Comprehensive Business Plan—cont'd

Metric	Deal Stand-Alone Financial Impact	Deal Pro-Forma Financial Impact
NPV	Deal/project value	N/A
EPR	Deal/project EPR	Effect on business's total IFO
IFO	Stand-alone IFO	Effect on business's total IFO
EBITA	Stand-alone EBITA and EBITA margin	Effect on business's total EBITA and margin

8. Risk assessment: risks, contingencies, and sensitivities
    a. Primary risks that could affect success of the project
        (1) Economic
        (2) Market
        (3) Competitive
        (4) Regulatory
        (5) Technology related
    b. Risk scenarios
        (1) Create up to three scenarios and indicate the severity, probability, and likely financial impact
        (2) Identify the three assumptions with the greatest potential impact
    c. Risk mitigation
        (1) Develop mitigation plans for the identified scenarios
        (2) Identify measures or indicators that can alert the team to a developing risk scenario
9. Preliminary implementation plan
    a. Business management plan
        (1) Key milestones, checkpoints
        (2) Translation of individual steps to create the product or service
        (3) Key dependencies
        (4) Estimated dates for start and completion of each step
    b. Resource requirements
        (1) Personnel
        (2) Financial
10. Next steps
    a. Critical unanswered questions
    b. Action items required to obtain answers to critical questions
    c. Resources required to carry out all action items

CONCLUSION

Finally, as the rapid pace of change in health care continues to come to light, more and more opportunities will become available to nurses who are interested in becoming entrepreneurs. Every CNS, by virtue of having a CNS skill set, has a whole assortment of entrepreneurial opportunities just waiting to emerge. In addition to refining the CNS skill set, it is important for the CNS to continuously expand his or her knowledge in the areas of health care reimbursement and health care policy and to keep abreast of the clinical research that relates to his or her clinical areas of expertise. Successful nurse entrepreneurship can provide both great personal satisfaction and a positive endorsement for the profession of nursing.

References

AACN. (2005). The AACN Synergy Model for Patient Care. *American Association of Critical-Care Nurses.* Retrieved April 6, 2006 from www.aacn.org.

Ayanian, J.Z., Weissman, J.S., Schneider, E.C., Ginsburg, J.A., & Zaslavsky, A.M. (2000). Unmet health needs of uninsured adults in the United States. *Journal of the American Medical Association, 284*(16), 2061-2069.

Benner, P. (1982). From novice to expert. *American Journal of Nursing, 82*(3), 402-407.

Bixby, M. (2004). Multidiscipinary approach to protocol development. *Clinical Nurse Specialist, 18*(3), 160-162.

Bryant, J. (2004). *Hospitals go overseas for nurses.* Retrieved January 22, 2006, from www.nurse-town.com.

Coile, R.C. (2005). Futurescan: Healthcare trends and implications, 2004-2008. *Society for Healthcare Strategy and Market Development*, American Hospital Association: Chicago, IL.

Dayhoff, N.E., & Moore, P.S. (2003). You don't have to leave the hospital system to be an entrepreneur. *Clinical Nurse Specialist, 17*(2), 19-21.

ENGN. (2006). *ENGN Pressbox.* Entrepreneurial Networking Group for Nurses. Retrieved January 21, 2006, from www.engn.org/pressbox.html.

Ginsburg, P. (2004). Controlling healthcare costs. *New England Journal of Medicine, 351*(16), 1591-1593.

Giuliano, K.K., & Adams, D. (2000). The clinical nurse specialist in non-traditional roles. *Clinical Nurse Specialist, 14*(4), 155, 157.

Harris Interactive, Inc. (2004). Cost and coverage are top health care issues in election 2004. Retrieved January 21, 2006 from the Internet: *Wall Street Journal Online, 21*(3), www.wsj.com.

Hecker, D.E. (2004). Occupational employment projections to 2012. Retrieved January 21, 2006 from the Internet: *Monthly Labor Review, 127*(3), www.bls.gov.

Ieong, S.L. (2005). Clinical nurse specialist entrepreneurship. Retrieved January 21, 2006 from the Internet: *The Internet Journal of Advanced Nursing Practice, 7*(1), www.ispub.com.

JCAHO. (2005). Health care at the crossroads: Strategies for addressing the evolving nursing crisis. *Joint Commission on Accreditation of Healthcare Organizations.* Retrieved January 21, 2006 from the Internet, www.aacn.nche.edu.

Kohn, L.T., Corrigan, J.M., & Donaldson, M.S. (2000). *To err is human: Building a safer health system.* Washington, D.C.: National Academies Press.

McLean, B. (2006). How does your garden grow? The fertile fields of accountability in practice. *Critical Care Medicine, 34*(2), 558-559.

National Association of Clinical Nurse Specialists. (2004). *Statement on clinical nurse specialist practice and education* (ed. 2). Harrisburg, PA: Author.

Thompson Business Intelligence (2005). Retrieved January 21, 2006 from the Internet: *Thompson Business Intelligence Report*, www.research.thompsonbusinessintelligence.com.

Vollman, K. (2004). Nurse entrepreneurship: Taking an invention from birth to marketplace. *Clinical Nurse Specialist, 18*(2), 68-71.

Walston, S., Burns, L., & Kimberly, J. (2000). Does reengineering really work? An examination of the context and outcomes of hospital reengineering initiatives. *Health Services Research, 34*(6), 1363-1388.

Wolfe, A. (2001). Crossing the quality chasm: A new health care system for the 21st century. *Policy, Politics and Nursing Practice, 2*(3), 233-235.

15

Current Issues and Future Trends

Karla A. Knight
Connie Barden
Gladys M. Campbell

A practicing critical care clinical nurse specialist (CNS) and a nursing administrator discuss the current challenges of the CNS role and share their vision for the future. Based on more than 50 years of collective experience, their perspectives on change, quality, role confusion, leadership, and practice articulate the importance of the role of the CNS in critical care and what it will take to keep the CNS role viable and energized in an ever-changing health care environment.

Karla Knight (KK): Consider the CNS role in acute and critical care when you started your career. What has stayed the same? What has changed?

Gladys Campbell (GC): Over 100 years ago, Florence Nightingale spoke to our need as nurses and leaders to remember that our duty and responsibility are our patients and the outcomes of their care. In this same vein, our licensure is a statement of public trust, and this license obligates us to put patients first in the work that we do as nurse leaders. This need for focus on the patient has not changed since the inception of the CNS role. What has changed is the complexity of the care environments in which we work. There are serious concerns today about the costs of health care and subsequently on the affordability of health care for the consumer.

Errors in care delivery and the dangers inherent in our acute care settings have led to national patient safety goals and publicly accessible databases that contrast costs of care, patient volumes, and care outcomes. An emphasis on evidence-based practice and the use of national guidelines or standards for care require that the CNS has extensive knowledge of the scientific literature. The CNS should ensure that hospital-based care standards are validated by the literature. The expectation that national standards are met and that we allow the public to hold us accountable to those standards places fresh pressure on those in the CNS role. The high cost of the nursing labor force requires that the CNS be able to economically justify the role to hospital administration. To verify the value of their role, CNSs must demonstrate cost savings in improved practice, error reduction, and a higher quality of patient outcomes.

Connie Barden (CB): It's really not the role that's changed—it's the environment in which we practice, and it's changed tremendously. The demands of the health care environment have changed, and this has altered how people "do" their CNS role. There's a bigger focus on evidence-based practice, on outcomes and outcomes management; and "throughput"—getting patients in and out. In the past, depending on the environment, patients may have been hospitalized for 2 weeks at a time. Today, if managed care or the insurance company says patients have to go out the door in 4 days, there's a push to get them out the door. Depending on where you practice, patients might not be older, but they certainly might be sicker than they would have been 20 years ago. People are also living longer—and living longer with chronic diseases that used to kill them sooner. Part of the reason that they are staying alive longer is that we have the technologies with which to keep them alive—so we have a whole new phenomenon, which is the chronically critically ill person. Outcome measurements are also being reported to the public, making us all more accountable for what we do.

KK: What do you see as the biggest change in the CNS role and how does that change what CNSs do?

GC: The biggest change in the CNS role is the migration of CNSs to the role of the acute care nurse practitioner (NP) with a subsequent loss of volume of available CNSs and a loss of a strong and vital presence of the CNS role within our acute care hospitals. It is not uncommon now for a large hospital to have no CNSs or only one or two for the entire facility. With this loss of volume and presence, the CNS role is increasingly less understood and thus easily devalued. The loss of CNS positions within our hospitals places an almost impossible burden on those who remain. To be successful, the CNS must often focus on only one or two components of the CNS role— most generally education. The CNS also faces increased pressure to be responsive to day-to-day organizational crises and has less ability to be strategic in focusing on activities that will advance practice, improve overall patient outcomes, or create sustainable practice efficiencies. In this environment it is more essential than ever before that the CNS be a good strategist. CNSs must be able to consistently aim their efforts in areas in which practice improvements can be realized, especially those that result in improved safety and clinical care or cost savings.

KK: Why is there increased demand for CNSs?

CB: When there wasn't a place for the CNS at many tables, people felt the negative consequences of that empty seat. Part of the new demand is related to this backlash of fewer practicing CNSs. I hope the current push for more CNSs will continue because they are key to great patient outcomes. However, I don't trust that the push will be sustained. There are too many pressures in this health care business, and so many things could distract decision makers from making decisions to hire CNSs. The increased demand for CNSs can be attributed to the quality gaps left by the absence of CNSs when there was a shift to NP roles.

GC: The nursing shortage has pushed our experienced and tenured nurses harder. With an influx of novice nurses into the profession, there is a need for more clinical mentorship and oversight. At the same time we are also pushing patients hard and fast. The average patient has a length of stay of about 3 days, and with such a short time frame there is a huge concern that clinical needs may be missed. At the same time we have increased public accountability related to safety, cost of care, and adherence to best practices. The proliferation of public websites calls us all to meet quality outcomes. The need for public accountability will only get greater. Who will the hospitals use to meet the needs? Who is going to be the leader in creating efficient, high-quality patient care when there are fewer and fewer nurses and other employed clinicians? There is also an increasing requirement for capacity management or patient "throughput." Although hospitals feel very threatened by all of these demands, the CNS is positioned to effectively address these areas of need.

KK: Are there unique knowledge and skills that the CNS brings to the health care arena?

CB: CNSs must be certain that they have unique and extensive clinical knowledge, as well as the ability to work within systems and to create change. It's really very unique to have a person who has in-depth clinical knowledge and skills together with those other abilities.

For example, a lot of very knowledgeable staff nurses have great skills and knowledge but may not be adept at participating in or leading a meeting effectively. They may not know how to create change, manage a project, and see it through to completion—all things that are needed to make sustained clinical improvements. Ideally the CNS brings both pieces—a huge amount of clinical knowledge but also the ability to sit in a meeting with a CEO and explain the importance of a certain project for a group of patients. The CNS's blend of clinical knowledge and the ability to work creatively within systems is relatively uncommon, unique, and very valuable.

GC: The CNS role is the only role that includes research as a part of its scope of practice. With research as a formal component of the CNS role, the CNS brings leadership to the initiation of evidence-based practice, the establishment and use of practice standards, and the creation of the structures and processes that guide excellence in clinical practice. It is the CNS who ensures that patient care is guided by contemporary, evidence-based standards of practice across a specialty domain, regardless of where the patient is cared for within the organization.

KK: Advanced practice nurses are often lumped together. How would you explain the differences between the CNS and the NP roles? Why are the roles misunderstood?

CB: Many things are complementary; but the roles, tasks, and expectations are really very different. These are two distinct practice roles with different educational preparation and role expectations. The constituency is clear for NPs—it is the patient and handling multiple care and assessment needs, as well as interventions needed to help manage the course of the illnesses. NPs provide direct patient management for a specific population group. But as a CNS, the beneficiary or "target" of my role is both the nursing staff and the patient. I have a completely different practice, and, while I may not direct the care of the patient, I absolutely impact it by helping nurses immediately and appropriately intervening with patients. My constituency includes the nurses, the patients, the units, and the systems within which I operate. I'm looking at the overall population of patients and the environments in which we care for them. My colleagues as NPs are looking more at the day-to-day management of patients. CNSs and NPs are as different as apples and oranges, and yet they are totally complementary. Some of the confusion may stem from the fact that some universities no longer have the CNS track. A nurse studies to be an NP but takes a job as a CNS. This is problematic because the roles are very different, just as it would be inappropriate for someone to come out of a CNS program and practice as an NP. How wise is it to study one thing and practice another? This inevitably creates confusion about the two distinct roles.

KK: What kind of day-to-day "real work" is important to the role of the CNS?

GC: In all nursing roles there is routine, responsive, and strategic work. Effectiveness in the CNS role is highly dependent on an incumbent's ability to be responsive to the staff nurses in their specialty areas, as well as to physicians, patients, and their families and to the priorities of the organization, while still being strategic in ensuring that patient care outcomes are improved in a meaningful and sustained way. The power of the role is attained through influence, and because of this, CNSs must attend to the fact that their ability to be influential is most often gained when others see their ability to respond to real-time clinical situations and make a difference. The practice of the CNS must then be present in the domain of care delivery. The CNS must be able to impact the intersection where the caregiver meets the patient in a way that improves patient care outcomes and assists the care provider in being more efficient and effective. The danger of the CNS role is that, in being responsive, it is easy for CNSs to focus on "sweat equity" or "how hard am I working today" rather than on strategically focusing their work to achieve long-term, sustainable improvements in practice, care delivery, and clinical outcomes.

CB: A CNS must be present on the unit and accessible to the nursing staff. There it's a hands-on, troubleshooting, thinking, analyzing, helping-to-figure-out-what's-going-on interaction with the bedside nurse when a clinical problem arises. This presence is the critical piece to ensure that the best care gets delivered to the patient. These interactions at the bedside also contribute to the growth and development of nursing staff. Nothing teaches like live action—as it happens at the bedside. The real work of the CNS involves helping the nurse to act and think appropriately so that the patient receives the best care.

KK: Organizationally, where can CNSs have the most power?

GC: A focus on clinical outcomes, evidence-based practice, and the push for Magnet status has increased the potential power of the CNS role. The nursing shortage and predicted worsening of that shortage is also forcing nursing administrators to look at care delivery models with skill mix ratios that require fewer RNs but require more oversight of clinical practice. This oversight and the assurance that practice standards are known and adhered to is a natural extension of the CNS role. Finally, the CNS is the only role in which involvement in research is a formal part of the scope of practice of the role. Given that Magnet facilities must show staff involvement with and a commitment to research, the CNS is uniquely positioned to lead a nursing department's initiatives to integrate evidence-based practice and to promote staff nurse involvement in clinical research. For all nurses, our power is in our practice.

CB: The CNS's power lies in three domains: improving patient outcomes, developing the thinking and analytical abilities of the nursing staff, and providing clinical leadership for a unit/department/division. These are the three main areas in which the value and power of the CNS can shine. Few others in health care systems have the unique ability to impact all three of these areas, and, if left "undiluted" in the role (i.e., not pulled to do other tasks), CNSs can create major improvements in all three of these domains. The presence of a CNS really helps to set the tone and create the "thinking culture" of a unit.

KK: How is the power of the CNS role related to excellence?

GC: The term "excellence" is used somewhat loosely in most organizations' mission statements as a buzzword without definition. I believe that excellence is the ability to stand firmly on known contemporary practice standards and to then lean into the unknown. Excellence is the discovery and application of new knowledge, and the journey of discovery begins by questioning what is known—by leaning into the unknown from the point of what is known. This opportunity sits squarely within the domain of the CNS role. The CNS is actually at the center of the most powerful place of practice.

CB: The crux of the CNS role is excellence; that's the CNS's reason to be—to impact/improve patient care and clinical outcomes by influencing the way nursing care is delivered.

KK: What are the major challenges a CNS faces? How can a CNS successfully address these challenges? Are there untapped opportunities for a CNS?

CB: One of the most important challenges is role confusion. The challenge is to be clear about what one does and have others be clear about it, too. Another challenge is that, if CNSs are not visible or able to make visible their value to an organization, at any time they could be seen as "extra"; those salary dollars could be allocated for other resources. Some CNSs are chronically pulled into the staff nurse pool to deliver direct patient care or constantly assigned tasks not related to the CNS role. Justification of the CNS role as separate and distinct from the staff nurse and other roles is a chronic challenge in many institutions. On the other hand, the opportunities for the CNS are endless because improvements can always be made in clinical outcomes and nurses' abilities to think, analyze, understand, and grow. The challenge is to allow the CNS to practice the fundamental elements of the role without being pulled in many other, often non-clinical directions.

GC: A big opportunity for the CNS lies in the area of collective professional leadership. At a national level the need for voice and focus for the role (i.e., the need to create a universal understanding related to what the CNS has to offer hospitals that are facing crushing challenges) could not be greater. It is said that in challenge lies opportunity; this is so true for the CNS role now. To embrace this opportunity, individually the CNS needs to develop skills and ability in strategic and systems thinking and change management and transformational leadership. The CNS should not wait for recognition or role understanding from others but should create it. The CNS should not wait to be directed toward areas of need but should independently embrace the national priority needs of our hospitals and pioneer a path to success. The CNS should create vision rather than waiting for enlightenment.

KK: Are challenges actually tied to untapped opportunities?

GC: Yes. Unfortunately I do not see our CNSs collectively aligned around a national vision that capitalizes on current opportunities. I also see many individual CNSs who seem paralyzed by the challenges in the health care environment coupled with the threat of being misunderstood in their role and in their work settings. I think that CNSs (and many others) are experts at problem identification, and what we need are experts in problem resolution. If I could give our CNS colleagues one thing, it would be the gift of mentorship. When so many of our hospitals are experiencing a scarcity of CNSs, the opportunity for a novice CNS to link with a role-based mentor is rare. The individual CNS often has not had the experience of being guided and mentored in leadership, priority setting, change management, strategic thinking, problem solving, group or team leadership, conflict mediation, research, quality improvement, or how to demonstrate and market the value of the role. Novice CNSs need time in dialogue; they need affirmation and time to be heard. They often need someone who can help them dissect issues and problems and then strategically advance a resolution process so that the resolution is sustained and systematized. Sometimes it is so much easier to be a "doer" rather than a thinker. It is often easier and takes less discipline

to take action than to be still and really think through an issue. The paradox of "slower is faster" applies to many system-based problems in our hospitals, but it feels counterintuitive to be still in a crisis. I often see unmentored CNSs as action junkies. They are very busy. They work very hard, but they are not effective in creating sustained improvement or change. I would emphasize that the CNS role is a leadership role and that leaders need to be "meaning makers." Leaders set context and in that context surround an issue, concern, or problem with meaning. Leaders connect seemingly disconnected points of data and in that connection create understanding for others. The power for change is not in taking action but in the creation of meaning and shared understanding that compels and directs action. Finally I would say that, for CNSs to evaluate their effectiveness, they must look at what happens when they are NOT present. They must ask, "How have I influenced practice or changed practice such that improved practice is the norm even when I am not on duty?"

KK: What is happening today to prepare CNSs for change? And conversely, what is happening today to block CNSs from being prepared?

CB: External forces are going to continue to impact the CNS because these same forces impact health care—they may not prepare the CNS for change, but they certainly demand it. Academicians preparing nurses for the role are in a pivotal position to be able to send new CNSs to the workplace who are clear about their role and ready to make an impact in this demanding environment. But, to do this, faculty needs to be current in their experience with today's health care workplace and understand the challenges to the very viability of the CNS role. CNSs are making a comeback right now; but, even so, nurses have more opportunity to be educated as NPs than they do as CNSs. This blocks CNSs from entering the marketplace. That means that RNs who want to be CNSs may have to pick up and move, which is not possible for everyone. There is room for all advanced practice nurses at the health care table, but nurses need schools that will give them the educational preparation they need.

KK: Do you think that professional organizations play a part in preparing for future changes to the CNS role?

GC: Our professional organizations have an obligation to prepare our CNSs and our care environments for changes to the CNS role. The preparation should focus on defining the universal threats in the current national health care environment and the opportunities inherent in those threats. Professional organizations can also align the CNS role with nursing management and administrative roles, NP roles, and the emerging clinical nurse leader role. There should be clarity of domains and understood points of collaboration without conflict over territory. To address the need for CNS mentors, our professional organizations could work with specific schools of nursing or known hospital sites of excellence to establish fellowship programs with both advanced didactic content and support for placements for one-on-one mentorships with known CNS role models.

CB: The challenge to specialty nursing organizations is that advanced practice nurses of any kind are often a very small percentage of their membership; thus it's difficult to put huge resources in that direction. The American Association of Critical-Care Nurses (AACN) does a really good job of focusing on advanced practice nurses in acute and critical care even though they make up only about 4% of the total membership. During the National Teaching Institute (NTI), there is a whole other "institute" called the Advanced Practice Institute (API) dedicated to furthering the education and skills of both NPs and CNSs. Few professional organizations put that much time and that many dollars toward advanced practice preparation. Any place where advanced practice nurses can get more information and networking opportunities, such as the API, is a good place to prepare for change.

KK: The American Association of Colleges of Nursing (AACN-Colleges) has proposed the development of a new role, the clinical nurse leader (CNL). What do you see as its

likely impact on the CNS role in acute and critical care?

CB: Keeping in mind that this new role of the CNL is just being created and studied, I'll make my comments like everyone else, without yet having data on the impact this role may have. I am concerned that new advanced practice roles are being created before we're clear about CNS practice and the entry-level issue in nursing. The role of the CNS has not been optimized, maximized, or used to its full potential. Now a new role is being suggested. It makes no sense to me. I'm fearful that this will lead us to decades and decades of debate between many people who have interests on both sides. Frankly, I feel that it is irresponsible of nursing to leave the entry into practice debate unsolved and create another debate that is going to be just as divisive in the long run on the advanced practice end. Even the name (CNL) is a perfect set-up for total confusion.

GC: Sometimes I think all of us in nursing are just going to die from role confusion in our tendency to address new and emerging challenges with a new role. With that being said, I am aware of our need to refocus bedside nursing onto the coordination of patient-focused care and the creation of safe passage for patients as they transition through the continuum of care. It is that "needful thing" again. I would love to see the CNL be the force to reinvigorate the true intent of the primary nurse role—a bedside role focused on accountability to the patient and family for the outcomes of nursing care. The CNL must be a bedside care provider because another fixed position in nursing will only layer more labor costs onto care delivery. We cannot afford to move in this direction. The CNL will most certainly create more role confusion related to the domain and role of the CNS. My greatest fear is that our administrators will use a CNL-prepared nurse as a CNS when they do not have CNS-prepared leaders readily available. Our history tells us this is sure to happen unless state licensure or credentialing regulations prevent it.

KK: What should the educational preparation for CNSs look like? The American Association of Colleges of Nursing has

proposed the Doctorate of Nursing Practice (DNP), a new degree that, by 2015, would be required for advanced practice in clinical areas, education, administration and policy, including anesthesia and midwifery. How will this impact the CNS role in acute and critical care?

CB: I'm watching this topic and its evolution closely. There are people on both sides of the issue whom I respect very much. As a practicing CNS, I don't think a doctorate is necessary as an automatic entry-level criterion to function as a CNS today. I have not seen evidence that CNSs are less effective because they lack a doctorate in clinical practice. Huge impacts are being made with the current master's preparation, and, when CNSs are not effective, I have no evidence that doctoral level education is the missing piece that would make the difference. Thus I'm not convinced that adding another layer with further debate and divisiveness is necessary. I'm very interested in this debate because I don't yet understand it. Practice today is nothing like it was just 10 or 15 years ago. We need to be very careful and certain that the major practice and academic changes we make are relevant to the reality of today's health care system.

GC: Nursing and nurses have hurt themselves and our collective credibility by not keeping pace with the education and credentialing patterns of other professions. I do believe our CNSs should be doctorally prepared with a DNSc or a DNP. To achieve this credential though, we need to be realistic. Logical and reasonable pathways for degree achievement that are focused on the needs of the student and user of information must be established, or we will not have *any* CNSs at exactly the time when our nursing workforce shortage hits its peak. I hope that these doctoral programs have a dual focus on expertise in the practice domain and leadership within organizational structures so that graduates can be creative, strategic systems thinkers and agents for positive change. Potentially a fellowship model of practice rotations could also address the need for mentorship in the CNS role. This type of model would allow CNS students to establish lifelong mentoring relationships. Ironically, doctoral

preparation for the CNS would also distinguish this role from the CNL and diminish the role conflict that is already emerging between these two professional groups.

KK: What about prescriptive authority? Should it be included in CNS educational preparation?

GC: CNSs should have access to a pathway for prescriptive authority, but it does not need to be part of the generic CNS role. Some CNSs are in positions in which the ability to prescribe is critically important, but for the general CNS in an acute care setting, it is not. Universal prescriptive authority would create overlap and role confusion with the NP. Prescriptive authority should be an option but not a necessity for basic CNS practice.

CB: Prescriptive authority is not critical for the majority of nurses practicing in the CNS role. The education and regulation needed for this should be available, but it doesn't need to be a fundamental part of curriculum for all CNSs.

KK: What changes in credentialing for CNSs do you foresee? Should credentialing be mandatory? What organization or group should be doing the certification?

GC: Credentialing should be mandatory and consistent. This is difficult because there is not consistency across all states on this issue. The more we can be consistent, the less confusion there will be around the CNS role. AACN is the appropriate certification body for the critical care CNS and for many other acute care and progressive care CNSs.

CB: Credentialing via certification in the CNS role is important. Although there are other clinical certifications that are meaningful to CNS practice, certifying the role component is of value. For example, I have my CCRN and CCNS. I do enough hands-on care to recertify for CCRN, which is a bedside credential. I carefully track my hours in order to recertify. However, when I took the CCNS examination, which is specific to my role, I found that it reflected the full picture of what I do as a practicing CNS. The CCRN certification is not a credential that was designed for CNS practice, and this is reflected in the content of the examination. The CCNS (for critical care) should be mandatory after a certain number of years of practice. Ideally specialty nursing organizations should handle their own CNS certification; however, there needs to be collaboration with state boards of nursing so that these credentials can be readily recognized in those states where they are required for practice. The CCNS examination through the AACN is very much focused on critical care scenarios and is specifically designed to test the CNS's knowledge of critical care. The examination is based on the AACN Synergy Model for Patient Care, so that all of the Synergy Model characteristics are tested (e.g., clinical inquiry, clinical judgment, collaboration, advocacy). Perhaps not all examinations need to be based on the Synergy Model, but the most ideal situation is to have specialty organizations testing their own. The role is clinical nurse *specialist*, not clinical nurse generalist.

KK: Are there professional development considerations that are vital to the success of the CNS role?

CB: CNSs certainly are leaders and major influencers of practice and the total care of patients. Because of this, one of the most important growth trajectories for CNSs is to continually develop leadership skills. We also have to look at systems in general, because we all operate as little specks in this great big hospital system. The more we can augment knowledge about big systems work, the more effective we can be in the CNS role. Leadership development, creating change, and measuring outcomes should be the focus of ongoing and never-ending learning for the CNS.

GC: Beyond the need to be a clinical expert in your domain, the big development areas have to do with leadership, systems thinking, change management, team leadership, conflict mediation, being a meaning maker, understanding the job roles versus accountability to the profession, and finally the need for mentorship of those coming into the role.

KK: CNSs fulfill various functional roles alone or in combination. For example, case

manager, inpatient care coordinator, specialty-focused educator. Do these roles limit or expand the influence of the CNS or do they merely create more confusion?

CB: Each of these roles is completely distinct from the CNS role, adding to the confusion. The person, even if prepared as a CNS, really needs to be clear about what they're doing in the role and call it that. Otherwise it's total continuing confusion. Many skills that the CNS has can be brought to these other roles. But none of those things is the same as being a CNS. A common source of confusion is when nurses are called CNSs and yet are doing nonspecialty (but very important) educational tasks, which could be handled by the people who don't have CNS preparation. When you look at the wide variety of roles that continue to carry the label of CNS, it's no surprise that there is confusion about the role. On this issue, we need to learn to be more "purist."

GC: People learn about a role by watching the people in that role. If a nurse calls himself or herself a CNS but is not doing the work of a CNS (i.e., if he or she is an educator, a case manager, a risk or quality manger), it creates role confusion. CNSs continue to fill other nursing roles and still call themselves CNSs. Frequently you see people who define themselves as holding a dual CNS/manager position. The roles of manager and CNS are distinct, and the person holding this "dual" role is a manager and not a CNS. To call oneself a CNS when not fulfilling the obligations of the role does a disservice to the CNS role title and to every other role in which the individual is engaged. In the workplace people must be clear about what work role they hold and then define themselves by that role. For example, a CNS on my staff made a decision to accept the role of our stroke coordinator. This is not a CNS role. Does she bring all of her neurosciences knowledge and experience to bear on the stroke coordinator role? Of course she does. But she does not define herself in the workplace as a CNS, she defines herself as a stroke coordinator. Professionally she defines herself as a CNS when she is engaged in outside professional activities, and that is highly appropriate.

KK: What contributes to CNSs' inability to articulate their role?

GC: Many nurses, CNSs and others, do not seem to be clear about the unique domain of nursing practice. What is it that nurses do that no one else does? What is it that nurses do that, if they do not do it, will not get done? What is the nurse's unique contribution to patient well-being? When Florence Nightingale talked about focus, this is what she was talking about. She referred to this place as "our needful thing." Many nurses do not know what our needful thing is. Nursing leaders and CNSs as the leaders of bedside nursing practice must be clear about their needful thing and must be able to role model that focus to others. Many nurses also do not understand the difference between their profession and their job. Our place of employment is just the environment where we practice our profession. It is a place where, if you will, our knowledge, skills, and abilities are purchased for the good of a particular practice setting. Our profession is the larger national and international domain in which our scope of practice and the obligations of licensure and patient protections are defined and maintained. The obligation of the CNS role, in the purest sense, is defined by the profession, not the employer. It is through this distinction that the employer actually gains the greatest "value added" from the CNS role. When CNSs understand and can articulate their professional obligation, they inherently protect the organization from losing focus of the core business of the hospital, which is excellence in patient care delivery. It takes courage for a professional who is also an employee to ensure that the patient remains the organization's focus, and it also takes a full understanding of what it means to be a licensed professional nurse.

KK: How does the CNS promote evidence-based practice?

CB: CNSs are often the ones driving the implementation of evidence-based practice at the bedside. Learning the literature backward and forward, both the medical and the nursing literature, on a particular clinical issue, devising a plan, and looking at what's workable: this is the change agent piece. CNSs look at clinically relevant changes and sometimes "go out on the skinny branches" by taking risks to create the change that needs to happen. CNSs must know the politics of the place and work not only through nursing but also medicine, pharmacy, and sometimes even legal circles to implement a change in practice. This is one of the fundamental areas in which the CNS can make a huge difference. Knowing how to do these things successfully is vital to the role.

GC: The CNS has a very important role in promoting evidence-based practice. For the past 25 years, I have been working with my CNS colleagues to develop models for unit-based clinical research to promote the ability of staff to question their practice scientifically. This model uses teams of staff nurses at the bedside, guided by a CNS research mentor, to uncover practice questions or inconsistencies that are ripe for study. The model is based on fostering a culture of clinical inquiry. With this approach, research is driven from practice and from the needs of the patient versus being driven by the needs or interests of the researcher. The model creates research that is clinically relevant and user friendly. If we are ever going to bring home evidence-based practice and best practice, the research that we do must be based on the needs of the patients and valued by the bedside clinician. In 1946 Lewin stated, "for research to be useful it must meet the needs of the user." That statement challenges us today, 60 years later. The CNS is uniquely positioned to lead a patient-focused research process and to allow us to develop science that truly enriches our practice in useful ways. For the CNS, the greatest power can be in the strategic application of evidence-based practice and the advancement of relevant clinical research.

KK: How do reimbursement and regulation affect the CNS role in acute and critical care?

GC: Hospitals are always looking for ways to identify the value added. Since there is no direct reimbursement to CNSs, they must articulate how an implemented intervention they have put into place has reduced either length of stay or complications. They must tie their practice to cost savings. States have specific education credentials that they require for the CNS role. Many people have been functioning in the CNS role and have advanced practice preparation. But they cannot get a CNS credential from a specific state board of nursing. In that way the CNS role is impacted by regulation. I'm a purist, so I'm glad that we have standards that we must meet to use a certain professional title; however, these standards don't always seem practical.

CB: Changes in reimbursement are affecting everyone in health care, either directly or indirectly. Although CNSs aren't directly reimbursed, they are impacted because the entire system is so severely impacted. The changes affect most aspects of "life" in the health care system (for example shorter lengths of stay, placement after discharge, and the ability of patients to obtain specialist care). Because the CNS role is so vitally intertwined with patients and their outcomes, these issues impact how we approach patient care from A to Z—everything from how quickly patient education is done to coordinating what procedures take place at which point in the hospitalization. And, because the system is so squeezed from a financial standpoint, the necessity for CNSs to be able to articulate their "worth" to that system is all-important. The regulation issue is paramount as well. Because our system allows individual states to regulate practice, the varied requirements for CNS practice make mobility from state to state quite a challenge. There is a need for a universal credential or certification and educational requirements for advanced practice that allows CNSs to move from one location to another. Health care does not need or have the time to be encumbered by such varied regulations. The need for talented clinicians in health care is too great.

KK: Are there particular outcome measures that are useful in validating the role of the CNS in acute and critical care?

CB: CNSs have impacts in so many spheres that sometimes it's overwhelming to think of how to measure that impact. But, it is important, not as a survival tactic, but as a benchmark to ensure that progress is being made and goals are being met. One of the most important areas in which CNSs have value is in helping to ensure that evidence-based interventions are put into place in the care of patients. In critical care, insulin therapy to tightly control blood glucose is an example, as are oral care protocols for decreasing ventilator-associated pneumonia. CNSs can follow measures put into place and their impact on patient outcomes. A CNS may impact patient and family satisfaction and nurse retention—two things that are harder to measure but need to be considered as well. Although a sharp CNS impacts a staff nurse's ability to think critically, I don't know of a reliable measure with which to really prove that particular outcome.

GC: If there is any area of universal CNS focus, it should be the nurse-sensitive outcomes of care. These outcomes (e.g., patient falls, ventilator-associated pneumonias, skin ulceration rates) carry with them a tremendous opportunity to reduce length of stay, reduce hospital costs, and improve the outcomes and quality of life of our patients while emphasizing the value of expert nursing care. The CNS impacts these outcomes by working through the bedside staff and influencing their practice. Once practice protocols are implemented, it is the role of the CNS to monitor that practice, evaluate the outcomes of that practice, modify process or practice when improvements are needed, and ensure that positive change is maintained and advanced. The CNS makes sure that the change is "stuck, sustained, and spread."

KK: If you look to the future, what do you predict will stay the same in the CNS role? What will change and how?

GC: The regulation and public oversight of health care is not going to go away. The pressure and demand that this places on our hospitals, coupled with an aging nursing workforce and the influx of many novice and new graduate nurses into the profession, may actually strengthen the perceived value of the CNS role and lead to its resurgence.

Currently hospitals are looking for systems, processes, and roles that will help meet the demands for oversight and training of a novice nurse workforce; new partnerships with schools of nursing to increase the volume of available nurses; ways to increase patient safety; methods to reduce length of stay and increase patient capacity; improvements and change in practice models that reduce labor costs; assurance that quality and safety metrics are achieved; improvement in practice partnerships between physicians and nurses and an increase in physician and nurse satisfaction; initiation of evidence-based practice protocols, guidelines, and standards; and continual Joint Commission for the Accreditation of Healthcare Organizations (JCAHO) readiness. The CNS role is potentially well positioned to help hospitals in their struggle to meet all of these demands. To be successful in confronting these issues, the professional leadership of our CNS groups and individual CNSs themselves must demonstrate strategic leadership and the ability to articulate the value of the CNS role. If CNSs do not step up to address these very serious hospital needs, another group will, or another role will be created.

CB: The external regulation of health care is not going away. The nursing shortage and all of its inherent challenges certainly won't subside for quite a while. But the CNS has the potential to be one of the forces that creates stability at the bedside. The CNS also has the skills and abilities to "grow" new nurses and instill the confidence that comes with solid education and the ability to function efficiently within the system. Societal trends, too, such as folks not trusting the health care system, not trusting that we will do the right thing for them, and coming into the health care system thinking that the dollar sign is the bottom line, will continue to impact everyone in health care. The pressures from the outside, such as demanding quality, excellence, and outcomes, could actually help to strengthen the CNS role. CNSs who understand their role and are able to clearly articulate that role will most likely survive and thrive. We must seize the opportunity to make the quality impact and be willing to talk about it and demonstrate its importance.

KK: How will the necessary changes in the role occur?

CB: The CNS is one of the quality creators in the hospitals. Smart, forward-thinking administrative people are always looking for a way to get great outcomes and a well-qualified staff in this demanding world. Enlightened administrators see that CNSs are the way to go and a means of meeting a higher standard with fewer resources. You've got to find smarter ways to meet higher standards; the CNS is a way to get there. The CNS can be seen as an avenue toward attaining quality, even with fewer resources. Envisioning the CNS in this way speaks to future job security. This is particularly true in critical care, where I've spent my career. Although there is a focus on minimally invasive interventions—trying to get more things done quickly and in the outpatient setting—there is still a fundamental need to care for critically ill patients in the hospital setting. Trauma isn't going away; neither is heart disease or many other illnesses that still require the expertise of skilled critical care clinicians within the walls of an intensive care unit. Patients are going to be older and sicker. Advances in technology will help save many and prolong the lives of those with chronic illnesses. The CNS will still be vital to producing top-notch outcomes and keeping nurses willing to work at the bedside in acute and critical care.

KK: How would you characterize the future for the CNS?

CB: CNSs are an often misunderstood, untapped resource—the resource that people know the least about and are quick to eliminate. They are also one of the critical links to quality, which is more important than ever, now and in the future because patients are sicker and the demands of the health care system are greater. CNSs are critical to the future of nursing because they are key to ensuring quality and outcomes. They have the big picture of nurses, patients, families and the issues affecting their specialty.

They develop nurses to be the best they can be. They ensure that the latest approaches to nursing care are put into place. They intervene directly with patients and families to facilitate their "journey" through the complex health care system. They advocate not only for patients but for nurses at all levels of the system. They create certainty and direction, yielding the best possible environments in which patients and families can be cared for and where nurses can practice optimally. CNSs are such a valuable clinical asset that no hospital should be without them.

GC: I'm a harsh critic of CNSs because I value their role so much. I worry that CNSs have not stepped up to the plate in the right way. Those who have stepped up have changed practice dramatically. In many ways these CNSs are our practice exemplars and heroes. They represent what the role can and should be. Everyone doesn't have to be a nationally known practice expert, but we need CNS leaders who are grounded in nursing, not just in medicine, and who understand the unique contribution of nursing to patient well-being. These CNS leaders are nurses who have taken areas of practice that are not sexy, jazzy, or exciting (i.e., areas such as hand-washing, skin care, pain management, and family presence) and have made these practice areas visible, important, vital, and exciting to nurses and others. The courage, vigilance, and commitment that this takes is unbelievable. Again, I would remind us all of Florence Nightingale's words of caution, "Let us not forget our needful thing." What she meant by that was that, in the midst of it all, with our credentials, tasks, expectations, and pressures, we should not forget why we are here. She is really talking about the irreducible essence of nursing. I think the best and brightest CNSs are in touch daily with the needful thing. That is the heart and soul of the CNS—it is the power they can have—it is their brass ring, ready for the taking.

KK: The National Council of State Boards of Nursing (NCSBN) has issued a proposed change in state regulations that would no longer classify CNSs as advanced practice nurses.

For the purposes of regulation, the "advanced practice nurse" designation would be limited to nurse anesthetists, certified nurse-wives, and nurse practitioners. If this proposal were implemented, what are the implications for CNS practice?

CB: This proposed change in regulations highlights many of the issues that either enhance or complicate the CNS's ability to practice, move from state to state, and influence health care. CNSs are so important to outcomes and quality in hospitals that they will continue to exist, regardless of how this current debate is resolved; however, the regulatory discussion has arisen because of the significant role confusion around CNS practice. It is a perfect example of "when we don't fix something ourselves, someone else will fix it for us." As previously outlined, many nurses function in roles called CNS, and yet their role consists predominantly of non-CNS behaviors. At the other end of the spectrum, some CNSs incorporate activities such as prescriptive authority into their practice, whereas the majority of CNSs do not. It is no wonder that the health care community, and even many CNSs, remain confused.

When studying the impact of this proposal, a number of points should be considered. First, the NCSBN does not control state regulatory processes. Although the organization's constituents are the state boards of nursing and their representatives, regulatory authority for each state still rests in the hands of individual state boards. Second, the vision statement is a 10-year vision, and as such we still have time—if we are skillful and not reactionary—to work together on solutions to this issue. Third, input and dialogue have been invited.

This is a critical time for leaders, regardless of their opinion on this issue, to come forward with respect, openness, and a willingness to continue the dialogue, regardless of how difficult or uncomfortable. Continuing in a polarized and contentious state is destructive and will result in a fractured and ineffective profession. Discussions must be grounded in a common vision—providing the best care and outcomes for patients and families—and nothing else. This vision must drive the dialogue.

CNSs will remain in health care no matter how this issue is resolved. They are needed, and there is room for many roles at the health care table. Hopefully this challenge will be resolved in a way that strengthens nursing practice and our ability to influence patient care and nurses' thinking and systems outcomes, while finally clarifying the "who's who" of advanced nursing roles. Although it is well disguised and seems to be an insurmountable barrier, this challenge actually represents a huge opportunity for the growth of our profession.

Standards of Practice and Performance for the Acute and Critical Care CNS

STANDARDS OF PRACTICE

I. Assessment

The acute and critical care CNS collects data relevant to 3 spheres of influence: the patient and family members, nursing personnel, and organizational systems.

Measurement Criteria
1. Develops and uses data collection tools that have been established as reliable and valid.
2. Includes the patient, family members, and other health care providers in the data collection process to develop a holistic picture of the patient's needs.
3. Obtains data from multiple sources that reflect sensitivity to ethnic and cultural differences of individuals (patient, family members, nursing personnel, and systems).
4. Collects data on an ongoing basis that reflect the dynamic nature of patients and systems.
5. Collects data in all 3 spheres and prioritizes according to immediate conditions and needs.

6. Identifies factors that influence outcomes during the data collection process (e.g., financial and regulatory requirements and effectiveness of interdisciplinary collaboration) and classifies them as facilitators or barriers to proposed changes.
7. Synthesizes the data and documents in a retrievable form.
8. Uses and designs appropriate tools and methodologies to identify the clinical and professional development needs or gaps in knowledge, skills, and competencies of nursing personnel.

II. Diagnosis

The acute and critical care CNS analyzes the assessment data to determine the needs of patients, family members, nursing personnel, and organizational systems.

Measurement Criteria
1. Formulates differential diagnoses by systematically comparing and contrasting assessment findings.

2. Derives diagnoses from the assessment data.
3. Discusses, validates, and prioritizes diagnoses in collaboration with patients, family members, nursing personnel, and systems.
4. Prioritizes and documents diagnoses to facilitate development of a plan of care and to achieve expected outcomes.
5. Reevaluates and revises diagnosis when additional assessment data become available.
6. Identifies and analyzes factors that enhance or hinder the achievement of desired outcomes for patients, family members, nursing personnel, and systems.

III. Outcome Identification

The acute and critical care CNS identifies expected outcomes for patients, family members, nursing personnel, and organizational systems.

Measurement Criteria
1. Formulates expected outcomes with patients, family members, and the multidisciplinary health care team that are based on current clinical and scientific knowledge.
2. Identifies expected outcomes by considering associated risks, benefits, and costs.
3. Modifies expected outcomes and plan of care or actions based on changes in condition or needs.

IV. Planning

The acute and critical care CNS develops and facilitates a plan that prescribes interventions to attain the expected outcomes for patients, family members, nursing personnel, and organizational systems.

Measurement Criteria
1. Develops a plan that is individualized, dynamic, and can be applied across the continuum of acute and critical care services.
2. Develops the plan in a collaborative manner, promoting each individual's

contributions toward achieving the expected outcomes.
3. Identifies interventions within the plan of care that reflect current scientific knowledge and practice and promote continuity of care.
4. Documents the plan in a format easily accessible to, and understandable by, all team members involved.

V. Implementation

The acute and critical care CNS effectively implements the interventions identified in the plan(s) for patients/family, nursing personnel, and organizational systems.

Measurement Criteria
1. Prescribes, orders, and/or implements pharmacologic and nonpharmacologic interventions, treatments, and procedures for patients and family members, as identified in the plan of care, within the framework of state licensure and hospital privileges.
2. Performs evidence-based interventions consistent with the needs of the patient and family.
3. Delivers interventions in a safe and ethical manner that promotes health and stability and that minimizes complications.
4. Documents interventions in a manner that is appropriate, retrievable, and effective, as well as facilitates patient care, quality improvement, and administrative initiatives.
5. Promotes implementation of the plan of care collaboratively with patients, family members, and the health care team.

VI. Evaluation

The acute and critical care CNS evaluates progress toward attainment of expected outcomes for patients, family members, nursing personnel, and organizational systems.

Measurement Criteria
1. Performs evaluation in a systematic and ongoing manner.

2. Bases the evaluation process on the analysis of risks, benefits, and cost-effectiveness.
3. Includes interdisciplinary collaboration and multiple sources of data in the evaluation process.
4. Bases the evaluation process on advanced knowledge, practice, and research.
5. Documents the evaluation process in an appropriate, retrievable, and effective manner.
6. Revises the diagnoses, expected outcomes, and plan of care based on information gained in the evaluation process.
7. Establishes, monitors, and evaluates the *effect* of interventions on patient care, organizational and nursing personnel outcomes, and cost.
8. Incorporates the use of quality indicators and benchmarking in evaluating the progress of patients, family members, nursing personnel, and systems toward expected outcomes.

STANDARDS OF PROFESSIONAL PERFORMANCE

I. Quality of Care

The acute and critical care CNS systematically develops criteria for and evaluates the quality and effectiveness of nursing practice and organizational systems.

Measurement Criteria
1. Assumes a leadership role in establishing criteria for and monitoring quality of care initiatives within the 3 spheres of influence.
2. Assesses the need for, plans, and implements quality-improvement programs.
3. Evaluates quality improvement data and formulates evidence-based recommendations to improve quality of care and nursing practice.
4. Participates in interdisciplinary efforts to address costs, duplication, and barriers to goal attainment.

II. Individual Practice Evaluation

The acute and critical care CNS evaluates his or her practice in relation to professional practice standards and relevant regulations.

Measurement Criteria
1. Evaluates own clinical and professional performance according to the standards of the appropriate professional and regulatory bodies, and takes action to improve practice.
2. Assists in the development and evaluation of criteria for evaluation of CNS practice within the 3 spheres.
3. Seeks feedback regarding own practice and role performance from peers, professional colleagues, patients and their family members, and others.

III. Education

The acute and critical *care* CNS acquires and maintains current knowledge and competency *in* the 3 spheres of influence in acute and critical care nursing.

Measurement Criteria
1. Proactively seeks and participates in experiences and learning opportunities that will advance his or her knowledge of interventions, therapeutics, and clinical skills on a regular basis.
2. Pursues and participates in formal and independent learning activities to enhance skills in promoting the professional development of nursing personnel.
3. Pursues and participates in educational and mentoring opportunities to increase effectiveness as a change agent.
4. Pursues and participates in formal and independent learning activities to enhance skills in proactive problem solving for system issues.

IV. Collegiality

The acute and critical care CNS contributes to the professional development of peers, colleagues, and others.

Measurement Criteria
1. Identifies and participates in opportunities to share skills, knowledge, and strategies for patient care and system improvement with colleagues and other health care providers.
2. Promotes a learning environment that enables nursing and other health care personnel to make optimal contributions and systems to function most effectively.
3. Participates in professional organizations to address issues of concern in meeting patients' needs and improving nursing practice and system effectiveness.

V. Ethics

The acute and critical care CNS's decisions and actions are made on behalf of patients and their family members, nursing personnel, and organizational systems and are determined in an ethical manner.

Measurement Criteria
1. Fosters the establishment of an ethical environment that supports the rights of all participants.
2. Contributes to the resolution of ethical dilemmas by enhancing the responsiveness of individuals as well as organizational systems.
3. Serves as a mentor and role model by participating in the resolution of ethical and clinical dilemmas.

VI. Collaboration

The acute and critical care CNS collaborates with patients and their family members and health care personnel in creating a healing and caring environment.

Measurement Criteria
1. Provides consultation and initiates referrals to facilitate optimal care.
2. Optimizes the collaboration and coordination of the interdisciplinary team to enhance the environment of patient care.
3. Provides mentoring to nursing students, specifically in the area of critical care and CNS preparation in collaboration with schools of nursing.
4. Collaborates with other disciplines in teaching, consultation, management, and research activities to improve outcomes in nursing practice and enhance the health care environment.

VII. Research

The acute and critical care CNS utilizes, participates in, and disseminates research to enhance practice.

Measurement Criteria
1. Critically evaluates existing practice based on current research findings and integrates changes into practice.
2. Chooses, applies, or withholds interventions in a manner that is substantiated by relevant research and appropriate to the needs of the patient or system.
3. Utilizes the research process to improve patient outcomes and enhance the environment of care.
4. Collaborates with senior investigators and/or members of the interdisciplinary team in conducting research relevant to practice.

VIII. Resource Utilization

The acute and critical care CNS influences resource utilization in order to promote safety, effectiveness, and fiscal accountability in the planning and delivery of patient care.

Measurement Criteria

1. Evaluates factors related to safety, effectiveness, availability, and cost to design and implement best practices.
2. Advocates for patients and their family members and nursing personnel, and supports policy and services that advocate for patient rights and optimal environments of health care.
3. Facilitates access for patients and their family members to appropriate health care services.
4. Serves as a resource to various populations for the purpose of influencing the delivery of health care and the formation of policy.

CCNS Examination Blueprint

ADULT PROGRAM

I. Clinical Judgment (22%)

A. *Cardiovascular*
1. Acute coronary syndromes/unstable angina
2. Acute heart failure/pulmonary edema
3. Acute inflammatory disease (e.g., myocarditis, endocarditis, pericarditis)
4. Acute myocardial infarction/papillary muscle rupture
5. Acute peripheral vascular insufficiency (e.g., acute arterial occlusion, carotid artery stenosis, endarterectomy, peripheral stents)
6. Cardiac surgery (e.g., valve replacement, coronary artery bypass graft)
7. Cardiac tamponade
8. Cardiac trauma (blunt and penetrating)
9. Cardiogenic shock
10. Cardiomyopathies (e.g., hypertrophic, dilated, restrictive, idiopathic)
11. Cardiovascular pharmacology
12. Conduction defects, blocks, and pacemakers
13. Dysrhythmias/automatic internal cardiac defibrillators
14. Heart failure
15. Hemodynamic monitoring
16. Hypertensive crisis
17. Hypovolemic shock and volume deficit
18. Pulmonary hypertension (e.g., valvular defects, aortic stenosis, mitral stenosis)
19. Ruptured or dissecting aneurysm (e.g., thoracic, abdominal)

B. *Pulmonary*
1. Acute pulmonary embolus, fat embolus
2. Acute respiratory distress syndrome
3. Acute respiratory failure, hypoxemia
4. Acute respiratory infections
5. Air leak syndromes (e.g., spontaneous pneumothorax, pneumopericardium, pneumomediastinum, pulmonary interstitial emphysema)
6. Aspirations (e.g., aspiration pneumonia, hospital-acquired pneumonia, foreign body aspiration)
7. Chronic lung disease
8. Pulmonary pharmacology
9. Pulmonary trauma (e.g., pulmonary hemorrhage, tracheal perforation)
10. Respiratory distress (e.g., emphysema, bronchitis)
11. Status asthmaticus, exacerbation of chronic obstructive pulmonary disease, emphysema
12. Thoracic surgery (e.g., lung contusions, fractured ribs, hemothorax, pulmonary hemorrhage, lung reduction, pneumonectomy, lobectomy, tracheal surgery)
13. Thoracic trauma (e.g., lung contusions, fractured ribs, hemothorax, pneumothorax from trauma, pulmonary hemorrhage)

14. Ventilator management and arterial blood gas interpretation, mixed venous gases, continuous positive airway pressure, volutrauma and barotraumas

C. *Endocrine*
 1. Acute hypoglycemia
 2. Diabetes insipidus
 3. Diabetic ketoacidosis
 4. Hormones and endocrine anatomy and physiology
 5. Hyperglycemic hyperosmolar nonketotic coma

D. *Hematology*
 1. Hematology, anatomy and physiology, blood products and plasma
 2. Immunosuppression-acquired (e.g., HIV, AIDS, neoplasms)
 3. Life-threatening coagulopathies (e.g., idiopathic thrombocytopenia, disseminated intravascular coagulation, hemophilia, heparin-induced thrombosis thrombocytopenia syndrome, abciximab-induced) and nonlife-threatening coagulopathies
 4. Organ transplantation (e.g., liver, bone marrow, kidney, heart, pancreas, lung)
 5. Sickle cell crisis

E. *Neurology*
 1. Aneurysm, arteriovenous malformation
 2. Encephalopathy (e.g., hypoxic ischemic, metabolic, edema, infectious)
 3. Head trauma (blunt, penetrating), skull fractures
 4. Intracranial hemorrhage/intraventricular hemorrhage (e.g., subarachnoid, epidural, subdural)
 5. Neurologic infectious diseases (e.g., meningitis, Guillain-Barré syndrome, West Nile virus)
 6. Intracranial pressure monitoring
 7. Neurosurgery (e.g., evacuation of hematoma, tumor resection)
 8. Seizure disorders

9. Stroke (e.g., embolic events, hemorrhagic)

F. *Gastrointestinal*
 1. Acute abdominal trauma
 2. Acute gastrointestinal hemorrhage (e.g., esophageal, upper and lower)
 3. Bowel infarction, bowel obstruction, bowel perforation
 4. Gastrointestinal surgeries (e.g., Whipple procedure, esophagogastrectomy, gastric bypass)
 5. Hepatic failure/coma (e.g., portal hypertension, cirrhosis, esophageal varices, fulminant hepatitis)
 6. Pancreatitis
 7. Gastroesophageal reflux

G. *Renal*
 1. Acute renal failure (e.g., acute tubular necrosis, hypoxia, dialysis)
 2. Chronic renal failure and dialysis
 3. Life-threatening electrolyte imbalances (e.g., potassium, sodium, phosphorus, magnesium, calcium)
 4. Fluid balance concepts, renal anatomy, and physiology
 5. Renal trauma

H. *Multisystem*
 1. Multisystem trauma
 2. Septic shock/infectious diseases (e.g., viral, bacterial, line sepsis, nosocomial infections, immunosuppression)
 3. Systemic inflammatory response syndrome, sepsis, multiorgan dysfunction syndrome
 4. Toxic exposure (e.g., chemicals, radiation, anaphylaxis)
 5. Toxic ingestions and inhalations (e.g., drug/alcohol overdose, poisoning)

II. Professional Caring and Ethical Practice (78%)

A. Advocacy/moral agency (7%)
B. Caring practices (11%)

C. Collaboration (14%)
D. Systems thinking (8%)
E. Response to diversity (4%)
F. Clinical inquiry (13%)
G. Facilitation of learning (21%)

PEDIATRIC PROGRAM

I. Clinical Judgment (22%)

A. *Cardiovascular*
   1. Acute heart failure/pulmonary edema
   2. Acute inflammatory disease (e.g., myocarditis, endocarditis, pericarditis)
   3. Cardiac surgery
   4. Cardiac trauma (blunt and penetrating)
   5. Cardiogenic shock
   6. Cardiomyopathies (e.g., hypertrophic, dilated, restrictive, idiopathic)
   7. Cardiovascular pharmacology
   8. Conduction defects, blocks, and pacemakers
   9. Congenital heart defect/disease
   10. Dysrhythmias
   11. Hemodynamic monitoring
   12. Hypertensive crisis
   13. Hypovolemic shock and volume deficit
   14. Pulmonary hypertension (e.g., aortic and mitral stenosis and regurgitation)

B. *Pulmonary*
   1. Acute respiratory distress syndrome
   2. Acute respiratory failure, hypoxemia
   3. Acute respiratory infections (e.g., pneumonia, croup, streptococcal pneumonia, respiratory syncytial virus, bronchiolitis)
   4. Air leak syndromes (e.g., spontaneous pneumothorax, bronchofistula, emphysema, pulmonary interstitial emphysema, pneumopericardium, pneumomediastinum)
   5. Apnea of prematurity
   6. Aspirations (e.g., aspiration pneumonia, hospital-acquired pneumonia, foreign body aspiration)
   7. Chronic lung disease (e.g., bronchopulmonary dysplasia)
   8. Congenital anomalies
   9. Persistent pulmonary hypertension
   10. Pulmonary trauma (e.g., pulmonary hemorrhage, tracheal perforation)
   11. Pulmonary pharmacology
   12. Respiratory distress (e.g., epiglottitis, bronchitis)
   13. Status asthmaticus
   14. Thoracic surgery (e.g., lung contusions, fractured ribs, hemothorax, pulmonary hemorrhage, lung reduction, pneumonectomy, lobectomy, tracheal surgery)
   15. Thoracic trauma (e.g., lung contusions, fractured ribs, hemothorax, pulmonary hemorrhage)
   16. Ventilator management and arterial blood gas interpretation, mixed venous gases, continuous positive airway pressure, volutrauma, and barotraumas

C. *Endocrine*
   1. Acute hypoglycemia
   2. Diabetes insipidus
   3. Diabetic ketoacidosis
   4. Hormones, anatomy and physiology
   5. Inborn errors of metabolism
   6. Syndrome of inappropriate secretion of antidiuretic hormone

D. *Hematology*
   1. Hematology, anatomy and physiology, blood products and plasma
   2. Hyperbilirubinemia
   3. Immunosuppression (e.g., congenital [severe combined immunodeficiency syndrome], acquired [HIV, AIDS, neoplasms])
   4. Life-threatening coagulopathies (e.g., disseminated intravascular coagulation, idiopathic thrombocytopenia purpura, hemophilia)
   5. Organ transplantation (e.g., liver, bone marrow, kidney, heart, pancreas, lung)
   6. Sickle cell crisis

E. *Neurology*
1. Acute spinal cord injury
2. Congenital neurological abnormalities (e.g., spina bifida, myelomeningocele, anencephaly, encephalocele)
3. Encephalopathy (e.g., hypoxic ischemic, metabolic, edema, infectious)
4. Head trauma (blunt, penetrating) including shaken baby
5. Hydrocephalus
6. Intracranial pressure monitoring
7. Intracranial hemorrhage/intraventricular hemorrhage (e.g., subarachnoid, epidural, subdural), including stroke
8. Neurologic infectious diseases (e.g., meningitis, congenital infections, viral infections, West Nile virus)
9. Neuromuscular disorders (e.g., muscular dystrophy, Werdnig-Hoffman disease)
10. Neurosurgery (e.g., evacuation of hematoma, tumor resection)
11. Seizure disorders
12. Space-occupying lesions (e.g., brain tumors)
13. Spinal fusion

F. *Gastrointestinal*
1. Acute abdominal trauma
2. Acute gastrointestinal hemorrhage
3. Bowel infarction /obstruction/ perforation (e.g., necrotizing enterocolitis)
4. Gastroesophageal reflux
5. Gastrointestinal abnormalities at birth (e.g., Hirschsprung's disease)
6. Gastrointestinal surgeries
7. Hepatic failure/coma (e.g., portal hypertension, fulminant hepatitis, biliary atresia, hyperbilirubinemia)

G. *Renal*
1. Acute renal failure (e.g., acute tubular necrosis)
2. Chronic renal failure and dialysis
3. Congenital renal-genitourinary abnormalities (e.g., polycystic kidneys, exstrophy of bladder, hydronephrosis)

4. Fluid balance concepts, renal anatomy, and physiology
5. Life-threatening electrolyte imbalances (e.g., potassium, sodium, phosphorus, magnesium, calcium)
6. Renal trauma

H. *Multisystem*
1. Asphyxia (e.g., near-drowning, traumatic)
2. Burns
3. Hemolytic uremic syndrome
4. Multisystem trauma
5. Septic shock/infectious diseases (e.g., congenital viral, bacterial, line sepsis, nosocomial infections)
6. Systemic inflammatory response syndrome, sepsis, multiorgan dysfunction syndrome
7. Toxic exposure (e.g., fetal exposure to drugs/alcohol, drug withdrawal, anaphylaxis)
8. Toxic ingestions and inhalations (e.g., drug/alcohol overdose, poisoning)

II. Professional Caring and Ethical Practice (78%)

A. Advocacy/moral agency (7%)
B. Caring practices (11%)
C. Collaboration (14%)
D. Systems thinking (8%)
E. Response to diversity (4%)
F. Clinical inquiry (13%)
G. Facilitation of learning (21%)

NEONATAL PROGRAM

I. Clinical Judgment (22%)

A. *Cardiovascular*
1. Acute heart failure/pulmonary edema
2. Acute inflammatory disease (e.g., myocarditis, endocarditis, pericarditis)
3. Cardiac surgery
4. Cardiovascular pharmacology
5. Congenital heart defect/disease

6. Hemodynamic concepts
7. Pulmonary hypertension
8. Shock states (e.g., cardiogenic, hypovolemic), volume deficit

B. *Pulmonary*
1. Acute respiratory failure, hypoxemia
2. Acute respiratory infections
3. Air-leak syndromes (e.g., spontaneous pneumothorax, bronchofistula, emphysema, [pulmonary interstitial emphysema], pneumopericardium, pneumomediastinum)
4. Apnea of prematurity
5. Aspirations (e.g., aspiration pneumonia, meconium aspiration)
6. Chronic lung disease (e.g., bronchopulmonary dysplasia)
7. Congenital anomalies
8. Pulmonary hypertension in newborns
9. Respiratory distress syndrome
10. Respiratory pharmacology
11. Thoracic surgery (e.g., lung contusions, fractured ribs, hemothorax, pulmonary hemorrhage, lung reduction, pneumonectomy, lobectomy, tracheal surgery)
12. Transient tachypnea of the newborn
13. Ventilator management and arterial blood gas interpretation, mixed venous gases, continuous positive airway pressure, volutrauma, and barotrauma

C. *Endocrine*
1. Acute hypoglycemia
2. Hormones, anatomy and physiology
3. Inborn errors of metabolism
4. Infant of diabetic mother

D. *Hematology*
1. Anemia of prematurity
2. Hematology, blood products and plasma
3. Hyperbilirubinemia
4. Immunosuppression (e.g., Rh incompatibilities, ABO incompatibilities, hydrops fetalis)

5. Life-threatening coagulopathies (e.g., idiopathic thrombocytopenia purpura, disseminated intravascular coagulation) and nonlife-threatening coagulopathies

E. *Neurology*
1. Congenital neurological abnormalities (e.g., spina bifida, myelomeningocele, anencephaly, encephalocele)
2. Encephalopathy (e.g., hypoxic ischemic, metabolic, edema, infectious)
3. Hydrocephalus
4. Intracranial pressure monitoring
5. Intracranial hemorrhage/intraventricular hemorrhage
6. Neurologic infectious diseases (e.g., meningitis, congenital infections, viral infections, TORCH complex)
7. Seizure disorders

F. *Gastrointestinal*
1. Bowel infarction/obstruction/perforation (e.g., necrotizing enterocolitis, adhesions, short gut syndrome)
2. Gastroesophageal reflux
3. Gastrointestinal abnormalities at birth
4. Hepatic failure/coma

G. *Renal*
1. Acute renal failure (e.g., acute tubular necrosis, hypoxia)
2. Congenital renal-genitourinary abnormalities (e.g., polycystic kidneys, exstrophy of bladder, hydronephrosis)
3. Fluid balance concepts, renal anatomy, and physiology
4. Life-threatening electrolyte imbalances (e.g., potassium, sodium, phosphorus, magnesium, calcium)

H. *Multisystem*
1. Asphyxia (e.g., neonatal-perinatal)
2. Life-threatening maternal-fetal complications (e.g., birth trauma and birth-related injuries, genetic disorders, maternal-fetal

transfusion, placental abruption, placenta previa)
3. Low birth weight/prematurity
4. Septic shock/infectious diseases (e.g., congenital, viral, bacterial, line sepsis, nosocomial infections)
5. Toxic exposure (e.g., fetal exposure to drugs/alcohol, drug withdrawal, anaphylaxis)

II. **Professional Caring and Ethical Practice (78%)**

A. Advocacy/moral agency (7%)
B. Caring practices (11%)
C. Collaboration (14%)
D. Systems thinking (8%)
E. Response to diversity (4%)
F. Clinical inquiry (13%)
G. Facilitation of learning (21%)

AACN Standards for Establishing and Sustaining Healthy Work Environments: A Journey to Excellence*

ABOUT THE STANDARDS

Each day thousands of medical errors harm the patients and families served by the American health care system. Work environments that tolerate ineffective interpersonal relationships and do not support education to acquire necessary skills perpetuate unacceptable conditions. So do health professionals who experience moral distress over this state of affair, yet remain silent and overwhelmed with resignation. Consider these all-too-familiar situations:

- A nurse chooses not to call a physician known to be verbally abusive. The nurse uses her judgment to clarify a prescribed medication and administers a fatal dose of the wrong drug.[1]
- Additional patients are added to a nurse's assignment during a busy weekend because on-call staff is not available

and back-up plans do not exist to cover variations in patient census. Patients are placed at risk for errors and injury, and nurses are frustrated and angry.
- Isolated decision making in one department leads to tension, frustration, and a higher risk of errors by all involved. Whether affecting patient care or unit operations, decisions made without including all parties places everyone involved at risk.
- Nurses are placed in leadership positions without adequate preparation and support for their roles. The resulting environment creates dissatisfaction and high turnover for nurse leaders and staff as well.
- Contentious relationships between nurses and administrators heighten when managers are required to stretch their responsibilities without adequate preparation and coaching for success.[2] Only 65% of hospital managers are held accountable for employee satisfaction.[3]

Each situation characterizes poor and ineffective relationships. Attention to work relationships is often dismissed as unworthy of resource allocation in health care today, especially when those resources are aimed at supporting education and development of essential skills. This is because of the mistaken perception that effective relationships do not affect an organization's financial health. Nothing could be further from the truth. Relationship issues are real obstacles to the development of work environments in which patients and their families can receive safe, even excellent, care. Inattention to work relationships creates obstacles that may become the root cause of medical errors, hospital-acquired infections and other complications, patient readmission, and nurse turnover.

Adequately addressing the reputedly "soft" issues that involve relationships is the key to halting the epidemic of treatment-related harm to patients and the continued erosion of the bottom line in health care organizations. Indeed, the Institute of Medicine has reported that safety and quality problems exist in large part because dedicated health professionals work within systems that neither prepare nor support them to achieve optimal patient care outcomes.[4] Addressing these issues aligns with nurses' ethical obligations, specifically the obligations to establish, maintain, and improve health care environments and employment conditions conducive to providing quality care consistent with the values of the profession and maintain compassionate and caring relationships with "a commitment to fair treatment of individuals and integrity-preserving compromise."[5]

For more than two decades, AACN has advocated for principles such as interdisciplinary collaboration and effective leadership that are essential to healthy work environments.[6] The standards continue this legacy and respond to the Institute of Medicine's call for professional groups to serve as advocates for change.[7] A nine-person panel developed the standards, drawing from extensive published and unpublished reports from individual nurses and other experts in health care organizations across the United States.

Representing a wide range of roles, acute and critical care settings, and geographic locations in which nursing care is provided, 50 expert reviewers validated the standards, critical elements, and explanatory text.

Essential Standards

The American Association of Critical-Care Nurses (AACN) recognizes the inextricable links among quality of the work environment, excellent nursing practice, and patient care outcomes. The AACN Synergy Model for Patient Care further affirms how excellent nursing practice is that which meets the needs of patients and their families.[8] The AACN is strategically committed to bringing its influence and resources to bear on creating work and care environments that are safe; healing; humane; and respectful of the rights, responsibilities, needs and contributions of all people, including patients, their families, and nurses.

Six standards for establishing and sustaining healthy work environments have been identified. The standards represent evidence-based and relationship-centered principles of professional performance. Each standard is considered essential because studies show that effective and sustainable outcomes do not emerge when any standard is considered optional. The standards align directly with the core competencies for health professionals recommended by the Institute of Medicine. They support the education of all health professionals "to deliver patient-centered care as members of an interdisciplinary team, emphasizing evidence-based practice, quality improvement approaches, and informatics."[9] With these standards, AACN contributes to the implementation of elements in a healthy work environment articulated in 2004 by the 70-member Nursing Organizations Alliance. The standards further support the education of nurse leaders to acquire the core competencies of self-knowledge, strategic vision, risk taking and creativity, interpersonal and communication effectiveness, and inspiration identified by the

Robert Wood Johnson Executive Nurse Fellows Program.[10]

The standards are neither detailed nor exhaustive. They do not address dimensions such as physical safety, clinical practice, clinical and academic education, and credentialing—all of which are amply addressed by a multitude of statutory, regulatory, and professional agencies and organizations. The standards are designed to be used as a foundation for thoughtful reflection and engaged dialogue about the current realities of each work environment. Critical elements required for successful implementation accompany each standard. Working collaboratively, individuals and groups within an organization should determine the priority and depth of application required to implement each standard.

The standards for establishing and sustaining healthy work environments are as follows:

- *Skilled communication*: Nurses must be as proficient in communication skills as they are in clinical skills.
- *True collaboration*: Nurses must be relentless in pursuing and fostering true collaboration.
- *Effective decision making*: Nurses must be valued and committed partners in making policy, directing and evaluating clinical care, and leading organizational operations.
- *Appropriate staffing*: Staffing must ensure the effective match between patient needs and nurse competencies.
- *Meaningful recognition*: Nurses must be recognized and must recognize others for the value each brings to the work of the organization.
- *Authentic leadership:* Nurse leaders must fully embrace the imperative of a healthy work environment, authentically live it, and engage others in its achievement.

Adoption and Implementation

The standards provide a functional yardstick for performance and development of individuals, units, organizations, and systems. They reaffirm that safe and respectful environments are imperative and require systems, structures, and cultures that support communication, collaboration, decision making, staffing, recognition, and leadership.

These standards support the provisions of the American Nurses Association Code of Ethics for Nurses and provide a framework to assist nurses in upholding their obligation to practice in ways consistent with appropriate ethical behavior.[5] Properly implemented, the standards will ensure that acute and critical care nurses have the skills, resources, accountability, and authority to make decisions that ensure excellent professional nursing practice and optimal care for patients and their families. Implementation of the standards demonstrates an organization's ethical responsibility. The standards can lead to excellence only when they have been adopted at every level of the organization—from the bedside to the boardroom. Adoption requires creating the systems, structures, and cultures that provide the ongoing collaborative education necessary to enhance and support the effort. This requires recognition by the organization that people often create and support unhealthy work environments because they lack the knowledge, skills, and experience to do otherwise.

Success will be further ensured when individuals are afforded the programs to acquire needed skills and willingly embrace implementation of the standards as a personal obligation, holding themselves and others accountable. This requires a committed partnership between nurses and their work environment. For example, safe staffing cannot be accomplished when a fatigued nurse works excessive overtime hours and perhaps attempts to maintain a second job. Careful scrutiny of these six standards (Figure C-1) immediately reveals the interdependence of each standard. For example, effective decision making, appropriate staffing, meaningful recognition, and authentic leadership depend on skilled communication and true collaboration. Likewise, authentic leadership is imperative to ensure sustainable implementation of the other behavior-based standards.

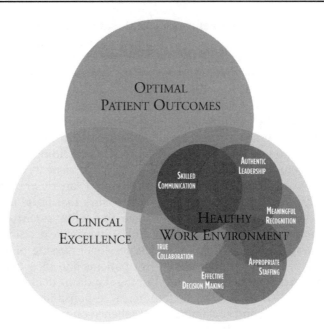

FIG C-1 Interdependence of health work environment, clinical excellence, and optimal patient outcomes.

SKILLED COMMUNICATION

Nurses must be as proficient in communication skills as they are in clinical skills.

Optimal care of patients mandates that the specialized knowledge and skills of nurses, physicians, administrators, and multiple other professionals be integrated. This integration will be accomplished only through frequent, respectful interaction and skilled communication. Skilled communication is more than the one-way delivery of information; it is a two-way dialogue in which people think and decide together.

A culture of safety and excellence requires that individual nurses and health care organizations make it a priority to develop among professionals communication skills—including written, spoken, and nonverbal—that are on a par with expert clinical skills.[1,2] This culture expects civility and respects nurses who speak from their knowledge and authority.[3] Patients in the care of clinically expert professionals suffer medical errors with alarming frequency.[4] Nearly three in four errors are caused by human factors associated with interpersonal interactions.[5] In addition, according to data from the Joint Commission on Accreditation of Healthcare Organizations, breakdown in team communication is a top contributor to sentinel events.[6]

Intimidating behavior and deficient interpersonal relationships lead to mistrust, chronic stress, and dissatisfaction among nurses. This unhealthy situation contributes to nurses leaving their positions and often their profession altogether. More than half of nurses surveyed report they have been subject to verbal abuse, and more than 90% have witnessed disruptive behavior.[1] Nurses can encounter conflict in every dimension of their work. Whether the conflict is with others or between their own personal and professional values, skilled communication supports the ethical obligation to seek resolution that preserves a nurse's professional integrity while ensuring a patient's safety and best interests.[7] Ensuring that nurses are provided the education, competency mastery, and rewards to effectively negotiate these conflict-laden conditions would itself dramatically alter the environment.

Critical Elements of Skilled Communication

- The health care organization provides team members with support for and access to education programs that develop critical communication skills, including self-awareness, inquiry/dialogue, conflict management, negotiation, advocacy, and listening.
- Skilled communicators focus on finding solutions and achieving desirable outcomes.
- Skilled communicators seek to protect and advance collaborative relationships among colleagues.
- Skilled communicators invite and hear all relevant perspectives.
- Skilled communicators call upon goodwill and mutual respect to build consensus and arrive at common understanding.
- Skilled communicators demonstrate congruence between words and actions, holding others accountable for doing the same.
- The health care organization establishes zero-tolerance policies and enforces them to address and eliminate abuse and disrespectful behavior in the workplace.
- The health care organization establishes formal structures and processes that ensure effective information sharing among patients, families, and the health care team.
- Skilled communicators have access to appropriate communication technologies and are proficient in their use.
- The health care organization establishes systems that require individuals and teams to formally evaluate the impact of communication on clinical, financial, and work environment outcomes.
- The health care organization includes communication as a criterion in its formal performance appraisal system, and team members demonstrate skilled communication to qualify for professional advancement.

TRUE COLLABORATION

Nurses must be relentless in pursuing and fostering true collaboration.

True collaboration is a process, not an event. It must be ongoing and build over time, eventually resulting in a work culture in which joint communication and decision making between nurses and other disciplines and among nurses themselves become the norm. Unlike the lip service that collaboration is often given, in true collaboration the unique knowledge and abilities of each professional are respected to achieve safe, quality care for patients. Skilled communication, trust, knowledge, shared responsibility, mutual respect, optimism, and coordination are integral to successful collaboration.[1]

Without the synchronous, ongoing collaborative work of health care professionals from multiple disciplines, patient and family needs cannot be optimally satisfied within the complexities of today's health care system. Extensive evidence shows the negative impact of poor collaboration on various measurable indicators, including patient and family satisfaction, patient safety and outcomes, professional staff satisfaction, nurse retention, and cost.[2,3] The Institute of Medicine points to "a historical lack of interprofessional cooperation" as one of the cultural barriers to safety in hospitals.[4]

Nearly 90% of the AACN's members and constituents report that collaboration with physicians and administrators is among the most important elements in creating a healthy work environment.[5] Further, nurse-physician collaboration has been found to be one of the three strongest predictors of psychological empowerment of nurses.[6] Mutual respect between nurses and physicians for each other's knowledge and competence, coupled with a mutual concern that quality patient care will be provided, are key organizational elements of work environments that attract and retain nurses.[1,7,8] In addition, an unresponsive bureaucracy generates organizational stress, which is significantly more predictive of nurse burnout and resignations than emotional stressors inherent in the work itself.[9]

Collaboration requires constant attention and nurturing, supported by formal processes and structures that foster joint communication and decision making. Evidence documenting differing perceptions about the importance and effectiveness of nurse-physician collaboration among nurses, physicians, and health care executives points to a mandate that effective methods be developed to improve working relationships between nurses and physicians.[10]

Critical Elements of True Collaboration

- The health care organization provides team members with support for and access to educational programs that develop collaboration skills.
- The health care organization creates, uses, and evaluates processes that define each team member's accountability for collaboration and how unwillingness to collaborate will be addressed.
- The health care organization creates, uses, and evaluates operational structures that ensure that the decision-making authority of nurses is acknowledged and incorporated as the norm.
- The health care organization ensures unrestricted access to structured forums such as ethics committees and makes available the time needed to resolve disputes among all critical participants, including patients, families, and the health care team.
- Every team member embraces true collaboration as an ongoing process and invests in its development to ensure a sustained culture of collaboration.
- Every team member contributes to the achievement of common goals by giving power and respect to each person's voice, integrating individual differences, resolving competing interests, and safeguarding the essential contribution each must make to achieve optimal outcomes.
- Every team member acts with a high level of personal integrity.

- Team members master skilled communication, an essential element of true collaboration.
- Each team member demonstrates competence appropriate to his or her role and responsibilities.
- Nurse managers and medical directors are equal partners in modeling and fostering true collaboration.

EFFECTIVE DECISION MAKING

Nurses must be valued and committed partners in making policy, directing and evaluating clinical care, and leading organizational operations.

To fulfill their role as advocates, nurses must be involved in making decisions about patient care.[1] A significant gap often exists between what nurses are accountable for and their ability to participate in decisions that affect those accountabilities. Evidence suggests that physicians, pharmacists, administrators, and nurses assign primary responsibility for patient safety to nurses. However, only 8% of physicians recognize nurses as part of the decision-making team.[2] Other research reports that a majority of nurses feel relatively powerless to change things they dislike in their work environment.[3] This autonomy-accountability gap interferes with nurses' ability to optimize their essential contribution and fulfill their obligations to the public as licensed professionals.

As the single constant professional presence with hospitalized patients, nurses uniquely gather, filter, interpret, and transform data from patients and the system into the meaningful information required to diagnose, treat, and deliver care to a patient. This data management role of nurses is a vital link in the decision-making activities of the entire health care team.[4-6] Failure to incorporate the experienced perspective of nurses in clinical and operational decisions may result in costly errors, jeopardize patient safety, and threaten the financial viability of health care organizations.

Nurses believe that they provide high-quality nursing care and are accountable for their own practice.[7,8] Nurses who do not have control over their practice become dissatisfied and are at risk for leaving an organization. Health care organizations recognized for attracting and retaining nurses have successfully implemented professional care models in which nurses have the responsibility and related authority for patient care along with formal operational structures that support autonomous nursing practice. Their success is recognized by national programs such as the AACN Beacon Award for Critical Care Excellence, the Magnet Nursing Services Recognition Program, and the Baldrige National Quality Program.[9-11]

Critical Elements of Effective Decision Making

- The health care organization provides team members with support for and access to ongoing education and development programs focusing on strategies that ensure collaborative decision making. Program content includes mutual goal setting, negotiation, facilitation, conflict management, systems thinking, and performance improvement.
- The health care organization clearly articulates organizational values, and team members incorporate these values when making decisions.
- The health care organization has operational structures in place that ensure that the perspectives of patients and their families are incorporated into every decision affecting patient care.
- Individual team members share accountability for effective decision making by acquiring necessary skills, mastering relevant content, assessing situations accurately, sharing fact-based information, communicating professional opinions clearly, and inquiring actively.
- The health care organization establishes systems such as structured forums involving all departments and health care disciplines to facilitate data-driven decisions.
- The health care organization establishes deliberate decision-making processes that

ensure respect for the rights of every individual, incorporate all key perspectives, and designate clear accountability.
- The health care organization has fair and effective processes in place at all levels to objectively evaluate the results of decisions, including delayed decisions and indecision.

APPROPRIATE STAFFING

Staffing must ensure the effective match between patient needs and nurse competencies.

Inappropriate staffing is one of the most harmful threats to patient safety and to the well-being of nurses. Evidence suggests that better patient outcomes result when a higher proportion of care hours is provided by registered nurses as compared with care by licensed practical nurses or nursing assistants.[1] The likelihood of death or serious complications after surgery increases when fewer nurses are assigned to care for patients.[2] Further research supports a relationship between specialty certification and clinical nursing expertise.[3,4]

Because nurses intercept 86% of all medication errors made by other professionals, an increase in these errors will likely occur when nurses are overworked, overstressed, and in short supply.[5] Inadequate staffing leads to nurse dissatisfaction, burnout, and turnover.[2] Nurse turnover jeopardizes the quality of care, increases patient costs, and decreases hospital profitability.[6] Staffing is a complex process with the goal of matching the needs of patients at multiple points throughout their illness with the skills and competencies of nurses. Because the condition of critically ill patients rapidly and continuously fluctuates, flexibility of nurse staffing that goes beyond fixed nurse-to-patient ratios is imperative.[7] Relying on staffing ratios alone ignores variance in patient needs and acuity.

Organizations must engage in dramatic innovation to devise and systematically test new staffing models. All staffing models require methods for ongoing evaluation of staffing decisions in relation to patient and system outcomes.[8] This evaluation is essential to provide accurate trend data from which targeted improvement tactics—including technologies to reduce the demand and increase the efficiency of nurses' work—can be undertaken.

Critical Elements of Appropriate Staffing

- The health care organization has staffing policies in place that are solidly grounded in ethical principles and support the professional obligation of nurses to provide high-quality care.
- Nurses participate in all organizational phases of the staffing process from education and planning—including matching nurses' competencies with patients' assessed needs—through evaluation.
- The health care organization has formal processes in place to evaluate the effect of staffing decisions on patient and system outcomes. This evaluation includes analysis of when patient needs and nurse competencies are mismatched and how often contingency plans are implemented.
- The health care organization has a system in place that facilitates team members' use of staffing and outcomes data to develop more effective staffing models.
- The health care organization provides support services at every level of activity to ensure that nurses can optimally focus on the priorities and requirements of patient and family care.
- The health care organization adopts technologies that increase the effectiveness of nursing care delivery. Nurses are engaged in the selection, adaptation, and evaluation of these technologies.

MEANINGFUL RECOGNITION

Nurses must be recognized and must recognize others for the value each brings to the work of the organization.

Recognition of the value and meaningfulness of one's contribution to an organization's work is a fundamental human need and an essential requisite to personal and professional development. People who are not recognized feel invisible, undervalued, unmotivated, and disrespected. A majority of nurses are dissatisfied with the recognition they receive from their employer.[1] This lack of recognition leads to discontent, poor morale, reduced productivity, and suboptimal care outcomes. Inadequate recognition is cited as a primary reason for turnover among employees and is linked to decreasing nurse satisfaction.[2-4]

Three out of four members and constituents of the AACN rank recognition for their contributions as a central element of a healthy work environment.[5] Hospitals recognized for attracting and retaining nurses emphasize personal growth and development and provide multiple rewards for expertise and opportunities for clinical advancement.[6] Like true collaboration, meaningful recognition is a process, not an event. It must be ongoing and build over time, becoming a norm within the work culture. Recognition has meaning only when it is relevant to the person being recognized. Recognition that is not congruent with a person's contributions or comes in tandem with emotionally charged organizational change is often perceived as disrespectful tokenism. Effective programs of recognition will not occur automatically and require formal structures and processes to ensure desired outcomes.

Critical Elements of Meaningful Recognition

- The health care organization has a comprehensive system in place that includes formal processes and structured forums that ensure a sustainable focus on recognizing all team members for their contributions and the value they bring to the work of the organization.
- The health care organization establishes a systematic process for all team members to learn about the institution's recognition system and how to participate by recognizing the contributions of colleagues and the value they bring to the organization.
- The health care organization's recognition system reaches from the bedside to the

board table, ensuring that individuals receive recognition consistent with their personal definition of meaning, fulfillment, development, and advancement at every stage of their professional career.

- The health care organization's recognition system includes processes that validate that recognition is meaningful to those being acknowledged.
- Team members understand that everyone is responsible for playing an active role in the organization's recognition program and meaningfully recognizing contributions.
- The health care organization regularly and comprehensively evaluates its recognition system, ensuring effective programs that help to move the organization toward a sustainable culture of excellence that values meaningful recognition.

AUTHENTIC LEADERSHIP

Nurse leaders must fully embrace the imperative of a healthy work environment, authentically live it, and engage others in its achievement.

Less than half of members of the AACN rank their relationships with their managers and administrators as positive, yet more than 90% identify effective leaders as an important element of a healthy work environment.[1] A multitude of reports and white papers issued by leaders in all sectors of the health care community document the issue of inadequately positioned and prepared leaders in nursing and strongly call for effective measures to strengthen nursing leadership.[2]

Nurse leaders—including managers, administrators, advanced practice nurses, educators, and other formal and informal clinical leaders—seldom have the support resources commensurate with their scope of responsibilities and often do not have access to key decision-making forums within health care organizations. Nurse managers in particular are key to the retention of satisfied staff yet all too often receive little preparation, education, coaching, or mentoring to ensure success in their role. Nurse leaders must be skilled communicators, team builders, agents for positive change, committed to service, results oriented, and role models for collaborative practice.[3] This requires skill in the core competencies of self-knowledge, strategic vision, risk taking and creativity, interpersonal and communication effectiveness, and inspiration.[4] Healthy work environments require that individual nurses and organizations commit to the development of nurse leaders in a systematic and comprehensive way. Nurse leaders must be positioned within key operational and governance bodies of the organization to inform and influence decisions that affect nursing practice and the environment in which it is practiced.[2,3]

Critical Elements of Authentic Leadership

- The health care organization provides support for and access to educational programs to ensure that nurse leaders develop and enhance knowledge and abilities in skilled communication, effective decision making, true collaboration, meaningful recognition, and ensuring resources to achieve appropriate staffing.
- Nurse leaders demonstrate an understanding of the requirements and dynamics at the point of care and within this context successfully translate the vision of a healthy work environment.
- Nurse leaders excel at generating visible enthusiasm for achieving the standards that create and sustain healthy work environments.
- Nurse leaders lead the design of systems necessary to effectively implement and sustain standards for healthy work environments.
- The health care organization ensures that nurse leaders are appropriately positioned in their pivotal role in creating and sustaining healthy work environments. This includes participation in key decision-making forums, access to essential information, and the authority to make necessary decisions.

- The health care organization facilitates the efforts of nurse leaders to create and sustain a healthy work environment by providing the necessary time and financial and human resources.
- The health care organization provides a formal co-mentoring program for all nurse leaders. Nurse leaders actively engage in the co-mentoring program.
- Nurse leaders role model skilled communication, true collaboration, effective decision making, meaningful recognition, and authentic leadership.
- The health care organization includes the leadership contribution to creating and sustaining a healthy work environment as a criterion in each nurse leader's performance appraisal. Nurse leaders must demonstrate sustained leadership in creating and sustaining a healthy work environment to achieve professional advancement.
- Nurse leaders and team members mutually and objectively evaluate the impact of leadership processes and decisions on the organization's progress toward creating and sustaining a healthy work environment.

References

About the Standards

1. Greene, J. (2002). The medical workplace: No abuse zone. *Hospital Health Network, 76,* 26,28.
2. American Association of Critical-Care Nurses. (2003). *Strategic market research study.* Aliso Viejo, CA: Author.
3. University Health System Consortium. (2003). *Successful practices for workplace of choice employers.* Oak Brook, IL: UHC.
4. Institute of Medicine. (2001). *Crossing the quality chasm: A new health system for the 21st century.* Washington, D.C.: National Academy Press.
5. American Nurses Association. (2001). *Code of ethics for nurses with interpretive statements.* Washington, D.C.: American Nurses Publishing,
6. Adler, D., Ayres, S., Disch, J., Greenbaum, D., Lavandero, R., Millar, S. (1983). The organization of human resources in critical care units. *Focus on Critical Care, 101,* 43-44.

7. Kohn, L., Corrigan, J., Donaldson, M. (Eds). (2000). *To err is human: Building a safer health system.* Washington, D.C.: National Academy Press.
8. Hardin, S., Kaplow, R. (2004). *Synergy for clinical excellence: The AACN Synergy Model for Patient Care.* Sudbury, MA: Jones & Bartlett.
9. Greiner, A.C., Knebel, E. (Eds.). (2004). *Health professions education: A bridge to quality.* Washington, D.C.: National Academy Press.
10. Robert Wood Johnson Executive Nurse Fellows Program. Accessed December 3, 2004, from website http://www.futurehealth.ucsf.edu/rwj/.

Skilled Communication

1. Joint Commission on Accreditation of Healthcare Organizations. Health care at the crossroads: Strategies for addressing the evolving nursing crisis. Accessed October 4, 2004, from website http://www.jcaho.org/about+us/public+policy +initiatives/health+care+at+the+crossroads.pdf.
2. Institute for Safe Medication Practices. (March 11, 2004.) *Intimidation: Practitioners speak up about this unresolved problem: Part I. ISMP Medication Safety Alert!*
3. Buresh, B., Gordon, S. (2000). *From silence to voice: What nurses know and must communicate to the public.* Cornell University Press Services, Ithaca, NY.
4. Kohn, L., Corrigan, J., Donaldson, M. (Eds.). (2000). *To err is human: Building a safer health system.* Washington, D.C.: National Academy Press.
5. Schaefer, H.G., Helmreich, R.L., Scheidegger, D. (1994). Human factors and safety in emergency medicine. *Resuscitation, 28,* 221-225.
6. Joint Commission on Accreditation of Healthcare Organizations. Root Causes of Sentinel Events 1995-2003. Accessed December 17, 2004, from website: http://www.jcaho.com /accredited+ organizations/ambulatory+care/sentinel+events/ root+causes+of+sentinel+ event.htm.
7. American Nurses Association. (2001). *Code of Ethics for Nurses With Interpretive Statements.* Washington, D.C.: American Nurses Publishing,

True Collaboration

1. American Hospital Association Commission on Workforce for Hospitals and Health Systems. (2002). *In our hands: How hospital leaders can build a thriving workforce.* Chicago: Author.
2. Knaus, W.A., Draper, E.A., Wagner, D.P., Zimmerman, J.E. (1986). An evaluation of outcome from intensive care in major medical centers. *Annals of Internal Medicine, 104,* 410-418.

3. Page, A. (Ed.). (2003). *Keeping patients safe: Transforming the work environment of nurses.* Washington, D.C.: Institute of Medicine Committee on the Work Environment for Nurses and Patient Safety.

4. Kohn, L., Corrigan, J., Donaldson, M. (Eds.) (2000). *To err is human: Building a safer health system.* Washington, D.C.: National Academy Press.

5. American Association of Critical-Care Nurses. (2003). *Strategic market research study.* Aliso Viejo, CA: Author.

6. Larrabee, J.H., Janney, M.A., Ostrow, C.L., Withrow, M.L., Hobbs, G.R. Jr., Burant, C. (2003). Predicting registered nurse job satisfaction and intent to leave. *Journal of Nursing Administration,* 33, 271-283.

7. American Organization of Nursing Executives. *Healthy work environments: Striving for excellence.* vol 2. (2003). Chicago, IL: McManis & Monsalve Associate.

8. VitalSmarts. (2005). *Silence kills: The 7 crucial conversations in healthcare.* Provo, Utah: Available at http://www.vitalsmarts.com.

9. Scott, R.A., Aiken, L.H., Mechanic, D., Moravcsik, J. (1995). Organizational aspects of caring. *Milbank Quarterly,* 73, 77-95.

10. Rosenstein, A.H. (2002). Original research: Nurse-physician relationships: Impact on satisfaction and retention. *American Journal of Nursing,* 102, 26-34.

Effective Decision Making

1. American Nurses Association. (2001). *Code of ethics for nurses with interpretive statements.* Washington, D.C.: American Nurses Publishing.

2. Greene, J. (2002). The medical workplace: No abuse zone. *Hospital Health Network,* 76, 26, 28.

3. Freeman-Cook, A., Hoas, H., Guttmannova, K., Joyner, J.C. (2004). An error by any other name. *American Journal of Nursing,* 104, 32-42.

4. Kimball, B., O'Neil, E. (2002). *Healthcare's human crisis: The American nursing shortage.* Princeton, NJ: The Robert Wood Johnson Foundation.

5. Fruth, R. (1995). *Organizational technology and professional communications in a hospital setting.* [dissertation]. Chicago: University of Illinois at Chicago.

6. Nutt, P. (2002). *Why decisions fail.* New York: Berrett-Koehler Publishers.

7. American Hospital Association Commission on Workforce for Hospitals and Health Systems. (2002). *In our hands: How hospital leaders can build a thriving workforce.* Chicago, IL: Author.

8. American Organization of Nursing Executives. (2003). *Healthy work environments: Striving*

for excellence. vol 2. Chicago, IL: McManis & Monsalve Associates.

9. American Association of Critical-Care Nurses Beacon Award for Critical Care Excellence. Accessed December 17, 2004, from website: http://www.aacn.org.

10. Magnet Nursing Services Recognition Program. Accessed December 17, 2004, from website: http://www.ana.org/ancc/magnet.html.

11. Baldrige National Quality Program. Accessed December 17, 2004, from website: http://www.baldrige.gov.

Appropriate Staffing

1. Needleman, J., Buerhaus, P., Mattke, S., Stewart, M., Zelevinsky, K. (2002). Nursing staffing levels and the quality of care in hospitals. *New England Journal of Medicine,* 346, 1715-1720.

2. Aiken, L., Clarke, S., Sloane, D.M., Sochalski, J., Silber, J. (2002). Hospital nurse staffing and patient mortality, nurse burnout, and job dissatisfaction. *Journal of the American Medical Association,* 288, 1987-1993.

3. Foley, B.J., Jennings, B.M., Kee, C.C., Minick, P., Harvey, S.S. (2002). Characteristics of nurses and hospital work environments that foster satisfaction and clinical expertise. *Journal of Nursing Administration,* 325, 273-282.

4. American Association of Critical-Care Nurses, AACN Certification Corporation. Safeguarding the patient and the profession: The value of critical care nurse certification. Accessed January 4, 2005, from website http://www.aacn.org/certcorp/certcorp.nsf/vwdoc/BenefitsofCert.

5. Bates, D.W., Cullen, D.J., Laird, N., et al. (1995). Incidence of adverse drug events and potential adverse drug events: Implications for prevention. ADE Study Group. *Journal of the American Medical Association,* 274, 29-34.

6. VHA. Shortages impacting: Quality of care, patient satisfaction, and market share. Accessed October 4, 2004, from website: https://www.vha.com/news/releases/public/ 021111.asp.

7. Snyder, D.A., Medina, J., Bell, L., Wavra, T.A. AACN Delegation Handbook. (2004, second edition). Accessed December 17, 2004 from website: https://www.aacn.org./__8825651000134c1b.n8.f/0/b37a82e9fcc3c1cf882567530067ed9e?OpenDocument&Highlight=2,DELEGATION.

8. American Association of Critical-Care Nurses. Position statement: Maintaining patient-focused care in an environment of nursing staff shortage and financial constraints. Accessed December 17,

2004, from website: http://www.aacn.org/pdfLibra. NSF/Files/burson/$file/burson.pdf.

Meaningful Recognition

1. United States General Accounting Office. Nursing workforce: Recruitment and retention of nurses and nurse aides is a growing concern. Accessed October 6, 2004, from website: http://www.gao.gov/new.items/d01750t.pdf.
2. Cronin, S.N., Bechrerer, D. (1999). Recognition of staff nurse job performance and achievements. *Journal of Nursing Administration,* 29, 26-31.
3. McConnell, C.R. (1997). Employee recognition: A little oil on the troubled waters of change. *Health Care Supervision,* 15, 83-90.
4. Blegen, M.A., Goode, C.J., Johnson, M., Maas, M.L., McCloskey, J.C., Moorhead, S.A. (1992). Recognizing staff nurse job performance and achievements. *Research in Nursing Health,* 15, 57-66.
5. American Association of Critical-Care Nurses. (2003). *Strategic market research study.* Aliso Viejo, CA: Author.
6. American Hospital Association Commission on Workforce for Hospitals and Health Systems. (2002). *In our hands: How hospital leaders can build a thriving workforce.* Chicago: Author.

Authentic Leadership

1. American Association of Critical-Care Nurses. (2003). *Strategic market research study.* Aliso Viejo, CA: Author.
2. Kimball, B., O'Neil, E. (2002). *Healthcare's human crisis: The American nursing shortage.* Princeton, NJ: The Robert Wood Johnson Foundation.
3. American Hospital Association Commission on Workforce for Hospitals and Health Systems. (2002). *In our hands: How hospital leaders can build a thriving workforce.* Chicago: Author.
4. Robert Wood Johnson Executive Nurse Fellows Program. Accessed December 17, 2004, from website:http://www.futurehealth.ucsf.edu/rwj/.

Index

Page numbers followed by f indicate figure(s); t, table(s); b, box(es).